Revised and updated version of the classic
Financial Management text by Bruce R.
and James D. Suver

FINANCIAL MANAGEMENT

Concepts and Applications
for Health Care Organizations

Fourth Edition

Bruce R. Neumann, Ph.D.
Professor of Accounting and Health Administration
Graduate School of Business
Graduate Programs in Health Administration
University of Colorado at Denver

Jan P. Clement, Ph.D.
Associate Professor
Department of Health Administration
Medical College of Virginia Campus
Virginia Commonwealth University

Jean C. Cooper, Ph.D.
Associate Professor
School of Accountancy
C.M. Gatton College of Business and Economics
University of Kentucky

KENDALL/HUNT PUBLISHING COMPANY
4050 Westmark Drive   Dubuque, Iowa 52002

Contents

4 Cost Definitions and Cost Behavior —————————— 132

5 Short-Term Decision-Making —————————— 163

6 Cost Allocation _____ 215

7 Costing of Outputs _____ 240

8 Budgeting _____ 267

12 Managing Current Assets _____ 391

13 The Capital Investment Decision _____ 420

14 Sources of Financing: Debt and Equity _____ 444

This book is dedicated to the memory of James D. Suver, DBA

Foreword

For the reader who hopes to become a general manager in the health care field, there is no more important knowledge to be found than what is available in this book. You should come to know the content of this book as well as you know your own language. This topic is not for skimming, but for complete mastery.

I learned the importance of finance a long time ago, when I was treasurer of a college organization. The president could do anything he wanted without my approval except spend money. When money was to be spent, I was the one who said if there was any money available, and others did not question me. Fortunately, I made decisions in the very best interests of the organization. If you become a general manager who is ignorant of finance, you may have a title without power because you will need a dedicated financial officer to do the real job.

It is said that the world is made up of quantitative and qualitative personalities, that is, those who like numbers and those who don't, those who emphasize the left brain over the right brain, or those who run organizations by the numbers versus those who emphasize interpersonal skills. If such divisions have any meaning, presumably, the quantitative types feel more comfortable with finance. Good general management, however, needs a balance between qualitative and quantitative styles. No health care organization can be run purely "by the numbers," and it can't be run without keeping track of the numbers. Even if you see yourself as more on the qualitative side, the content of this book is the minimum financial knowledge you need for being a general manager in health care.

Now consider another meaning to quality, as in quality of care. Costs of care and quality of care are too often seen as separate compartments in medical care organizations. Professional managers deal with the dollars, while nurses, physicians, and other providers deal with the quality of the services provided. Dollars are easily counted, but the quality of care is tougher to measure. There are many methods of quantifying quality in health care, such as patient satisfaction scores, waiting times, error rates, adjusted mortality rates, and completed medical records. None of these are perfect, but health care organizations continue to work harder and harder to demonstrate to the world that the quality of the service they provide is better.

It is easier to understand key cost concepts using measures such as costs per admission, cost per outpatient visit, or cost per diagnosis related group, and appropriately, this book considers such measures. However, keep in mind that one can conduct the same kind of analysis on quality-adjusted production units.

Health care organizations invest in quality and the analytic techniques used here are needed to make such investment decisions. Will a change in patient monitoring by the nursing staff and costs associated with this change be justified by a reduction in the frequency of patient falls? You can't answer such questions without knowing the techniques described in this book.

Health care financial managers should understand the cost and revenue implications of medical decision-making. This is a plea that financial thinking should not be separated from patient care decisions. We need financial managers who think about quality of care and providers of care who think about the financial implications of their decisions. This is simply another way of saying that financial reasoning needs to be pervasive in high performance medical care organizations.

Duncan Neuhauser, Ph.D.
Co-Director—Health Systems
Management Center
Case Western Reserve University
Cleveland, Ohio 44106

Preface

An understanding of basic financial management concepts and techniques is necessary for health care providers, such as nurses, physicians, and physical therapists, as well as for managers of a variety of health care organizations that produce health care services and insurance, pharmaceutical, information and other health and medical care products. This text addresses the needs of these diverse audiences. It is ideally structured for a first course in graduate health care administration or nursing administration since it surveys basic financial management techniques and develops the necessary background for more advanced courses.

Each chapter provides thorough coverage of a specific topic with examples of practical applications. Questions and problems at the end of each chapter highlight important aspects of the material and challenge students to apply it to a variety of situations. Each chapter also includes references for additional reading for more depth or on related topics. A glossary defines terms frequently used in financial management and health care.

The text is divided into three major sections: financial accounting (Chapters 2 and 3), managerial accounting (Chapters 4 through 10) and finance (Chapters 11-14). Chapter 2 develops the basic methods and statements of financial accounting. Chapter 3 builds upon Chapter 2, showing how to analyze financial statements. Chapter 4 develops the basic managerial concepts of cost. In Chapters 5-10, the relevant cost concepts are applied to specific types of decisions. Chapters 11 and 12 overview short-term financial management. Chapter 13 describes long-term decision-making tools. Finally, Chapter 14 summarizes financing sources for health care organizations.

The appearance of this revised edition (Fourth Edition) reflects our excitement about the challenges health care financial management faces as the health care industry continues to evolve into the next century. Although the target is ever moving and changing, we have attempted to address recent changes in organization, payment, and financing. We have broadened our focus to include a variety of provider as well as payer organizations. We hope you find the material in this text useful in furthering the objectives of an improved health care system and in developing health care professionals who are caring, ethical and financially astute.

The appearance of this edition is also marked by great sadness. The sadness is for the loss of one of the original authors of the text, James D. Suver, DBA, FACHE, who died in 1995. Jim was one of the founding fathers of the academic field of health care financial management. His pioneering efforts in the classroom, in journals and in books demonstrated the relevance of financial management to health care in the 1970s, when many practitioners and academics paid little attention to it. Through his teaching and extraordinary mentorship, he also stimulated the involvement of many young professionals in health care financial management. Personally, he taught each of the current authors so much on both professional and personal levels. He enriched our lives through his friendship and love. We miss him tremendously.

Our students and faculty colleagues deserve many thanks and much praise for helping us make this book a long-term success. Special thanks are extended to Matt Moore and John (Jay) Moore for their contributions to this edition.

As always, the authors remain responsible for any and all errors and omissions. We welcome your continued calls that help us to improve the text. You may contact us as follows

Bruce R. Neumann, Ph.D.
Phone: (303) 556-5884
E-mail: BNEUMANN@CASTLE.CUDENVER.EDU

Jan P. Clement, Ph.D.
Phone: (804) 828-1886
E-mail: JCLEMENT@GEMS.VCU.EDU

Jean C. Cooper, Ph.D.
Phone: (606) 257-1876
E-mail: ACC224@POP.UKY.EDU

1 The Financial Management Function and the Health Care Environment

The Financial Management Function

Financial management can be viewed both as a body of knowledge and as a set of activities that management performs. As a subject matter, financial management has its major roots in three separate academic disciplines: **financial accounting, managerial accounting,** and **managerial finance**. As can be seen in Table 1-1, these three disciplines have certain areas of commonality and divergence in their purpose, scope, time orientation, and outputs that help determine their impact on financial management. For example, the primary purpose of financial accounting is to produce standardized statements, such as the balance sheet, for persons outside of the organization. To do so, financial accountants record past and present transactions and follow procedures that enable them to communicate information reliably to a variety of users. In contrast, using managerial accounting tools, managers identify the firm's objectives and relevant data, financial and nonfinancial, to assist insiders in making short-term decisions and evaluating performance.

Together, these three disciplines furnish a body of knowledge and a set of tools and techniques that can be used to improve managerial decision-making for an organization's acquisition, utilization, and control of resources. In this vein, it is useful to define management from the point of view of the three stages of activity involved in task accomplishment: planning, implementing, and controlling. In the health care field these three stages involve: (1) deciding which customers to serve, what products and services to produce, how to provide these products and services, and how to obtain needed resources (planning); (2) obtaining resources and managing the production of products and services (implementing); and (3) monitoring resource use, services, and outcomes and taking corrective action where appropriate (controlling). The financial management function can be viewed from the same perspective as a subset of the management of health care organizations.

Planning

In the **planning** stage, financial management is concerned with examining the long- and short-range financial implications of alternative courses of action identified in the firm's strategic planning process. Analyses of long-term investments in product lines, including the value of cash flows they generate, are undertaken using managerial finance concepts and tools. Sources of financing for the plans may be identified as a part of the planning process. Short-term decisions about annual resource needs, contracting with payers or providers, determining the cost of outputs and their prices, and motivating employees to accomplish the firm's plan use tools from managerial accounting and are part of the planning process as

1

Table 1-1 Characteristics of Disciplines Contributing to Health Care Financial Management.

	Financial Accounting	Managerial Accounting	Managerial Finance
Purpose	Producing standardized statements for outside users	Assisting management in short-term decision-making	Assisting management in long-term decision-making and managing short-term and long-term financing
Major Foci	Monitoring and recording transactions Protection of assets Reliably communicating to a variety of outside users	Identifying objectives and relevant financial information Planning, budgeting and evaluating performance Short-term decision making Behavioral effects of information Costing and pricing of outputs	Evaluating long-term (capital investment) decisions Determining value of physical and financial assets Financing decisions Identifying relevant cash flows
Time Orientation	Past and present	Largely present and future, Some past	Future
Common Reports	Balance Sheet, Income Statement, Statement of Cash Flows	Budget, Budget variance report	Capital budgets, Cash flow analyses, Investment performance
Other Types of Reports	Financial statement analysis, Billing, Payroll, Inventory, Accounts receivable analyses	Cost reports, Reimbursement analyses, Output statistics	

well. The results of such decisions are represented in budgets and projected financial statements reflecting anticipated revenues, expenses, cash flows, and the financial position of the provider if certain actions are taken (managerial and financial accounting).

Examples of long-range decisions currently facing many health care payers and providers include whether to remain not-for-profit or to become a for-profit entity; whether to continue self-management or contract out for management of all or part of the organization; whether to move into new or different product lines such as surgical-centers, home health care, hospice care, insurance, and physician group practice management; and whether to invest in new (and usually expensive) capital equipment such as new information systems or imaging equipment. Examples of short-term decisions being considered by various health care providers include whether to make changes in case mix; whether to make changes in salaries and/or scheduling of professionals; whether to implement direct contracting with employers rather than contracting through third party payers; and whether to make changes in service delivery.

Implementing

After it has planned, the health care firm must **implement** its plans. In this stage, health care financial management is concerned with acquiring and utilizing cash and other resources in order to accomplish effectively the financial and service goals of the organization. As discussed in detail in Chapter 14, in addition to revenues derived from providing services and related businesses, there are two other major sources of funds: debt and owners' equity. Debt is money borrowed or credit obtained by an organization. Owners' equity consists of funds received from owners or stakeholders of the firm and profits retained by the organization.

Once a health care organization has acquired cash, often through external financing (managerial finance), it must convert the cash to the various resources needed to provide products and services. It must implement its budgets and carefully consider the behavioral effects of its financial goals and plans on its employees (managerial accounting). The firm must also implement systems to protect its assets, such as separation of financial functions, which is an example of how financial accounting is involved in implementing plans.

Controlling

In addition to the planning and implementing stages, there is a third stage of management called controlling. **Controlling** is the term used to describe management's attempts to ensure that its procedures and outcomes are in line with its service and financial goals and objectives. Control is important on both a short-term basis, such as examining monthly or annual performance, as well as evaluating how well the firm's strategic plan has been implemented. With information gathered in the control stage, the firm may decide to continue what it is doing, or it may decide to change its operations and strategic plan.

As a part of the control of its operations, the firm must monitor and record transactions, prepare financial statements that reflect the organization's financial performance, and audit the internal control systems that safeguard its assets (financial accounting). In addition, the firm must evaluate its performance in achieving output and financial objectives on an ongoing basis and at the end of the year using managerial accounting reports for management.

Finally, the firm should evaluate the performance of its cash management and investments in light of the firm's overall strategic plan.

As can be seen from this summary of the financial management function, financial management specialists such as accountants, treasurers (who manage cash and arrange financing) and controllers (who oversee internal financial operations) have important roles in the firm's financial management. However, they are not the only managers who play an important role in the financial management in the firm. Managers from most areas of the organization have at least some role in financial management.

Financial management of health care organizations takes place within the broader health care environment. Next, we briefly discuss the size and range of the health care industry in the United States before returning to specific health care financial management concerns.

The Health Care Industry

National Health Care Expenditures

Health care is currently one of the largest industries in the United States. In 1993, health care expenditures in the United States totaled $884.2 billion[1] comprising 13.9% of the Gross Domestic Product (GDP). Table 1-2 summarizes total national health care expenditures and specific types of spending for selected years from 1960-1993. Total national health care expenditures are divided into health services and supplies, and research and construction. Health services and supplies, the largest component, are consumed during the year. Research and construction are expenditures that yield benefits beyond the current year.

Health services and supplies include various types of **personal health care services** consumed by patients, the cost of administration and net cost of private insurance, and the cost of public health activities of governments. The net cost of insurance for private insurance companies is the sum of profits and administrative costs. As can be seen from Table 1-2, hospital care has consistently been the largest personal health care expenditure followed by physician services.

Table 1-2 also shows that the health care industry has grown dramatically since 1960. Table 1-3 provides more data concerning this growth, showing the magnitude of the total national health expenditures, annual percentage growth rate, percent of gross domestic product (GDP) health care comprises, and per capita health care spending for selected years from 1960 to 1993.

Total health care spending has grown from 5.3% of GDP ($27.1 billion) in 1960 to 13.9% of GDP ($884.2 billion) in 1993, increasing at an average annual rate of 10% or more until recently. This rate of increase has been greater than the rate of growth in GDP. Per capita spending has also grown although not at quite as high a rate as total spending.

Also shown in Table 1-3 is the distribution of private and public, or governmental, funding of health care expenditures. Private spending includes payments made by consumers,

Table 1-2 Components of National Health Expenditures, 1960-1993.

Type	Amount in Billions of Dollars					
	1960	1970	1980	1985	1990	1993
Health Services and Supplies	**$25.4**	**$69.0**	**$239.4**	**$418.1**	**$672.2**	**$855.2**
Personal Health Care	23.9	64.8	220.1	380.5	612.4	782.5
Hospital Care	9.3	28.0	102.7	168.2	256.5	326.6
Physician Services	5.3	13.6	45.2	83.6	140.5	171.2
Dental Services	2.0	4.7	13.3	21.7	30.4	37.4
Other Professional Services	0.6	1.4	6.4	16.6	36.0	51.2
Home Health Care	0.0	0.2	1.9	4.9	11.1	20.8
Drugs and Other Medical Non-Durables	4.2	8.8	21.6	37.4	61.2	75.0
Vision Products & Other Medical Durables	0.8	2.0	4.5	7.1	10.5	12.6
Nursing Home Care	1.0	4.9	20.5	34.9	54.8	69.6
Other Personal Care	0.7	1.3	4.0	6.1	11.4	18.2
Program Administration & Net Cost of Private Insurance	1.2	2.8	12.1	25.3	38.3	48.0
Govt. Public Health Activities	0.4	1.4	7.2	12.3	21.6	24.7
Research & Construction	**1.7**	**5.3**	**11.6**	**16.4**	**24.3**	**29.0**
Research	0.7	2.0	5.5	7.8	12.2	14.4
Construction	1.0	3.4	6.2	8.6	12.1	14.6
Total National Health Expenditures*	**$27.1**	**$74.3**	**$251.1**	**$434.5**	**$696.6**	**$884.2**

Source: Levit, K.R., et al. "National Health Expenditures, 1993" *Health Care Financing Review* 16(1): 247-294, 1994.

* Because of rounding, not all columns sum exactly to totals.

Table 1-3 National Health Care Expenditures, 1960-1993.

	1960	1970	1980	1985	1990	1993
Total						
National Health Expenditures (in Billions)	$27.1	$74.3	$251.1	$434.5	$696.6	$884.2
Annualized Percent Change from Previous Year Shown	N/A	10.6	12.9	11.6	9.9	8.3
National Health Expenditures as a Percent of Gross Domestic Product	5.3	7.4	9.3	10.8	12.6	13.9
Per Capita						
National Health Expenditures per Capita	$143	$346	$1,068	$1,761	$2,686	$3,299
Annualized Percent Change from Previous Year Shown	N/A	9.2	11.9	10.5	8.8	7.1
Percent Distribution of National Health Expenditures						
Private	75.5	62.7	58.1	59.7	58.9	56.1
Public	24.5	37.3	41.9	40.3	41.1	43.9
Federal Government	*10.7*	*24.0*	*28.7*	*28.4*	*28.1*	*31.7*
State and Local Government	*13.8*	*13.4*	*13.3*	*11.9*	*13.0*	*12.1*

Source: Levit, K.R., et al. "National Health Expenditures, 1993" *Health Care Financing Review* 16(1): 247-294, 1994.

called **"out-of-pocket"** expenditures, spending by insurance companies, and other private spending. Public spending includes public health and research expenditures as well as payments made for care through the Medicare and Medicaid programs, which were enacted in 1966. **Medicare** is a federal program paying for care for the elderly. **Medicaid** is a federal and state partnership paying for care for the poor. In 1993, private spending constituted 56.1% and public spending was 43.9% of national health expenditures. However, the mix has changed steadily since 1960 when private spending was 75.5% and public spending was 24.5% of the total.

The ever increasing proportion of GDP and the rapid rate of growth of the health care industry have led to serious discussion concerning the appropriate amounts and rate of growth of such spending. As health care spending consumes a large part of the economy's resources, it may "crowd out" spending for other purposes such as education, economic growth and so on. Although there is no agreement about how much of GDP in the U.S. should be devoted to health care, there is agreement that the country cannot sustain such large increases indefinitely.

Several factors are responsible for the rapid growth in health care spending since 1960. Inflation in the general economy resulting in cost increases in non-medical inputs such as materials, non-medical supplies and the like is one factor that has contributed to the growth in health care expenditures. A second factor is inflation specific to the industry. This inflation occurs when firms must pay more for the same type of health care input, such as when nurses or physical therapists are in short supply and demand higher wages. A third factor is the increase in population in the United States. As more people consume health care, naturally, total spending increases. Population growth is why per capita health care expenditures shown in Table 1-3 have not grown as rapidly as total expenditures. Fourth, health care expenditures have increased because Americans have consumed more health care per person.

This last factor is thought to result largely from the expansion of private and public health insurance coverage and technology changes. Since 1960, both the number of individuals covered by health insurance and the benefits of the policies have expanded. A significant expansion in the number of individuals with insurance occurred in 1966 when Medicare and Medicaid were enacted to increase the access to care for the elderly and the poor, respectively. With time, the benefits of most health insurance policies and governmental programs have also expanded to cover more types of care.

Table 1-4 shows how the insurance as a source of payment for personal health services has increased from 1960 through 1993. While out-of-pocket spending has decreased as a percentage of total personal health expenditures, private health insurance and government payment, often through Medicare and Medicaid, have increased. Private health insurers and government programs that pay for medical care are often called **third party payers**. The other two parties are the patient and the provider. Third party payers reimburse providers for the care they deliver to patients.

Insurance increases health care expenditures by increasing the utilization of services. When third party payers pay medical bills, consumers tend to become less sensitive to the prices for individual services and to demand more volume and quality of services. Since many employers pay medical care insurance premiums for their employees, individuals are further insulated from the prices for health care services. The same is true of beneficiaries of governmental programs such as Medicare and Medicaid.

Payment to providers for services has often operated in concert with insurance coverage to increase expenditures. From the mid-1960s, through the early 1980s, most third party payers paid providers of health care services on the basis of either charges or actual costs incurred. As a result, providers, in addition to their patients, had few incentives to control utilization of services or to be efficient in producing each service. The provider received more

Table 1-4 Percent Distribution of Payment Sources for Personal Health Care Expenditures, 1960-1993.

	Percent* of Total Personal Health Care Expenditures					
	1960	1970	1980	1985	1990	1993
Private						
Out-of-Pocket	55.9	39.1	27.8	26.0	22.6	20.1
Private Health Insurance	21.0	23.6	29.1	31.5	33.8	33.0
Other Private	1.8	2.5	3.5	3.6	3.9	3.8
Public (Government)						
Federal	8.9	22.7	28.8	29.3	29.1	33.1
State and Local	12.5	12.0	10.7	9.6	10.7	10.0

Source: Levit, K.R., et al. "National Health Expenditures, 1993" *Health Care Financing Review* 16(1): 247-294, 1994.

* Because of rounding, not all columns sum exactly to 100%.

payment for providing more volume of services and more costly services. Efficiency was rewarded by decreased payment. Frequently, to attract patients, providers engaged in non-price competition by offering the latest technology, nicest surroundings, and cost-increasing amenities. This type of increased payment for producing more output is called **fee-for-service** payment.

New technology has also contributed to the rise in health care expenditures. New, costly procedures, such as transplants and coronary artery bypass grafts, and new equipment such as sophisticated imaging equipment have been developed. These have spread rapidly to many providers and their patients. Often the spread has resulted in duplication of services and excess capacity.

The escalation in health care costs has not gone unnoticed by those paying the bills—government, other third party payers, employers and individuals. The federal government has a long history of trying to control cost increases in health care. For many years, private third party payers simply passed on their cost increases to individuals or employers who paid health insurance premiums. During the last decade, these payers have also attempted to slow the escalation in health care expenditures.

Attempts to control spending have focused on regulation, altering payment methods, and managing care. Early attempts to control spending were primarily regulatory as in requiring approval for capital expenditures and setting of payment rates for all payers and providers in a state.

Payment method changes by third party payers have been numerous since the mid-1960s. Some have involved placing limits on the rate of increase in fee-for-service payments from year to year. Others have involved switching from paying on the basis of costs incurred to establishing uniform payment rates for particular types of services regardless of the cost, paying discounted charges, and contracting with a limited number of providers selected on the basis of competitive bidding. Recently, more payers have begun using methods that put providers at financial risk. These methods may involve uniform payment based upon the diagnosis of the patient not the consumption of resources, providing financial incentives to control the utilization of services, and paying a flat amount for the care of an enrolled member regardless of the utilization of services. Table 1-5 summarizes some of the payment changes the federal government has implemented for the Medicare program since 1966.

During the 1990s, **managed care,** the coordination of a patient's medical care by payers and providers, became one of the most popular methods of trying to controlling the rise in health care expenditures. Figure 1-1 shows how managed care grew in the early 1990s. The growth is expected to continue through the remainder of the decade.

Managed care firms may combine a variety of methods to coordinate care and to control costs including: (1) coordination of all of a patient's medical care by a primary care physician, (2) prior authorization by a payer for expensive care such as surgical procedures, (3) paying primary care physicians a set amount for each member of a health plan regardless of the actual use of services, (4) limiting patients' choice of physicians to those in a health plan's network because the physicians are efficient providers or accept a lower payment rate per service, (5) paying physicians on a discounted charge basis, and (6) providing other financial

Table 1-5 Major Federal Legislation and the Reimbursement Impact.

1966	Title XVIII (Medicare) and Title XIX (Medicaid) of the Social Security Act established reimbursement based on reasonable cost. A 2% plus factor was added to the reimbursable costs for hospitals.
1970	The 2% plus factor was eliminated but an 8 1/2% nursing differential was instituted to compensate for the increased nursing costs of Medicare patients.
1972	PL 92-603 established the concept of reimbursement at the lower of costs or charges for hospitals. Section 223 introduced the concept of cost limitations based on comparison with peer groupings of similar providers. Professional standard review organizations (PSROs) were authorized to review hospitals' utilization of services.
1974	PL 93-641, The Health Planning and Resource Development Act of 1974, reinforced the concept of areawide health planning. Health systems agencies (HSA) were established and certificate of need (CON) procedures were implemented.
1981	The Omnibus Budget Reconciliation Act of 1981 started the phaseout of federal support for the health planning systems and HSAs. CON thresholds were raised from $150,000 to $600,000 for capital expenditures, the 8 1/2% nursing differential was reduced to 5%, and the section 223 costs were reduced from 112% to 108% of the mean inpatient routine cost. Competition was encouraged by support for health maintenance organizations (HMOs) and restriction of freedom of choice for Medicare beneficiaries to providers deemed cost effective.
1982	The Tax Equity and Fiscal Responsibility Act of 1982 (TEFRA) placed a limit on all inpatient hospital costs while establishing a target rate which, if exceeded, would result in reduced reimbursement. In addition, reimbursement was to be computed on a per case (admission or discharge) basis and a case mix index established for all short-term hospitals to reflect the general mix of medical cases. Finally, the nursing salary differential was completely eliminated, and numerous other changes were made which would result in reduced reimbursement of Medicare and Medicaid patients.
1983	The Social Security Amendments of 1983 established a prospective payment system, effective October 1, 1983, based on a fixed price per diagnosis-related group (DRG) for inpatient services. It was noted that capital-related costs, outpatient care, and physician services, although not included in the initial prospective price, could be expected to be included as more experience with DRGs was gained.
1985	PL 99-272, the Consolidated Omnibus Reconciliation Act of 1985 (COBRA), reduced capital-related payments to hospitals through Medicare, established mandatory assignment for physician office laboratories, clarified reimbursement for graduate medical education, and established an inherent reasonableness test for physician reimbursement.
1986	PL 99-509, the Omnibus Budget Reconciliation Act of 1986 (OBRA), established payment criteria for ambulatory surgery procedures performed in hospitals, expanded the inherent reasonableness test for physician payments, and eliminated periodic interim cash payments (PIP) for hospitals.
1987	The Omnibus Budget Reconciliation Act of 1987 added over 100 Medicare and Medicaid provisions that reduced Medicare expenditures by almost $2 billion in FY 1988. Separate PPS rate update factors were determined for urban areas over 1 million in population, other urban areas and rural areas. Hospital capital payments continued on a reasonable cost basis minus

reduction of 12% in 1988 and 15% in 1989. There was also reduced reimbursement for physician services to Medicare beneficiaries.

1992   Medicare physician payment reforms included resource-based relative value scale (RBRVS) payments and prospective global budgeting for all physician payments. RBRVS payments are based upon a relative value scale reflecting resources needed to provide the service. Phased-in over a five-year period, payments to all physicians were expected to decrease, but especially to specialty services such as orthopedics, cardiology, psychiatry, surgery, gastroenterology and opthalmology. Payments to primary care physicians for "observation and management" services were expected to increase.

1993   As part of the Omnibus Reconciliation Act of 1993 (OBRA-93), also referred to as "Stark II," physicians were prohibited from making any Medicare or Medicaid referral to an entity with which the physician had a "financial relationship." A financial relationship means any ownership or investment interest, including those achieved through debt, equity, or any similar sources of financing, or any form of payment or remuneration.

Figure 1-1   Shift to Managed Care.

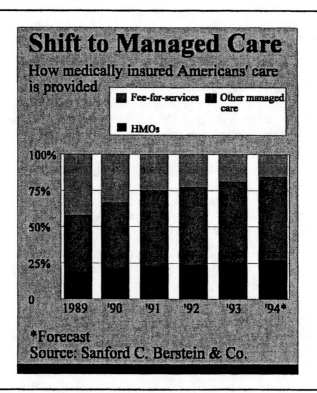

Source: "Dose of Reform" *The Wall Street Journal*, August 26, 1994, p.1.

incentives to providers and patients. The payment methods and other financial incentives used often involve putting providers of health care services "at risk." They are at risk for financial losses if they do not control the health care costs of enrollees in the managed care health plan. Although the "practice" of managed care is still evolving, there is some evidence of success in cost control.

Types of Health Care Organizations

The health care industry is inhabited by many types of organizations. Traditionally, these organizations have been divided into payers and providers.

Payers include medical care insurance companies, health maintenance organizations, preferred provider organizations and governmental programs such as Medicare and Medicaid. A **health maintenance organization** (HMO) is an organization that combines insurance and delivery of a broad range of comprehensive health services to an enrolled population. Members or enrollees pay a monthly fee or premium for access to services. A **preferred provider organization** (PPO) is an entity "through which employer health benefit plans and health insurance carriers contract to purchase health care services for covered beneficiaries from a selected group of participating providers. Typically, participating providers in PPOs agree to abide by utilization management and other procedures implemented by the PPO and agree to accept the PPO's reimbursement structure and payment levels."[2]

Providers include a range of organizations that actually provide services to patients or clients. Examples are acute care, psychiatric or rehabilitation hospitals, physician practices, home health care agencies, birthing centers, ambulatory surgical centers, hospices, and nursing homes.

Traditionally, payers have borne the risk of health care cost increases. They had fixed premiums for a period of time for enrollees or members. If costs exceeded the revenue generated by premiums during that time period, the payers lost money. Until recently, payers were able to limit their risk from year to year by passing increased costs along to employers or individuals in the form of higher premiums. Recently, employers have demanded better cost control and lower rates of increase in premiums. Another fairly recent change has been the transfer of risk to providers of health care services through various payment methods. Payers may make fixed payments for treatments regardless of the provider's cost; they may pay a fixed amount per enrollee who chooses to use a particular provider; or, payers may withhold a portion of the payment, "returning" it at the end of the year if specific utilization goals are met. Providers and payers may be freestanding entities or complex multiunit firms. Examples of freestanding organizations include unaffiliated hospitals, solo physician practices and local health plans. Increasingly, both providers and payers are consolidating to form larger firms. The consolidations may occur through outright purchase or merger or through alliances where ownership is not shifted. This phenomenon has occurred among hospitals, physicians, insurance companies and other health care organizations.

The larger firms may be **horizontally integrated**, as when the firm is comprised of many similar units. Examples include multihospital systems such as Columbia or Bon Secours Health System, physician group practices, firms that own many physician group practices, or firms that own many nursing homes such as Manor Care. They may also be **vertically integrated**, providing a continuum of care as when hospital firms provide physician, nursing home, home health, preventive and hospice care, too. Vertical integration of payer and provider firms, which has been relatively rare, is also gaining in popularity. Examples include the development of an insurance or HMO division of a hospital firm and the purchase of an insurance firm by a hospital system. Integration may be accomplished through common ownership of all subunits or through alliances with voluntary participation.

Ownership among health care firms also differs on another dimension. For-profit, not-for-profit and governmental ownership occur among provider and payer organizations. **For-profit firms** are owned by specific individuals or other firms. They exist to enhance the wealth of their owners and are often called investor-owned firms. The investors may be few, as in partnerships, or many as in firms that issue publicly traded stock. **Not-for-profit firms** are typically organized to serve a purpose other than wealth enhancement. The goals of not-for-profit firms are varied. Many such health care firms exist to further a charitable or educational purpose. Although they are not prohibited from generating profits, these firms cannot distribute profits to owners or other persons. Tax regulations differ for the many different types of not-for-profit firms. However, it is accurate to say that most receive at least some beneficial tax treatment from federal and state governments. For example, not-for-profit acute care hospitals are usually exempt from income and property taxes. Finally, health care organizations may be owned by various government entities. Veteran's Administration hospitals are owned by the federal government.

In the health care industry, there has always been a mixture of ownership types. Currently, the majority of acute care hospitals and hospices in the United States are not-for-profit organizations, but the majority of nursing homes and health maintenance organizations are for-profit firms. Why the disparity exists has not been resolved.

Ownership has become even more complex in recent history. Some state and local governments have challenged the exemption from income and property taxes of not-for-profit acute care hospitals claiming these organizations are not pursuing a charitable purpose. Formerly, one could label a firm as either for-profit or not-for-profit firm. Currently, many not-for-profit health care firms have for-profit subsidiaries as well. Another ownership issue is the conversion of not-for-profit firms to for-profit firms. The conversion may occur because a firm is bought by a for-profit firm, as is the case with several acute care hospitals. Or, the conversion may occur because the firm is seeking access to capital through issuing publicly traded stock. An example of the latter is Blue Cross of California's creation of WellPoint Health Networks, Inc.

Summary

This brief overview of the health care environment illustrates some of the complexity managers find in applying financial management concepts and tools in health care organizations. Managers face different types of organizations with different goals. They face pressures to be accountable for financial and medical care outcomes, to integrate disparate parts of their organizations, and to manage risk. As the health care environment continues to evolve, managers must deal with new challenges in realizing the financial and health care outcome goals of their firms.

There are many conflicting pressures on health care organizations today that have no definitive solutions. However, all key decision-makers in the health care field recognize an increasing need for financial resources and a greater emphasis on the financial management process. An effective financial management process is much more than an operating accounting system. It pervades all aspects of the managerial decision-making process. Indeed, in health care firms, the financial management function of all managers is assuming a greater importance. As a result, it is important for all health care managers to have a solid foundation of financial management knowledge and skills.

The goal of this book is to develop such a foundation. In this text, we develop concepts and tools that are useful for the range of health care organizations—providers, payers, and integrated delivery systems—and will continue to be useful as the health care environment continues to change.

Notes

1. Levit, K.R., et al. "National Health Expenditures, 1993" *Health Care Financing Review* 16(1): 247-294, 1994.

2. Kongstvedt, P.R. *Essentials of Managed Care.* Gaithersburg, MD: Aspen Publishers, Inc., 1995, p.26.

Bibliography

Boland, P. *Making Managed Healthcare Work: A Practical Guide to Strategies and Solutions.* New York: McGraw-Hill, 1991.

Hamburger, E., J. Finberg, and L. Alcantar. "The Pot of Gold: Monitoring Health Care Conversions Can Yield Billions of Dollars for Health Care" *Clearinghouse Review* (Aug.-Sept.): 471-504, 1995.

Kongstvedt, P.R. *Essentials of Managed Care.* Gaithersburg, MD: Aspen Publishers, Inc., 1995.

Kovner, A.R. (ed.) *Jonas's Health Care Delivery in the United States.* Fifth Edition. New York: Springer Publishing Co., 1995.

Lee, P.R. and C.L. Estes (eds.). *The Nation's Health.* Fourth Edition. Boston: Jones and Bartlett Publishers, 1994.

Levit, K.R., et al. "National Health Expenditures, 1993" *Health Care Financing Review* 16(1): 247-294, 1994.

Managed Care Assembly, Medical Group Management Association. "Glossary of Terms Used in Managed Care" *Medical Group Management Journal* (Sept./Oct.): 52-65, 1995.

Powell, W.W. (ed.) *The Nonprofit Sector: A Research Handbook.* New Haven: Yale University Press, 1987.

"The Disturbing Trend of Not-For-Profit Hospital Conversions" *Public Citizen Health Research Group Health Letter* 12(7): 1-7, 1996.

Terms and Concepts _____

controlling
fee-for-service
financial accounting
for-profit firm
health maintenance organization
horizontal integration
implementing
managed care
managerial accounting
managerial finance

Medicaid
Medicare
not-for-profit firm
out-of-pocket
payer
personal health services
planning
preferred provider organization
provider
third party payer
vertical integration

Questions _____

1-1   Why is the health care industry important to the economy of the United States?

1-2   What factors may explain the rapid rise in health care expenditures in the United States in the past 30 plus years? Explain.

1-3   Compare and contrast payers and providers. Why is the distinction less useful today than in the past?

1-4   How have payers tried to control inflation in the costs of personal health services?

1-5   How has the distribution of payments changed among consumers and third party payers?

1-6   Compare and contrast horizontally and vertically integrated firms.

1-7   What are the three academic disciplines that form the foundation for financial management?

1-8   What are the three stages of task accomplishment involved in financial management?

1-9   Give examples of some long- and short-term planning issues with which financial management is concerned.

1-10 Give some examples of implementation issues related to financial management.

1-11 Why is the controlling function important to the management of health care organizations?

1-12 How do not-for-profit and for-profit firms differ?

1-13 Why is "consolidation" heard frequently in discussions regarding the health care industry?

1-14 Identify some issues of current concern regarding for-profit and not-for-profit ownership of health care organizations.

2 Financial Accounting: The Language of Financial Management

Traditionally, financial accounting is concerned with the *recording* and *reporting* of the financial transactions of an organization. As such, it serves as a major foundation for understanding the financial management of health care organizations. This chapter explains the basic concepts of financial accounting and introduces three standardized financial statements. First, the methods for recording transactions are presented. Next, the financial statement reports are explained. Finally, some financial accounting concepts and current issues are discussed.

The Accrual Basis of Accounting

There are two accounting bases for recording economic events, or transactions "in the books" of organizations: the accrual basis and the cash basis. The accrual basis of accounting is the method required for most organizations by Generally Accepted Accounting Principles (GAAP). Although most authoritative sources recommend the accrual basis of accounting, the cash basis is still used by some small health care providers, physician practices and some community health care organizations that are under federal, state, or local governmental jurisdictions.

The **accrual basis of accounting** differs from the **cash basis of accounting** in several ways. The first difference concerns when revenues and expenses are recognized. **Recognized** means recorded in the books. In the cash basis of accounting, revenues are recognized when cash is received and expenses are recognized when cash is paid out. In the accrual method of accounting, revenues are recognized when they are earned and expenses are recognized when they are incurred (Figure 2-1). **Revenues** are **earned** when the good or service is delivered or provided. **Expenses** are **incurred** when assets, or resources, are used.

The second major difference between the two methods involves the fundamental accounting equation. This equation keeps the books in balance. The equations used for the accrual and cash methods are discussed below. The third difference is in how the financial statements for the accrual and cash bases are presented. This, too, will be discussed in a later section of the chapter.

The Fundamental Accounting Equations

The conceptual foundation for recording financial transactions consists of two equations. The first equation shows the **assets** (the economic resources) of the organization and the "claims" against those assets. Assets are provided by a variety of sources, and the other side of the equation is designed to identify these sources or claims against the assets. One type of

Figure 2-1   A Comparison of the Cash and Accrual Basis of Accounting.

	Revenue Recognition	**Expenses Recognized**
Cash	When received (When cash comes in)	When paid (When cash goes out)
Accrual	When earned (As they accrue)	When incurred (As they accrue)

"claim" is liabilities. **Liabilities** are the organization's legal obligations to pay for goods or services it receives from others. Liabilities represent the claims of outside parties against the assets of the business. Although they arise mainly as a result of the organization having borrowed money or having received goods or services in advance of having paid for them, they can also arise as a result of patients, clients, or third parties paying in advance. There is an additional type of residual claim that reflects the amount of assets remaining after the liabilities are satisfied. This type of residual claim highlights the difference between for-profit and not-for-profit organizations and is discussed shortly. The for-profit equations are discussed first.

For-Profit Organizations. For a commercial firm, or an investor-owned health care provider, the fundamental accounting equation is:

$$\text{Assets} = \text{Liabilities} + \text{Owners' Equity}$$

The term **owners' equity** or stockholders' equity represents the owners' claims against the assets of the firm. In a sale or bankruptcy, the owners would have legal claim to all the assets remaining after the liabilities were settled. In this event, of course, there may be nothing left for the owners to claim. The equity term in the accounting equation can always be interpreted as a **residual** amount; that is, the amount of assets that are "left over" after the liabilities have been satisfied.

This equation must always remain in balance. If assets are purchased (an increase to assets), then either another asset must decrease, for example, cash, or the right hand side of the equation must increase. The right hand side could increase due to a liability, as when the asset is purchased on credit.

The second fundamental accounting equation is:

$$\text{Revenues} - \text{Expenses} = \text{Income}.$$

The accrual basis of accounting **matches** the revenues earned with the expenses incurred to generate those revenues. Income can be viewed as a measure of efficiency because the fewer resources or expenses used for every dollar of revenues generated, then the higher the efficiency and the greater the profitability of the organization.

The two equations are related. Income can be distributed as dividends to stockholders or retained in the firm. The total amount retained is accumulated in **retained earnings,** which is a part of owners' equity. Thus, *increases* in revenue result in *increases* in retained earnings, but *increases* in expenses result in *decreases* in retained earnings.

Not-For-Profit Organizations. The fundamental accounting equation for not-for-profit NFP) firms is similar to that in the for-profit example:

$$\text{Assets} = \text{Liabilities} + \text{Net Assets} .$$

Net assets represent the residual or remaining interest in the assets of the organization after liabilities are considered. There are two sources of net assets. The first source is external to the organization, comprising money and other resources contributed by outside sources, such as foundations or governmental entities. The second source consists of net assets earned by the organization and retained or reinvested in the organization. Thus, the second fundamental equation, in a NFP setting, is:

$$\text{Unrestricted Revenues} - \text{Expenses} = \text{Change in Unrestricted Net Assets}$$

The same basic rule that applied to owners' equity applies to unrestricted net assets: *net assets increase when revenues increase, and decrease as expenses increase.*

Net assets are categorized as either restricted or unrestricted. The net assets provided by unrestricted donations or earnings (operating income) are **unrestricted net assets**, indicating that the organization is not constrained by donors to use these funds in a particular way. Net assets from donors, governments or foundation grants may be unrestricted or restricted. When donors or grants restrict the uses of funds they are called **restricted net assets.**

Double Entry Recording Method

Each time a transaction is recorded, at least two accounts are affected in the **double entry recording method**. These two entries ensure that the accounting equations discussed above stay in balance. For example, when cash decreases, another asset, such as supplies, increases. Or, if cash is borrowed from a bank, cash increases along with a corresponding increase in liabilities. If a foundation provides funds, then cash increases as does net assets. The following section provides examples of transactions and the double entry recording method for a NFP clinic.

Recording Transactions Using the Accrual Basis of Accounting

Figure 2-2 presents 11 sample transactions for CompClinic, a not-for-profit firm. CompClinic started with a donation of $100,000 in December. The following January was its first month of operations and the focus for this example. Thus, CompClinic begins operations

Figure 2-2 Transactions of CompClinic for the Month of January.

Assume CompClinic began business in December of 19X0. It started with a cash donation of $100,000. During the month of January, it has the following transactions:

(1)   The landlord is paid $3,000 for three months' rent in advance on January 1, 19X1.

(2) $5,000 of the money in the bank is used to purchase supplies. During the month, $500 worth of supplies are used.

(3)   CompClinic borrows an additional $50,000 from the bank.

(4)   The clinic purchases $75,000 worth of equipment on credit.

(5)   The clinic subsequently pays the equipment company $25,000 of the $75,000 it owes them.

(6)   Patients are billed for the $10,000 worth of services CompClinic has rendered.

(7)   Patients pay $6,000 of the $10,000 they were billed. They still owe the remaining $4,000.

(8)   CompClinic pays $2,000 for operating expenses (insurance, utilities, maintenance, etc.).

(9)   CompClinic earns $4,000 in interest on its money in the bank. However, the interest has not yet been received.

(10)   CompClinic owes its employees $700 for work they have done during this pay period.

(11)   CompClinic receives a cash donation of $1,000.

with $100,000 in assets (cash) and $100,000 in net assets. The fundamental accounting equation is in balance. Each transaction in Figure 2-2 is discussed below and its corresponding accrual basis of accounting treatment is shown in Table 2-1.

Rent Paid in Advance (1). The clinic pays for the next three months' rent in advance, which is called prepaid rent. This prepayment is an asset that will be "used up" over the next three months. *Cash* decreases and *prepaid rent* increases by $3,000. One asset account increases and another asset account decreases; the accounting equation remains in balance.

Supplies Purchased (2). The purchase of $5,000 of office supplies decreases *cash* by $5,000 and increases *supplies*, another asset account, by the same amount.

Cash Borrowed (3). The clinic borrows $50,000 from the bank, which increases *cash* and *liabilities* (for debt owed to bank) by $50,000. Both the asset and liabilities increase; the accounting equation remains in balance.

Equipment Purchased on Credit (4). The clinic purchases $75,000 of office and medical equipment on credit. Thus, the asset *equipment* is increased by that amount, and the second entry increases *liabilities* to reflect the $75,000 now owed to creditors.

Table 2-1 Recording of Financial Transactions in Figure 2-2 Using the Accrual Basis of Accounting.

Transaction	Cash	Accounts Receivable	Allowance for Doubtful Accounts	Interest Receivable	Supplies	Prepaid Rent	Equipment
			Assets				
Beginning Balance	$100,000	$0	$0	$0	$0	$0	$0
1. Paid rent in advance	(3,000)					3,000	
2. Purchased supplies (cash)	(5,000)				5,000		
3. Borrowed from bank	50,000						
4. Purchase equipment (credit)							75,000
5. Paid for equipment	(25,000)						
6. Patients billed for services		10,000					
7. Received from patients	6,000	(6,000)					
8. Paid for operating expenses	(2,000)						
9. Interest earned				4,000			
10. Wages payable							
11. Contribution donated	1,000						
Sub-totals	122,000	4,000	0	4,000	5,000	3,000	75,000
Adjustments:							
12. Operating expense					(500)		
13. Rent expense						(1,000)	
14. Depreciation							
15. Provision for bad debt			(400)				
Ending Balances, January 31, 19X1	$122,000	$4,000	($400)	$4,000	$4,500	$2,000	$75,000
Increase in net assets (net income)							

Table 2-1   continued

Transaction	Assets: Accumulated Depreciation	Assets: Total Assets	Liabilities: Wages Payable	Liabilities: Accounts & Notes Payable	Liabilities: Total Liabilities	Net Assets: Revenues	Net Assets: Expenses	Net Assets: Net Assets	Liabilities & Net Assets
Beginning Balance	$0	$100,000	$0	$0	$0	$0	$0	$100,000	$100,000
1. Paid rent in advance		100,000		0	0			100,000	100,000
2. Purchased supplies (cash)		100,000		0	0			100,000	100,000
3. Borrowed from bank		150,000		50,000	50,000			100,000	150,000
4. Purchase equipment (credit)		225,000		75,000	125,000			100,000	225,000
5. Paid for equipment		200,000		(25,000)	100,000			100,000	200,000
6. Patients billed for services		210,000			100,000	10,000		110,000	210,000
7. Received from patients		210,000			100,000			110,000	210,000
8. Paid for operating expenses		208,000			100,000		(2,000)	108,000	208,000
9. Interest earned		212,000			100,000	4,000		112,000	212,000
10. Wages payable		212,000	700		100,700		(700)	111,300	212,000
11. Donation contributed		213,000			100,700	1,000		112,300	213,000
Sub-totals	$0	$213,000	$700	$100,000	$100,700	$15,000	(2,700)	112,300	213,000
Adjustments:									
12. Operating expense		212,500			100,700		(500)	111,800	212,500
13. Rent expense		211,500			100,700		(1,000)	110,800	
14. Depreciation	(625)	210,875			100,700		(625)	110,175	210,875
15. Provision for bad debt		210,475			100,700		(400)	109,775	210,475
Ending Balances, January 31, 19X1	($625)	$210,475	$700	$100,000	$100,700	$15,000	($5,225)	$109,775	$210,475
Increase in net assets (net income)								$9,775	

Payment on Account (5). The clinic paid its creditors $25,000 of the $75,000 it owes for the equipment. It records decreases in both *cash* and *liabilities* of $25,000.

Patients Billed for Services (6). CompClinic bills $10,000 of services to patients, which increases *revenues* (recognized when service delivered). Since it has not yet received payment for the services it records a $10,000 increase in **accounts receivable**, an asset account that is used when money is owed to the clinic. Remember that revenues increase net assets. So, in this transaction, an asset, accounts receivable, and net assets increase; the accounting equation remains in balance.

Payment Received (7). Patients pay $6,000 of the receivables owed to the clinic. *Cash* is increased by $6,000 and *accounts receivable* is decreased by the same amount.

Operating Expenses Paid (8). The clinic pays $2,000 in cash for operating expenses. *Cash* decreases and *expenses* increase by $2,000. Expenses decrease net assets. The accounting equation remains in balance because cash and net assets both decrease.

Interest Earned (9). CompClinic earned $4,000 in interest, but it has not yet received the money. Under the accrual basis of accounting, revenues are recognized when earned. Thus, the clinic would record a $4,000 increase in *net assets* and a $4,000 increase in *interest receivable*, an asset account. When the cash is received, the interest receivable account will be decreased.

Wages Owed (10). The clinic owes its employees $700 in wages for work that the employees have performed. The $700 increases *liabilities (specifically, wages payable)*, since the clinic owes this money, and increases *operating expenses*, since the clinic used these labor resources. In the accrual method of accounting, expenses are recorded when the resources are used, regardless of when the cash is paid out.

Donation Received (11). On the last day of January, CompClinic received a donation of $1,000. This entry to the books is an increase to *cash* and an increase in other revenue.

On the last day of a month or year, the organization may need to adjust the books to record some revenues that have just been earned and some expenses that have just been incurred. These end-of-accounting-period entries are called **adjusting entries**. These adjustments are needed to bring the books up to date. The following four items are common adjusting entries.

Supplies Expense Recognized (12). In transaction (2), the clinic purchased $5,000 of supplies and recorded this transaction by decreasing cash and increasing the supplies account. No expense was shown at that time. Now, since $500 worth of supplies have been used in January, the clinic must record this supplies expense by decreasing the *supplies* account and increasing the *net assets* account. At the end of January, the supplies account has $4,500 of unused supplies in it.

Rent Expense Recognized (13). In transaction (1), the clinic paid for three month's rent in advance. One month has been used up at the end of January. To recognize January's rent expense, a decrease in *prepaid rent* is recorded as well as a decrease in *net assets*. The prepaid rent account now has two months' rent remaining.

Depreciation Expense Recognized (14). In transaction (4), the clinic purchased equipment and recorded an increase in the equipment account and an increase in a liability account. No expense was recorded. The expenses associated with plant and equipment are called depreciation. **Depreciation** is a means to systematically spread the cost of a long-lived asset over the years when it helps to earn revenues (called the **useful life**). Assume the equipment will be used for ten years and will have zero trade-in or resale value at the end of the ten years. The original cost of the equipment ($75,000) can be evenly spread over ten years ($7,500 per year), and further, the annual depreciation of $7,500 can be spread over each month of the year ($625 per month). When depreciation is spread evenly over the useful life of the asset it is called the straight-line method of depreciation. Other methods of depreciation are explained in financial accounting textbooks. The clinic would record an increase in *depreciation expense* and a decrease in the equipment asset. A special account, called a **contra-asset account**, is used to show this reduction in the asset amount on the books. Thus, the second entry would be an increase in **accumulated depreciation**, which is *subtracted* from the equipment account to show the reduction in recorded, or book, value. The accumulated depreciation will increase over time until, at the end of ten years, the accumulated depreciation will equal the original purchase cost of the asset, here $75,000. When that occurs, the equipment asset will have a net book value of zero. **Net book value** represents the original cost of the asset minus the accumulated depreciation amount for that asset.

Bad Debt Expense Recognized (15). Another contra-asset account is the allowance for doubtful accounts. This account reduces the amount of accounts receivable to recognize that some accounts receivable will never be collected. At the end of an accounting period (a month or a year), an estimate of bad debts is made. The entry recording this estimate is an increase in *provision for bad debts*, an expense account, and an increase in the **allowance for doubtful accounts**, a contra-asset account that reduces the amount of accounts receivable. **Net receivables** is the term used for accounts receivable minus the allowance for doubtful accounts. Assume that the provision for bad debts for January is $400. To recognize this expense, the *allowance for doubtful accounts* and the *provision for bad debt* are both increased by $400. The net receivables would be $3,600 (the $4,000 still owed minus $400 allowance for doubtful accounts). Although the clinic is owed $4,000, it expects to collect only $3,600 of this amount.

The Cash Basis of Accounting

Another way of recording transactions for financial purposes is on a "cash-in/cash-out" basis. The cash basis of accounting is similar to the method many people use for their personal finances. Revenues are recognized when money is received for services provided, and expenses are recognized when money is paid out for the resources used to provide those services. In the cash basis, expenses are called expenditures or disbursements. The double entry method is used with the cash basis, also.

The Fundamental Accounting Equation

Since only changes in cash are recorded, obligations or liabilities are *not* recognized under the cash basis of accounting. Each time a transaction is recorded, cash either increases or decreases because in the cash basis *only cash inflows or outflows trigger a double entry*. The equation is:

$$\text{Assets} = \text{Net Assets}$$

If cash increases, then revenues or net assets increase by that same amount. In the cash basis, revenues are recognized when cash is received by the organization. If cash decreases, then the expenditures of the organization increase and net assets decrease. An **expenditure** (analogous to an expense) is recorded only when cash is disbursed from the organization. Net assets increase with the amount of any cash brought into the organization and decrease by the amount of any cash disbursed.

Under the cash basis of accounting, profit represents the amount of money that came in for service-related items in excess of the money that went out. The cash basis provides no information on how much income was actually earned or how much of the organization's resources were consumed. Because income is dependent on the timing of cash flows under the cash basis of accounting, wide swings in reported income may occur. The distortion of expenses can affect the reported costs for patient or managed care services. These swings in cost may be mistakenly interpreted as the result of changes in the efficiency of management, but in fact they are only the result of cash flow patterns.

Recording Transactions Using the Cash Basis of Accounting

Table 2-2 shows the cash basis of accounting treatment for the first ten transactions in Figure 2-2. Each transaction is discussed below. To highlight the similarities and differences between the two methods of accounting, the cash basis treatment in Table 2-2 can be compared with the accrual basis treatment in Table 2-1. Recall that CompClinic started operations in January with a beginning balance of $100,000 in cash (an asset) and $100,000 in net assets.

Rent Paid in Advance (1). The clinic pays three months' rent in advance, which decreases *cash* by $3,000 and increases *expenditures* by $3,000. Recall that expenditures reduce net assets.

Supplies Purchased (2). The purchase of $5,000 worth of office supplies, is recorded by decreasing the *cash* account by $5,000 and showing a corresponding $5,000 increase in *expenditures*.

Table 2-2 Recording of Financial Transactions in Figure 2-2 Using the Cash Basis of Accounting.

TRANSACTION	Assets (Cash)	Net Assets		
		Increases	Decreases	Balance
Beginning Balances	$100,000			$100,000
1. Paid rent in advance	($3,000)		($3,000)	$97,000
2. Purchase supplies	($5,000)		($5,000)	$ 92,000
3. Borrowed from bank	$50,000	$50,000		$142,000
5. Paid for equipment	($25,000)		($25,000)	$117,000
7. Patients' payments	$6,000	$6,000		$123,000
8. Paid for operating expenses	($2,000)		($2,000)	$121,000
11. Donation contributed	$1,000	$1,000		$122,000
Totals	$122,000	$57,000	($35,000)	$122,000

Note: Transactions 4, 6, 9, and 10 are not recorded using the cash basis of accounting as they do not involve the exchange of cash. The differences between the revenues ($7,000) and expenditures ($35,000) represent the operating income for the period or a loss of $28,000 (Table 2-7).

Cash Borrowed (3). The clinic borrows $50,000 from the bank. *Cash* increases by $50,000, and *net assets* increase by $50,000.

Equipment Purchased on Credit (4). The clinic purchases $75,000 of office and medical equipment on credit. *Since no cash changed hands, this transaction is not recorded in the cash basis of accounting.*

Payment on Account (5). The clinic pays its creditors $25,000 of the $75,000 it owes for the equipment. It records a *cash* decrease of $25,000 and an *expenditure* of $25,000.

Patients Billed for Services (6). *Since no cash changed hands, this transaction is not recorded in the cash basis of accounting.*

Payment Received (7). When the patients pay $6,000 of the $10,000 they owed, CompClinic records that *cash* increases by $6,000 as does its *revenues*. Revenues increase net assets.

Operating Expenses Paid (8). CompClinic pays $2,000 for general operating expenses, reducing *cash* by $2,000 and increasing *expenditures* by the same amount.

Interest Earned (9). *Since no cash changed hands, this transaction is not recorded in the cash basis of accounting.* The transaction will occur when the cash is received for the $4,000 interest earned.

Wages Owed (10). *Since no cash changed hands, this transaction is not recorded in the cash basis of accounting.* The transaction is recorded when the employees are paid.

Donation Received (11). On the last day of January, CompClinic received a donation of $1,000. This entry to the books is an increase to *cash* and an increase in *net assets*.

Cash Versus Accrual Accounting

The difference between the cash and accrual bases of accounting rests primarily on when revenues and expenses are recognized (Figure 2-1). Under the cash basis of accounting, revenues are recognized only when cash is received from patients, clients, or others, whereas expenses are recognized only when the provider pays them. The major advantage of the cash basis of accounting is its simplicity. However, the cash basis of accounting has several disadvantages:

(1) It does not recognize liabilities the firm owes to creditors (payables);
(2) It does not recognize revenues that are earned, but not yet received (receivables);
(3) It does not recognize expenses as resources are used, but only when money is paid out (expenditures);
(4) It fails to match revenues with the expenses that helped earn them;
(5) Its income may differ greatly from that reported under the accrual basis of accounting; and
(6) Its financial statements are open to serious manipulation by management because, if an organization wants to make its costs look lower, it may try to delay paying some of its year-end bills.

The Journal, the Ledger, and the Chart of Accounts

For illustrative purposes, CompClinic's transactions were recorded chronologically in columns on a single sheet of paper (Table 2-1). This is possible because there are so few transactions. Many health care organizations record thousands of transactions during a single month. Therefore, to make sure that records are kept orderly, a standardized approach has been developed for recording financial transactions.

The financial accounting process begins when a document is created indicating that a transaction has occurred. Such documents for health care providers include receipts and service slips. A chronological summary of these transactions is recorded in a **journal**. The journal is also called the book of original entry. From this chronological listing, transactions are then recorded (posted) to a **ledger**, which keeps a running balance of the amounts in any of the asset, liability, owners' equity, revenue, and expense accounts of the organization. Thus, at any point in time, a health care organization is able to ascertain both a chronological record and the current balance of any account by referring to either the journal or the ledger, respectively.

Within the ledger are two types of accounts. The first, called **real accounts,** includes all asset and liability accounts as well as the net asset (owners' equity) accounts. These accounts are cumulative records of what has occurred since the organization began. The ending balance of these accounts, the amount reported on the balance sheet, is also the same amount that the organization begins with the following business day. For instance, CompClinic ended the month of January with $122,000 in cash. It will also begin business on February 1, 19X1, with the same amount (Table 2-3).

Nominal accounts are revenues and expenses. At the end of every period, these accounts are closed; that is, the expenses are subtracted from the revenues, and the increase (decrease) in net assets (net income or loss) is transferred to the unrestricted net assets (owners' equity) account. When the organization opens business the next day, the revenue and expense accounts begin with a zero balance. Thus, when the next financial statements are prepared, the ending amount in these accounts represents the revenues and expenses of the organization since the last financial statements were issued. In the case of CompClinic, the amounts in the revenue and expense accounts when it reports its February net income will be the amounts accumulated since the financial statements were prepared on January 31, 19X1.

Every health care organization uses a **chart of accounts**, which is a numbering system for all the accounts that a particular provider or payer is likely to use. For instance, all asset accounts may be assigned numbers between 1000 and 1999. The liability accounts may all be numbered in the 2000's. Similarly, the net asset (owners' equity), revenue, and expense accounts would likely be numbered in the 3000's, 4000's, and 5000's, respectively. Within each category, specific accounts have their own designations. For example, asset accounts may be categorized as cash (1100), marketable securities (1200), accounts receivable (1300), inventories (1600), and prepaid items (1800). Each of these categories might be further subdivided. A standardized chart of accounts has a number of advantages, including saving each organization the difficult task of developing its own, and standardizing the manner in which all organizations of similar types (e.g., health departments, hospitals, medical groups, insurance companies, etc.) record financial transactions. Many voluntary associations (e.g. American Hospital Association, Medical Group Management Association) have developed recommended charts of accounts for their members to use.

Financial Reporting Statements

There are three standardized financial statements: **the balance sheet, the income statement and the cash flow statement**. Whereas the income statement reports on the revenues and expenses of the organization for a *period of time,* such as over a month or a year, the balance sheet reports on the organization's assets, liabilities, and net assets (owners' equity) at a *point in time*, namely, at the conclusion of the last day of the accounting period, such as December 31. Thus, the balance sheet provides a snapshot of the organization at a single instant, whereas the income statement provides a summary of the revenues and expenses accumulated during the period being reported. The cash flow statement shows the sources and uses of cash by the organization for a *period of time*.

Table 2-3 Balance Sheet Prepared on the Accrual Basis of Accounting for Transactions in Table 2-1.

CompClinic
Balance Sheet
January 31, 19X1

Assets			Equities	
Current assets:			Current liabilities:	
Cash		$122,000		
Accounts receivable	4,000		Wages payable	$ 700
less: uncollectables			Current portion of	
and allowances	(400)	3,600	long-term notes payable	15,000
Interest receivable		4,000	Net current liabilities	15,700
Supplies		4,500		
Prepaid rent		2,000	Long-term debt, net of	
Total current assets		136,100	current portion	85,000
Assets limited as to use, net of amounts required to meet current obligations:			Total liabilities	100,700
			Net assets:	
Equipment, net		74,375		
			Unrestricted net assets	109,775
Net noncurrent assets		74,375		
Total assets		$210,475		
			Total liabilities and net assets	$210,475

Financial statement presentation may appear confusing. The accounting profession, notably the American Institute of Certified Public Accountants (AICPA), the Financial Accounting Standards Board (FASB), and the Government Accounting Standards Board (GASB), are all involved in trying to standardize these formats in an effort to make the statements more easily understood. In this text, we have adopted the financial statement formats indicated in the most recent (1996) audit guide issued by the Health Care Committee and the Health Care Audit Guide Task Force, Federal Government Division, of the American Institute of Certified Public Accountants (AICPA). It supersedes the previous edition of the *Audits of Providers of Health Care Services* and it contains the relevant sections of FASB Statement No. 117, *Accounting for Contributions Received and Contributions Made*, and FASB Statement No. 117, *Financial Statements of Not-for-Profit Organizations*. In the end-of-chapter materials, we have retained some variety in the financial statements illustrated.

The next sections discuss each of the financial statements. Unless otherwise noted, the accrual basis of accounting is presumed.

Balance Sheet

The balance sheet is sometimes called the statement of financial position or the statement of financial condition. The balance sheet is a *cumulative* record of the assets, liabilities, and net asset (owners' equity) accounts. The frequency of balance sheet preparation depends on the value of information obtained as compared to the cost of preparing the statement. Theoretically, the balance sheet could be prepared after every transaction. A balance sheet could be available, on demand, from a computer file. However, some accounting statements may require professional estimates or adjusting entries. Therefore, the "instantaneous" or "on-line" balance sheet might not be as useful as one that was prepared at year-end or at the end of a fiscal quarter.

Balance sheets provide a catalog or list of assets, liabilities and net assets (owners' equities). They document the amount of resources and sources of resources at a point in time. They provide a listing of all assets or resources controlled by the organization at that moment in time. Balance sheets always represent the fundamental accounting equation and must balance. Assets are listed on the left side (or top) of most balance sheets. Each line on the left side of a balance sheet indicates a different type of asset. Liabilities and equities are listed on the right side or bottom of the statement.

Some financial statements may contain a **statement of changes in net assets (owners' equity)**. This statement describes major reasons for the increases and decreases in the net assets or in owners' equity. Alternatively, this information may be shown in a separate statement, as is shown for CompClinic in Table 2-4. The statement's main purpose is to reconcile the beginning and ending balances of net assets and show how the net assets have changed during the period.

Assets. Assets represent future economic benefits that are owned or controlled by an organization. Assets typically represent economic resources that are tangible, like buildings or trucks. On the other hand, some economic resources or assets may not be tangible, like patent rights or copyrights. Assets may also be represented by promises of future payments, where the promises are made by customers who bought goods or services on credit. Assets are generally listed in order of liquidity, starting with cash. Most assets are recorded on the balance sheet at their historical acquisition cost.

Some providers of health care services, such as hospitals, show a separate listing of assets whose use is limited. These assets may include accounts for funds to pay principal on bonds, money to satisfy the requirements of third party payers or funds set aside for plant replacement. CompClinic has a zero balance for "assets limited as to use, net of amounts to meet current obligations" (Table 2-3).

Current Assets. Current assets include cash or other liquid resources that will typically become cash or cash equivalents in a short time period, usually a year or less. Cash equivalents are current assets because certificates of deposit or marketable securities can be turned into cash within several days.

Accounts receivable represent another typical current asset, showing resources due from customers or clients who have already bought goods or services and who have promised to

Table 2-4   Statement of Changes in Net Assets.

CompClinic
Statement of Changes in Net Assets
For the Period Ending January 31, 19X1

Unrestricted net assets:	
Excess of revenues over expenses	$8,775
Contributions from Comp Foundation	1,000
Increase in unrestricted net assets	9,775
Temporarily restricted net assets:	(N.A.)
Permanently restricted net assets:	(N.A.)
Increase in net assets	9,775
Net assets, beginning of month (including original contribution)	100,000
Net assets, end of month	$109,775

pay for such goods or services in the future. Accounts receivable are converted into cash as soon as the customers or clients pay their bills (their accounts). Credit terms will usually be stated explicitly on the customers' bills or accounts. Such terms may require payment in 30 days or less.

Supplies represent items that have been purchased for use by patients, or office supplies used in managing the organization. Supplies can be as prosaic as band-aids or aspirin, or they can be as exotic as silver recovered from x-ray films or artificial organs.

Prepaid expenses represent unexpired or unused assets such as insurance policies which have been purchased and paid for in advance. The unexpired portion, the portion of the policy paid for but not yet used, is shown as part of prepaid expenses. As the insurance is used, the prepaid expenses become actual expenses. Prepaids are usually minor elements of the balance sheet.

Most current assets turn over quickly, and their acquisition costs will be in terms of relatively current market values. In fact, marketable securities and supplies inventories are shown on the balance sheet at the lower of their historical cost or current market values.

Fixed Assets. Fixed assets are long-term assets that are used to produce goods or services. Hence, they relate to the organization's capacity to provide patient or other services. All fixed assets are recorded on the balance sheet at their historical acquisition costs, but many of these values are out-of-date in terms of current market values. They indicate little about the market value of the organization. They also indicate little about the future resources necessary to replace the fixed assets.

Most fixed assets are part of property, plant and equipment. Some balance sheets show these elements as separate categories, while others just list the types of fixed assets without any sub-totals or categories. Buildings and equipment represent the largest category of fixed assets in most health care organizations. Buildings may be used for offices or hospitals or health clinics. Equipment includes all of the desks and chairs, computers, x-ray and other scanners, operating room tables, surgical equipment, etc.

Since buildings and equipment are long-lived, their entire purchase costs are not charged or recorded as expenses during the first year, but are depreciated over their expected useful lives. Depreciation may be computed in a number of ways. Regardless of the depreciation method used, the net book values recorded on the balance sheet for each fixed asset decrease with the passage of time, due to the accountant's recognition of depreciation. Net book value is the difference between original cost and the depreciation that has been recorded. The depreciation that has already been recognized is called accumulated depreciation. In any balance sheet, the net book value of buildings and equipment is calculated by subtracting the accumulated depreciation from the original acquisition cost. For example:

Buildings & Equipment	$865,000
Less: Accumulated Depreciation	−313,000
Net Book Value (Bldgs. & Equip.)	$552,000

Land as an asset may be vacant land or it may be the land on which the office or hospital is situated. Since land is usually the oldest asset held by most organizations, it is often the most out-of-date in terms of current market values.

The current assets and fixed assets are added together to compute total assets. This total asset figure must equal the sum of the right hand side of the balance sheet equation.

Liabilities. There are two categories of liabilities, current and long-term. Each liability category has some attributes similar to the corresponding asset categories.

Current Liabilities. Current liabilities are short-term debts must usually be paid within a year. They often have no formal maturity date and includes the current portion of long-term debt. The first current liability shown on most balance sheets is called **accounts payable**. Accounts payable represent debts that the organization has incurred in the past—usually for the purchase of supplies. Accounts payable may be called "trade debt" because it occurs in the normal course of any trade or business.

Other typical current liabilities are related to short-term financing transactions, such as notes payable. Notes payable are more formal current liabilities than are the accounts payable because a formal legal document has usually been signed to acknowledge the outstanding debt.

Another category of current liabilities is accrued expenses. Accrued expenses are "the opposite" of prepaid expenses. Although both represent some previous transaction that also affects expenses. In the case of prepaid expenses, the cash outflow occurs prior to recognizing the expense, whereas in the case of accrued expenses, the expense is recognized prior to the cash outflow. Accrued expenses occur in the normal operations of most organizations and they usually represent liabilities for services already received, but not yet been paid for, such as wages payable.

Note that the term "expenses" has already been discussed twice in the context of the balance sheet, even though expenses themselves are shown on the income statement. This is an example of confusing and overlapping terminology that accountants often use. As a general guide, any expenses that are "prepaid" are an asset and any expenses that are "accrued" are a liability. In general, anything that is "accrued" or "payable" can be treated as a liability.

Taxes payable represent unpaid taxes that are owed to a governmental unit. Taxes payable may include unpaid employees' withheld taxes, unemployment taxes, workers' compensation, Social Security (FICA), or any number of other taxes that are incurred and accrued in the normal course of daily operations.

Long-Term Liabilities. Another major section of the balance sheet contains the long-term liabilities. The cycle of payment and maturity dates for long-term liabilities is usually longer than one year. Most long-term liabilities represent major contractual commitments by the organization. As such, they represent constraints on future operations because the original promises or commitments made to the lenders must be honored (or approval for changes must be obtained). Most balance sheets will also disclose (in the notes accompanying the financial statements) some of these constraints, especially in terms of expected future cash outflows for principal and interest payments.

A major type of long-term liability is the mortgage payable; a mortgage represents a legal agreement to repay the debt and it represents a pledge of certain assets that will revert to the lender if the debt is not paid. The problem with mortgages on physician offices and hospitals is that there are often very few buyers for specialized health care facilities. In such cases, a default on a mortgage represents more risk to the lenders and also indicates that most lenders will cooperate with the borrowers to find alternative solutions to avoid having to foreclose on the mortgage and seize the collateral property.

Bonds payable, pension liabilities, and malpractice liabilities are additional examples of long-term liabilities.

Both current and long-term liabilities are then summed to arrive at a new sub-total, called total liabilities.

Net Assets (Owners' Equities). The final category of information on the balance sheet represents resources provided by non-creditors. There are two general categories of net asset or owners' equity accounts, invested capital (for-profits) or donated capital (not-for-profits) and retained earnings.

For a commercial organization, this final section represents claims by owners, or stockholders, on the organization's residual resources. For a not-for-profit, this final section represents claims by a variety of external constituencies on the organizations net assets. A common misconception is that this section of the balance sheet represents money that could be taken out and spent. Net assets (or owners' equity) does *not* represent money that could be withdrawn. Actual funds are in the asset section. What net assets does represent is the *residual claims* on assets that have been invested or donated. And it also includes *residual claims* on resources that have been earned, but not yet withdrawn.

For NFP firms, net assets (or owners' equities) represent resources invested or contributed by donors or resources obtained from the organization's prior operating activities. The net assets include claims by the community-at-large, or, perhaps, claims that may be asserted by governmental agencies. These claims may be against restricted net assets or unrestricted net assets. For a not-for-profit organization, there is no invested capital from owners; yet, there are contributions and other grants that have been received in the past. Not-for-profit organizations and government agencies have an analogous category on their balance sheets, including terms such as Contributions or Grants Received or Founding Grants, Temporarily Restricted Net Assets, or Permanently Restricted Net Assets. Increases in net assets are used generically to represent all sources of resources not provided by creditors. Depending on the type of organization, this might also be called "Capital," "Shareholders' Equity," or "Fund Balance."

Invested capital in a corporation represents direct investments by owners in the organization. When the business was founded, someone invested cash, land, patents, or other resources. All of these original investments are capitalized as part of owners' equity. This section of the balance sheet often represents transactions and investments at earlier points in the history of the business. As such, the values shown as invested capital do not represent current market values. In fact, there is little relationship between invested capital on the balance sheet and the market value of a company's stock. Invested capital is a generic term that often encompasses several different equity accounts: Capital Stock, Common Stock, Preferred Stock, Paid-in-Capital or Capital in Excess of Par Value.

The other major element of owners' equity is called retained earnings. Both for-profit and NFP firms record retained earnings. Retained earnings represent accumulated earnings or net income from all prior periods that have not been withdrawn or used to pay dividends. In other words, retained earnings represents the accumulated, but not used, successes of the organization. Earnings that are distributed by a business are often paid in the form of dividends to shareholders or withdrawals by owners. Claims against resources represent earnings that were not distributed or "retained." Retained earnings does *not* represent cash that can be paid to owners. This is comparable to claims against net assets in a not-for-profit organization. The community (donors) or the government has a similar claim on all residual resources.

Retained earnings function as a balancing item, because changes in retained earnings summarize the effects of operations (revenues minus expenses). The balance sheet would not balance without an account like retained earnings or unrestricted net assets. Retained earnings include accumulated revenues in excess of expences.

The owners' equity or net assets accounts are summed to calculate the total owners' equity or total net assets. This total is then added to the total liabilities figure to compute the total amount on the right hand side of the accounting equation. It must equal the left hand side—total assets. Additional illustrations of the balance sheet accounts are found in Appendix 2A.

CompClinic's Illustrative Balance Sheet

The information for CompClinic's balance sheet (Table 2-3) comes from the row labeled "Ending Balances, January 31, 19X1" at the bottom of Table 2-1. All accounts are summarized on the balance sheet with the exception of revenues and expenses, which are presented on the income statement. The format of the balance sheet follows the fundamental accounting equation. Thus, in Table 2-3, the assets equal $210,475 and the liabilities and net assets (owners' equity) accounts together also equal $210,475.

Income Statement or Statement of Operations

The income statement prepared on the accrual basis of accounting has two major sections: revenues and expenses (Table 2-5). The revenues and expenses of CompClinic were recorded in the two right-hand columns of Table 2-1. CompClinic's income statement summarizes those revenues and expenses for interested parties. During January 19X1, CompClinic received $15,000 in revenues (Table 2-3). The income statement is designed to indicate the sources of these revenues.

Table 2-5   Income Statement Prepared on the Accrual Basis of Accounting.

CompClinic
Statement of Operations
For the Period Ending January 31, 19X1

Unrestricted revenues, gains and other support:		
Net patient service revenue		$10,000
Other, primarily interest income		4,000
Total revenues, gains and other support		14,000
Expenses:		
Operating expenses	3,200	
Depreciation	625	
Rent	1,000	
Provision for bad debts	400	
Total expenses		5,225
Excess of revenues, gains and other support over expenses		8,775
Contributions from Comp Foundation		1,000
Increase in unrestricted net assets		$ 9,775

Revenues. Revenues result from providing services or selling goods. The revenues are categorized as unrestricted revenues and other revenues. Each is discussed below. These types of revenues are then summed as total revenues, gains and other support.

Unrestricted revenues. The **unrestricted revenues** are revenues that are in the organization's main line of business. For providers in health care organizations, this is almost always the provision of health care. For payers and insurance companies and managed care organizations, revenues are generated in the form of fees or monthly premiums. Providers of health care services report net patient revenues. These are gross patient revenues less contractual allowances, charity care and administrative allowances. Gross revenues are revenues reported at full charges. However, many patients do not pay that amount. Contractual allowances reflect the difference between full charges and the amount third parties pay on their clients' behalf. This difference arises because of the contractual arrangement a health care provider makes with a third party in which the provider agrees to provide services to covered patients and accept a pre-negotiated, set, or "reasonable" amount in return. The amount by which the payment is below the full charge is the contractual allowance. Charity care occurs when the provider intends to provide services to patients at no cost. The provider's policy guides these decisions. Administrative allowances arise as a result of internal policies which allow deductions to certain categories of patients such as employees, clergy, and teachers. Such allowances might be included under the charity care category. Contractual allowances and charity care are now shown in the notes to the financial statements, and not as part of the income statement.

Other revenues. **Other revenues** are revenues that are earned from activities other than the organization's main line of business. Examples include interest and dividends from investments, cafeteria sales, and parking concessions. These other revenues are shown just below the net patient service revenue. (Alternatively, interest and dividends may be shown following expenses.) In the CompClinic example, other revenues, under the accrual basis of accounting are $4,000 (Table 2-5).

Expenses. Expenses reflect the cost of resources used to provide health care services. In addition, expenses include other costs of doing business such as the failure to collect receivables (bad debt expense). As with revenues, health care organizations used to divide their expenses into the two categories of operating and nonoperating expenses. However, expenses are now disclosed in a single category, that may be divided into a natural classification or a functional presentation. Many health care organizations report expenses in only two categories: (a) health services (including inpatient services, outpatient procedures, home health services, etc.) and (b) general and administrative. Expenses incurred in activities other than in the organization's main line of business are combined with other related expenses, and not separately disclosed. CompClinic's total expenses are $5,225 (Table 2-5) and are shown just below the list of expenses.

Other gains and losses. Any extraordinary losses, transfers, etc. are shown in later sections of the income statement. Operating results should also be reported separately from the following categories, which are not considered to be revenues or expenses but lead to changes in net assets:

- transactions with owners, acting in that capacity,
- equity transfers (involving other entities that control the reporting entity, are controlled by the reporting entity, or are under common control),
- receipt of contributions that are not recurring, which may be restricted or unrestricted (note that the contribution from Comp Foundation was not restricted),
- contributions of long-lived assets, and
- other items requiring separate disclosure (such as extraordinary items, the effects of discontinued operations, or the cumulative effect of accounting changes).

Although the distinction between operating and nonoperating expenses has been eliminated, the *separate disclosure* of many items that previously would have been shown as nonoperating items is still required.

Income. The statement of operations, or income statement, computes several different useful sub-totals. One of the most useful is the difference between total revenues and total expenses, which is called **net income** (or operating income) for for-profit firms. It is called the **excess of revenues, gains and other support over expenses** (or just **excess of revenues over expenses**) for not-for-profit firms. This sub-total provides an indication of the provider's efficiency.

Also included on the Statement of Operations for a not-for-profit firm is the **increase (decrease) in unrestricted net assets**. It is the excess of revenues over expenses plus or minus the other gains and losses. It shows the changes in unrestricted resources during the period. In either case, the bottom line increases or decreases retained earnings in for-profit firms or unrestricted net assets in NFP organizations.

Statement of Cash Flows

The **statement of cash flows** summarizes cash flows resulting from the three major financial management activities: operating, investing, and financing. A statement of cash flows for CompClinic can be found in Table 2-6. There are actually two different formats allowed for this statement, termed the direct and indirect methods. The format used in constructing Table 2-6 is the direct method, which is easier to understand and interpret. In addition to the actual statement itself, many organizations also provide a related schedule: Reconciliation of changes in net assets (net income) to cash provided by operating activities (indirect method). By including this supplementary information, health care organizations are essentially providing the information that would be contained under both the direct and indirect method. We have included this supplementary information in the bottom section of Table 2-6. In addition, the organization must present, in the notes, a disclosure of its accounting policies regarding how it calculates cash equivalents.

Table 2-6   CompClinic Statement of Cash Flows (Month ending 1/31/X1), Direct Method.

Cash flows from operating activities:		
Cash received from patients	$6,000	
Cash paid to suppliers	(5,000)	
Cash paid for operating expenses	(2,000)	
Cash paid for rent in advance	(3,000)	
Net cash used in operating activities		(4,000)
Cash flows from investing activities:		
Payments on equipment purchase	(25,000)	
Net cash used in investing activities		(25,000)
Cash flows from financing activities:		
Contributions	1,000	
Bank loan	50,000	
Net cash provided by financing activities		51,000
Net increase in cash and cash equivalents		22,000
Cash at beginning of month		100,000
Cash and cash equivalents at end of month		$122,000

Schedule of reconciliation of changes in net assets to net cash provided by operating activities (indirect method)

Cash flows from operating activities		
Changes in net assets		$ 9,775
Adjustments to reconcile change in net assets to		
Net cash provided by operating activities:		
Depreciation	625	
Increase in net accounts receivable	(3,600)	
Increase in inventory	(4,500)	
Increase in prepaid rent	(2,000)	
Increase in interest earned but not received	(4,000)	
Increase in wages payable	700	
Contribution	(1,000)	
Total Adjustments		(13,775)
Net cash provided (used) by operating activities		($4,000)

The first section of Table 2-6 presents CompClinic's cash flows from operating activities. Note that this section presents both the cash inflows and the cash outflows, it does not just present a net figure. This format is also required of the financing and investing sections of the statement. In this case, the cash flows from operating activities show that CompClinic received $6,000 in cash from its patients, but paid $5,000 in cash to its suppliers, $2,000 for miscellaneous operating expenses such as utilities and janitorial services, and $3,000 for three months of rent paid in advance. Thus, the cash flows resulting from operations were a negative $4,000.

CompClinic had only one investing activity: the purchase of equipment for $75,000. However, it only paid $25,000 in cash for these assets. Most purchases or sales of long-lived assets will result in cash inflows or outflows. In general, investing activities comprise buying and selling long-lived assets or other financial investments.

Financing activities, on the other hand, generally result from efforts designed to raise capital, such as issuing stock or making or paying-off loans. CompClinic's cash flows from financing include the $50,000 borrowed on a long-term basis, and the $1,000 contribution at the end of January. This results in $51,000 of cash inflows from financing activities during January. When all three categories are summed, they equal the $122,000 of cash shown at the bottom of the Statement of Cash Flows (Table 2-6). Note that this figure also equals the cash balance shown on the balance sheet, as it must.

Although the reconciliation of changes in net assets (net income) to cash provided by operating activities is a little more complicated to understand, its focus is to show the relationship between changes in net assets (net income) and cash provided by operating activities. It does this by making adjustments to changes in net assets (net income) for non-cash charges and adding back non-cash transactions that affect net assets (net income), such as depreciation.

This supplementary disclosure begins with changes in net assets (net income), which in the case of CompClinic is $9,775, the figure shown on the accrual-based income statement. Depreciation is added, because it affected net assets (net income), but did not require a cash out-flow. Then, changes in current assets are subtracted if they increased, or are added if they decreased, and vice-versa for current liabilities. To see why this is done, look at the inventory account: $5,000 of supplies were purchased and only $500 worth of supplies were used. Only the $500 was reflected on the income statement—the amount of supplies expense. The other $4,500 required cash, but was not used in determining changes in net assets (net income). Thus, it is necessary to subtract the $4,500 from the changes in net assets (net income) to show that $4,500 more in cash went out than is reflected for supplies on the income statement. The difference between the $4,500 and $500 arises solely because of the idiosyncrasies of the accrual basis of accounting. Along with other adjustments for current asset and current liability accounts and depreciation, the result is net cash provided (used) by operating activities, a negative $4,000 in the case of CompClinic.

Statements Under the Cash Basis of Accounting

Recording transactions under the cash basis of accounting allows an organization to summarize its revenues (cash inflows) and expenditures (cash outflows) for the period. In the cash basis, the reporting form that summarizes the revenues and expenditures for an accounting period may be called an operating statement, a statement of receipts and disbursements, or an income statement.

Table 2-7 presents an income statement on the cash basis for CompClinic. It summarizes the January cash-based transactions presented in Table 2-2. All revenues and expenditures made for patient-related items may be reported under categories that are labeled as **operating revenues** and **operating expenditures**, respectively.

For instance, in the CompClinic example, the net income reported on the cash basis of accounting is a $28,000 loss (Table 2-7), whereas the increase in unrestricted net assets reported on the accrual basis of accounting is $9,775 (Table 2-1). Incidentally, in comparing Tables 2-5 and 2-7, note that net income from operations is a negative $28,000 ($7,000 in revenues minus $35,000 in expenditures) using the cash basis of accounting, whereas on the accrual basis of operating income is a positive $8,775 ($14,000 total revenues minus $5,225 expenses). These two figures paint entirely different pictures. The former number represents cash flows, whereas the latter represents resource flows.

An illustration of these differences between the cash basis and the accrual basis, due to depreciation effects, is shown in Table 2-8. It illustrates how the choice of accounting basis

Table 2-7   Income Statement Prepared on the Cash Basis of Accounting.

CompClinic
Income Statement
For the Period Ending January 31, 19X1

Unrestricted revenues, gains and other support:		
Net patient service revenue		$6,000
Other		1,000
		7,000
Expenditures:		
Operating expenditures		
Supplies	5,000	
Equipment	25,000	
General and administrative	2,000	
Rent	3,000	
Net expenditures		35,000
Operating income		($28,000)

Changes in Net Assets, Cash Basis (only)

Beginning balance	$100,000
Add cash inflows	57,000
Deduct cash outflows	- 35,000
Ending balance	$122,000

Table 2-8 Reported Costs Per Unit Using the Cash and Accrual Bases of Accounting.

Transaction	Cash basis of accounting	Accrual basis of accounting
Year 1		
1. Purchased equipment for $99,000	$99,000	
2. Recognized depreciation for the year*		$33,000
Assume 1,000 units of service were delivered. The cost per unit is:	$99	$33
Year 2		
1. Recognized depreciation for the year		$33,000
Assume 1,000 units of service were delivered. The cost per unit is:	$0	$33
Year 3		
1. Recognized depreciation for the year		$33,000
Assume 1,000 units of service were delivered. The cost per unit is:	$0	$33

*Assume a useful life of three years with no salvage value.

Note: During year 1, the unit cost using the cash basis of accounting is three times the amount reported on the accrual basis of accounting. However, in years 2 and 3, the cost per unit for the organization appears to have decreased considerably using the cash basis, but remains the same using the accrual basis. The differences are solely due to the accounting method used, not to any differences in resource utilization or efficiency.

(cash versus accrual) causes per unit costs to vary from $99 per unit to $0 over a three-year period for the cash basis while the accrual basis indicates a constant $33 per unit for the same three-year period.

Financial Accounting Concepts _____

We have explained the accrual and cash bases for accounting, used sample transactions for each method, and presented financial statements. Now, we expand our discussion of some financial accounting concepts and present some additional topics that may prove helpful.

Revenue Recognition

Accountants must have some signal to determine when revenues should be recognized. The rules for determining how to recognize revenues are part of generally accepted accounting principles (GAAP). One of the first such determinations is to associate dollars of revenue with a particular event or time period. Such an association occurs when the revenue is earned—usually when the related services are provided to a patient or client.

In other words, revenue is earned and recognized when some benefit is provided to a patient or purchaser. In many cases, broader revenue recognition criteria can be used. Revenues are recognized when the seller has conducted most of the activities necessary to accomplish the sale and the amount of the revenue can be reliably estimated. Under GAAP, accountants have detailed rules that operationalize these basic revenue recognition criteria. Revenue recognition criteria are designed to give precedence to economic substance over legal form. When the risks of ownership pass from the seller to the buyer, then revenue recognition should occur. At least three timing options for revenue recognition are possible:

- at the time of sale,
- as production occurs, or
- at some time after sale or delivery (such as when cash is collected).

Recognizing revenue at the time of sale is the norm. In most cases, the firm has conducted most of its production or sales efforts at this time and the seller can estimate what it will collect from the customer or client. For most health care providers, recognition of revenue as services are provided would be the norm.

Recognizing revenue during production is only appropriate under multi-year contracts where the buyer can reasonably be expected to fulfill the contract terms. This might be most typical where an asset, such as a bridge, takes many years to construct. In health care, where managed care contracts might be in force for several years, it would be unreasonable and misleading to include all the revenue in the year the contract was signed. It would also be inappropriate to wait until all contract terms were met at the expiration of the contract. Under these circumstances, it is appropriate to recognize revenue each year, or each month, or each day, as the managed care services are provided. This method of spreading out the revenue over the contract period provides a better indicator of the resources used and controlled by the contractor—rather than lumping all of the revenues and expenses into any single year.

Another example is a capitated contract, where the patient pays a fixed monthly amount, and the health care plan agrees to pay for all necessary care. The revenue is recognized monthly as it is received by the health care plan. While the plan cannot evaluate its actual performance until long after the premiums have been received, it must have sufficiently accurate forecasts of the health care services that will be ultimately required, so it will have sufficient resources to pay for them as needed.

The third option for revenue recognition spreads out the timing until long after the goods or services have been delivered to the customer. This delay in recognizing revenue is most appropriate where the customer may return the item at any time or where long-term warranty or other obligations exist. Similarly, when the customer is given many years to pay for the goods or services and when great uncertainty exists regarding the amount of eventual payments, the recognition of revenue may be delayed until the time periods when cash is actually received. This situation usually involves an installment payment arrangement for real estate or other property where collectability from the purchaser is in question. It is not used for routine "time-purchase" plans or installment sales of household goods. The third option is only used in exceptional circumstances where great uncertainty exists or where the risks and benefits of ownership are not complete at the time of sale. It would not be typical in a health care setting.

Conservatism

GAAP incorporates conservatism as a guide to measuring revenues and expenses. Conservatism suggests that any possible measurement errors committed by accountants should be biased towards an understatement of income and assets, rather than an overstatement. Another way of saying this is to "anticipate all possible losses, but do not recognize any potential gains until they are realized (in cash)." A more rational way of interpreting conservatism is to view it as a means of coping with uncertainty and risk since accountants are not omniscient and cannot predict the future.

If income is understated in the current period, then it is likely to be overstated during a later period. In other words, conservatism is obtained at a cost of some overstatement in the future. A downward distortion now results in an upward distortion later. Consequently, conservatism is only an undercurrent in GAAP. It is not applied at maximal levels. Conservatism is applied when other measurement rules are unclear or when uncertainty is high.

Valuation

There are four valuation alternatives: historical acquisition costs, current replacement costs, net realizable values, and net present values (of cash flows to particular users). Accounting measurements, under GAAP, are generally based on historical costs. This may be called a *cost-based valuation* or a *cost basis*. Historical costs represent the amounts paid for an item at the time it is originally acquired. Generally, historical costs are measured from the original purchase invoices and include all of the incidental and related costs, such as installation, warranties, delivery costs, etc. For example, the historical cost of a new X-ray table might be $30,000. An older table, purchased 10 years ago, might have a historical acquisition cost of $12,500.

One market value is based on an asset's current replacement cost and might be called current cost or replacement cost. Replacement cost represents amounts of money that would be necessary to replace that asset or its equivalent level of services. Replacement costs are difficult to obtain because of technological changes. The replacement cost of the 10-year-old table might be difficult to measure because all new tables may be more comfortable, may have more accurately calibrated settings or adjustments and may include new electronic components. On the other hand, the services provided by the new table and the old table may be virtually identical, especially as viewed by both the patient and the physician. The X-ray technician, or the radiologist, may be able to differentiate between the two tables. In such cases, replacement costs represent an approximation of the costs necessary to acquire equivalent services from either table. Generally, replacement costs are not used under Generally Accepted Accounting Principles (GAAP).

Another type of market value that might be used under GAAP can be called net realizable values. Net realizable values are amounts of money that could be obtained by selling assets right now. Net realizable values would also include any costs necessary to put the asset into a saleable condition. The 10-year-old table might be saleable to a private clinic for $3,000, while a dealer may only pay $2,000 for the table. The private clinic may require that some part of the table be repaired at a cost of $200, while the dealer's offer may not require any further repairs on the part of the seller. The net realizable value associated with the private party buyer is, therefore, $2,800 ($3,000 minus $200). The net realizable value associated with the dealer's offer is $2,000 because there are no other costs that must be paid by the seller. Net realizable values depend on who is making the offer, or how the prices are obtained, and on how many additional costs must be incurred in order to sell the item. The estimates are based, in many cases, on auction or on appraisals. Often, a fee must be paid before an expert and unbiased opinion is rendered regarding net realizable values. Net realizable values are often used for certain types of assets, including accounts receivable.

The use of market values gives rise to a combination rule called the *lower of cost or market rule*. Accountants must determine whether an item's replacement cost or net realizable value is lower than its acquisition cost. If so, the asset's value is written down to the lowest market value for that item. This loss would be recognized within the income statement, separately reported if it is significant in amount or material to the predictability of the future income of the firm. The lower of cost or market rule is based on the perception that financial statements would be misleading if assets were reported or recorded at amounts higher than their potential selling prices. Valuation of inventory, such as supplies, is often determined under a lower of cost or market rule.

A final option for market values is based on future cash flows. Such values are only relevant to particular users and are often called values in use or user values. They are based on an economic principle called net present value (described in Chapter 13) and they reflect the economic benefits and costs of owning an asset. While this valuation basis is an important alternative to historical costs, it is generally only used to value certain long-term liabilities such as pensions and bonds.

Matching

Regardless of the valuation method chosen, accountants are very concerned about matching effort with accomplishment. Expenses are matched with revenues. Once the revenues are determined, the associated expenses must also be identified.

Expenses are matched on a transactional basis or on the basis of the time period associated with earning the revenues. In other words, expenses are accrued or recorded on the income statement in association with particular transactions where revenues are earned, or they are accrued or recorded on the income statement as a pro rata amount pertaining to a particular time period. Professional fees associated with interpreting laboratory tests or patient X-rays must be matched with costs of the test or X-ray. Each professional fee, paid to a physician, is also associated or matched with the revenue billed to the patient, or other purchaser. On the other hand, the cost of using the X-ray table is incurred each month and may not be associated with each patient, or each X-ray, or other related activities. The monthly cost of the table can be matched with the time period in which the table is used, rather than apportioned to each particular examination or patient. These two examples represent matching on the basis of a time period or on the basis of a transaction.

Three major matching criteria are used by accountants, but these criteria may not always be consistent with each other and they may affect the interpretation of the financial statements. One matching criterion requires a direct causal relationship between revenues and expenses. When the revenues and expenses are directly related to each other there is generally not much confusion or dispute regarding whether the expense is properly recognized. Professional fees for radiologists provide an excellent example of a direct linkage between revenues and related X-ray expenses.

A second matching criterion encompasses a systematic and predetermined allocation. When some assets are acquired, the allocation of costs to time periods is determined by a mathematical formula or table. Allocations are discussed in Chapter 6.

The third matching criterion can be called immediate or instantaneous expense recognition. In other words, there may be no deferral or waiting for some future signal to occur before the expense is recognized. In such cases, there may be no obvious future benefits relating to the expense, or the application of a causal or formula-based recognition criterion may not be useful or desirable. In other words, if neither a causal direct relationship exists, nor if a formula can be applied, then the expenses are immediately recognized. This is a typical "default option" when you don't know what else to do, then recognize the expense immediately. Examples include the medical director's salary or various marketing expenses. Each may have a causal relationship to many future revenues and each could be allocated by formula to future years, but in these cases the linkages are so tenuous that accountants just recognize the expenses immediately.

Audit Opinions and Practices of Health Care Organizations _____

The preparation of the financial statements is the responsibility of management. However, persons relying on these statements would like to have some assurance of their reliability. On audited statements, this is supplied by the external auditors.

External auditors begin their review of the financial statements by examining the internal control of the organization. The term internal control refers to how well management has developed and implemented plans, policies, and procedures to run the organization efficiently and effectively, to safeguard its assets, and to ensure the accuracy and reliability of its accounting records. The weaker the internal control of the organization, the more detailed the audit that has to be conducted.

As a result of their audit, the accounting firm issues a report which indicates the nature of the study they undertook and their opinion as to whether the financial statements fairly summarize the financial position (balance sheet), results of operations (income statement), cash flows (statement of cash flows) and net assets (or owners' equity) of the organization. The rendering of an opinion is called the attest function. Only if in the auditors' mind the financial statements do provide a fair picture is an unqualified opinion given.

Although it seems that the public generally interprets an unqualified opinion as indicating the auditor is giving the organization a "clean bill of health," in fact the opinion only attests to the fairness of the financial statements. Fairness in this case means that in the auditors' opinion there are no material errors—that is, no errors that would cause a reasonable person to make erroneous conclusions about the organization's financial condition. It does not necessarily mean the organization is well managed. In addition to their opinion, the auditing firm usually prepares a separate letter to the board detailing their observations concerning the health care organization's internal controls and recommendations for improvement.

External audits must be carried out under the auspices of a certified public accountant (CPA). There is a strong movement in this country to increase the burden on the external auditor to look more closely at the way the organization being audited is managed and to report in more detail to the public. The issues in this debate are numerous and complex, but they are beyond the scope of this book.

Summary _____

Health care managers increasingly rely upon financial information for various long- and short-run decisions. Financial accounting furnishes the basic tools and techniques for recording and reporting the transactions of financial substance that take place in the organization.

Transactions are originally recorded chronologically in a journal. The transactions are then summarized in a ledger, which summarizes the transactions by account. At the end of each accounting period, adjusting and closing entries are made and the financial statements are prepared.

There are two major approaches to recording and reporting transactions: the cash and accrual bases of accounting. The cash basis of accounting keeps records much as one does one's personal finances: on a cash-in/cash-out basis. The accrual basis of accounting was developed to overcome many of the problems of the cash basis of accounting. In order to match revenues and expenses, it recognizes the revenues when they are earned and expenses when they occur. Accrual accounting relies on the fundamental accounting equation:

Assets = Liabilities + Net Assets (Owners' Equity).

At the end of the financial period, the assets, liabilities, and net asset (owners' equity) accounts are summarized on the balance sheet and the statement of changes in net assets (owners' equity). The balance sheet provides a snapshot of the organization and is also called the statement of financial position. The income statement summarizes the revenues and expenses of the organization over the accounting period. The statement of cash flows summarizes cash flows resulting from the three major financial management activities: operating, investing, and financing. The preparation of these statements is the responsibility of management. However, these statements can be reviewed and their fairness attested to by CPAs after an independent external audit of the firm has been conducted.

APPENDIX, CHAPTER 2A

FURTHER EXAMPLES OF ACCOUNTING EQUATIONS

Expanded Balance Sheet Equation _____

An expanded balance sheet equation can be shown as:

CURRENT ASSETS + FIXED ASSETS = LIABILITIES + NET ASSETS

This expanded equation represents a useful version of the balance sheet equation because the two main categories of assets are separately stated. Each category can be examined separately and both liquidity and operating capacity can be considered individually by using this version of the balance sheet equation. The equation must balance, and when current and fixed assets are summed, their total must equal the sum of all liabilities and net assets (owners' equities). This numerical check for accuracy should always be made whenever some change is introduced into a balance sheet.

Now, consider what happens when another $1M is invested in a company that has the following initial balance sheet equation:

$$\$1,420,000 + \$637,000 = \$1,199,000 + \$858,000$$

After the $1M investment, the equation would be modified as:

$$+\$1,000,000 \qquad\qquad\qquad\qquad + \$1,000,000$$

$$\$2,420,000 + \$637,000 = \$1,199,000 + \$1,858,000$$

$$\$3,057,000 = \$3,057,000$$

In this circumstance, $1M is added to current assets and $1M to net assets. The totals on both sides of the equation also increase by $1M.

Now consider taking the $1M and buying new radiology equipment. Current assets are reduced by $1M and the $1M is transferred to fixed assets.

CURRENT ASSETS + FIXED ASSETS = LIABILITIES + NET ASSETS

$2,420,000 + $637,000 = $1,199,000 + $1,858,000

−$1,000,000 + $1,000,000
$1,420,000 + $1,637,000 = $1,199,000 + $1,858,000

$3,057,000 = $3,057,000

The balance sheet totals of $3,057,000 do not change as assets shift between different categories.

The liability section can also be separated into two categories, as shown below:

CURRENT ASSETS + FIXED ASSETS = CURRENT LIABILITIES + LONG-TERM
LIABILITIES + NET ASSETS

Assuming that the total liabilities from the preceding balance sheet example comprise $699,000 of current liabilities and $500,000 of long-term liabilities, then the balance sheet equation can be further decomposed as follows:

$1,420,000 + $637,000 = $699,000 + $500,000 + $858,000

$2,057,000 = $2,057,000

Consider what happens to this equation as a new mortgage and cash in amount of $2M is obtained:

+$2,000,000   =   + $2,000,000

3,420,000 + $637,000 = $699,000 + $2,500,000 + $858,000

$4,057,000 = $4,057,000

The new $2M mortgage is added to both sides of the equation as current assets (cash) and as a new mortgage payable. Current assets increase by $2M to $3,420,000 and mortgage payable increases from $500,000 to $2,500,000. At the same time, the balance sheet totals increase from $2,057,000 to $4,057,000. If a new balance sheet were constructed at this time, its sub-totals would correspond to the totals shown in the equation above.

To work through an example involving a new investment, using the expanded equation, assume that $4M is invested:

CURRENT ASSETS + FIXED ASSETS = CURRENT LIABILITIES + LONG-TERM
LIABILITIES + NET ASSETS

$1,420,000 + $637,000 = $699,000 + $500,000 + $858,000

+$4,000,000   =   + $4,000,000

$5,420,000 + $637,000 = $699,000 + $500,000 + $4,858,000

$6,057,000 = $6, 057,000

Current assets increase by $4M and net assets (owners' equity) increase by $4M. The totals on each side of the original balance sheet equation also increase by $4M to $6,057,000. This result would indicate more liquidity and more residual claims on the organization's resources. More capital was invested in this business and owners or donors have a larger claim on the organization's resources. While cash and current assets have increased as a result of this investment, most organizations will then invest the cash in other assets such as inventories and fixed assets, or they may use part of the $4M to pay-off some of the liabilities. The long-term effect of any new capital investment will affect many other parts of the balance sheet and will not remain in the cash or current assets section for very long.

Consider a final example where the business earns net income for the year of $100,000. Assume also that the impact on the left side of the balance sheet is an 80% increase in current assets and a 20% increase in fixed assets. The effect of net income of $100,000, in this case, on the expanded equation is as follows:

CURRENT ASSETS + FIXED ASSETS = CURRENT LIABILITIES + LONG-TERM
LIABILITIES + NET ASSETS

$1,420,000 + $637,000 = $699,000 + $500,000 + $858,000

+ $80,000 + $20,000 =   + $100,000

$1,500,000 + $657,000 = $699,000 + $500,000 + $958,000

$2,157,000 = $2,157,000

The totals on both sides of the balance sheet will increase by $100,000. The net assets section increases by the $100,000 increase in retained earnings. Current assets increase by $80,000 and fixed assets increase by $20,000. This example is highly aggregated and simplified because many individual transactions would be combined to produce these results. It does show the impact on each side of the balance sheet of a profitable year's operations and an increase in assets of various kinds to match the year's earnings.

Bibliography

Cheramy, S.J. and M. Garner. "Guidelines Clarify Managed Care Accounting Procedures" *Healthcare Financial Management* (August): 44-56, 1989.

Hay, L.E. and J.H. Engstrom. *Essentials of Accounting for Governmental and Not-for-Profit Organizations.* Homewood, IL: Irwin, 1987.

Health Care Committee and Health Care Audit Guide Task Force. Federal Government Division of the AICPA. *AICPA Audit and Accounting Guide Health Care Organizations.* Washington, DC: AICPA, June 1, 1996.

Titera, W. "FASB Proposes Changes in Not-for-Profit Reporting" *Healthcare Financial Management* (April): 39-49, 1993.

Terms and Concepts

accounts payable
accounts receivable
accrual basis of accounting
accumulated depreciation
adjusting entries
allowance for doubtful accounts
assets
balance sheet
cash basis of accounting
chart of accounts
contra-asset account
depreciation
double entry recording method
earned
expenses
excess of revenues, gains and other support over expenses
expenditures
income statement
incurred
invested capital
journal
ledger

liabilities
matching
net assets
net book value
net income
net receivables
nominal accounts
nonoperating items
operating expenditure
operating income
operating revenue
other revenue
owners' equity
real accounts
recognized
retained earnings
revenues
residual
restricted net assets
statement of cash flows
statement of changes in net assets
unrestricted net assets
unrestricted revenue
useful life

Questions and Problems _____

2-1   What is the fundamental accounting equation? How does it vary for a business vs. a not-for-profit organization?

2-2   What are the two components of net assets (owners' equities)?

2-3   What are the two sources of changes in net assets (equities)?

2-4   Which accounts would be affected if a health care center borrowed $10,000?

2-5   What are the differences between a journal and a ledger?

2-6   What is a chart of accounts?

2-7   What is the major difference between a balance sheet and an income statement?

2-8   What is the difference between current assets and long-term assets?

2-9   What is the difference between current liabilities and long-term liabilities?

2-10 What are three alternative names for the net assets account? What are the differences between the three?

2-11 What are the advantages and disadvantages of using the cash method of accounting?

2-12 Give an example of an expense that does not require a cash outlay.

2-13 What is the effect of an expense on net assets (owners' equity)?

2-14 What is the effect of revenues on net assets (owners' equity)?

2-15 What is the purpose of the allowance for bad debts? What kind of an account is it?

2-16 What is the purpose of recognizing depreciation?

2-17 Why was fund accounting developed for not-for-profit entities? Why do you suppose that it is becoming obsolete and losing favor?

2-18 Who is responsible for the preparation of an organization's financial statements?

2-19 What does it mean when financial statements have been "audited"?

2-20 How does an auditor know how extensive an audit needs to be?

2-21 At the end of July, 19XX the accounts for Dr. Stacie Zacharias's medical practice were as follows:

Cash	$25,000
Accounts receivable	$1,300
Allowance for doubtful account	$250
Supplies	$430
Prepaid rent	$5,000
Equipment	$25,000
Accumulated depreciation	$11,000
Accounts payable	$2,350
Notes payable	$2,430
Unrestricted net assets	$40,700

In August, Dr. Zacharias recorded the following transactions:

1.	Purchased medical supplies for cash	$750
2.	Received cash from patients who had already been billed	$1,000
3.	Delivered services for cash	$1,300
4.	Paid principle on bank note	$1,200
5.	Purchased lab equipment for	$2,500
	Paid cash in the amount of	$1,450
	She owes the remainder of	$1,050

At the end of the month, Dr. Zacharias recorded the following adjusting entries:

6.	Supplies used	$550
7.	Depreciation	$275
8.	Expired rent (which was prepaid)	$350

Prepare a balance sheet and a statement of operations (income statement).

2-22 At the end of April, 19XX the accounts for the Dahle Dental Clinic were as follows:

Cash	$15,000
Accounts Receivable	$17,000
Allowance for Doubtful Accounts	$1,500
Supplies	$950
Prepaid Rent	$5,400
Prepaid Insurance	$10,000
Equipment	$37,000
Accumulated Depreciation	$12,000
Accounts Payable	$5,280
Notes Payable	$6,000
Owners' Equity	$60,570

In May, the Dahle Dental Clinic recorded the following transactions:

1.	Purchased dental supplies on account	$450
2.	Performed dental work on patients (patients were billed—no cash received)	$10,000
3.	Received cash from patients who had already been billed (exams took place in April)	$11,000
4.	Paid interest on bank note	$300
5.	Purchased X-ray unit costing	$5,000
	-paid cash in the amount of	$3,200
	-remainder of the purchase was on credit	$1,800
6.	Paid utility bills	$250

At the end of the month, The Dahle Dental Clinic recorded the following adjusting entries:

7.	Depreciation	$1,500
8.	Supplies Used	$370
9.	Used one month of pre-paid insurance	$1,000
10.	Expired rent (which was prepaid)	$450

Prepare a balance sheet and income statement.

2-23   The infamous Hollywood liposuctionist, Dr. Tommy Tucker, has opened a new clinic in Beverly Hills. From the following transactions, prepare a statement of operations (income statement) and balance sheet.

1. Dr. Tucker put $100,000 of his own money into the clinic.
2. Dr. Tucker prepaid his advertising in the amount of $9,500.
3. Advertising expense for the month was $4,375.
4. He purchased equipment for $50,000 in cash.
5. Depreciation expense on the equipment was $400.
6. Dr. Tucker received a bill for $4,000 for remodeling.
7. He paid $2,000 of his remodeling bill.
8. He billed his patients for $87,205.
9. He recognized that $5600 of the amount billed would probably not be collected.
10. His patients paid $77,000 of the amount they were billed.
11. Salaries amounted to $26,000 of which he has paid $22,500.
12. Utility bills equaled $7,500, of which $5,675 has been paid.
13. Office supplies purchased equaled $450 of which $435 has been used.

2-24   In which year would Dr. Welby record the revenue or expense from each transaction below if the accounting records for his practice were kept on a cash basis? If they were kept on an accrual basis?

1. On January 3, 1998, Welby received and paid the December 1997 power bill.
2. On December 27, 1997, Welby (grudgingly) paid his malpractice insurance premium for the year 1998.
3. Welby paid property taxes on January 5, 1998. The taxes were assessed on his office property for the year 1997.
4. Dr. Welby received a $1,500 payment on January 9, 1998 for a liposuction procedure he performed on Ms. Barr on December 6, 1997.

2-25 Castle Clinic began the year with the following balances:

Cash	$45,000
Accounts receivable	$23,000
Allowance for doubtful account	$3,345
Supplies	$5,440
Prepaid rent	$4,500
Equipment	$1,550,000
Accumulated depreciation	$560,000
Accounts payable	$23,555
Notes payable	$155,895
Unrestricted net assets	

During the year they recorded the following transactions:

1. Patient revenue was $1,500,000.
2. Office supplies worth $5,650 were purchased on credit.
3. Salaries earned were $565,000.
4. Salaries paid were $495,895
5. Depreciation of $32,050 was recorded.
6. They received a loan of $240,000 in December.
7. Prepaid rent of $56,665.
8. Patients paid $995,000 of the amount they owed.
9. $35,000 of the amount owed was estimated to be uncollectable.
10. Paid $15,550 on the loan.
11. Recognized $44,750 rent for the year.
12. Recognized that $12,980 of the loan is due next year.

Prepare a statement of operations (income statement) and balance sheet.

2-26 The ending balances after recording the financial transactions for the Westgate Surgicenter for August are:

Cash	$54,000
Accounts receivable	$12,000
Allowance for doubtful account	$335
Supplies	$540
Prepaid rent	$2,555
Equipment	$133,235
Accumulated depreciation	$53,445
Accounts payable	$12,335
Notes payable	$122,775
Unrestricted net assets	

During the month of September they had the following transactions:

1. The owners contributed $43,500 each to the practice.
2. Supplies purchased with cash equaled $2,000.
3. Furniture purchased in the amount of $13,250, $565 paid in cash, the remainder due in 3 months.
4. Depreciation was recognized using straight-line depreciation, no salvage, 5 years.
5. Rent in the amount of $275 was recognized.
6. Tally of service slip—$3,600 worth of services were delivered in cash; $4,500 were delivered on credit.
7. An inventory was conducted, $320 worth of supplies remained. An entry was made to reflect this fact.
8. Wages payable in the amount of $2,465 was recognized.

Prepare a statement of operations (income statement) and balance sheet for the month of September.

2-27   After examining the books and records of Dr. Young's Pediatry Practice, you find the following data:

Salaries earned by employees	$145,000
Salaries Paid	140,000
Total revenue earned from all payer sources	625,000
Cash collected from all payer sources	470,000
Utility expense incurred	7,000
Utility bills paid	5,900
Purchased Supplies (paid 35,000 in cash)	40,000
Rent Paid in 1998	137,500
Rent expense incurred in 1998	150,000
Depreciation on equipment	35,000

1. Compute Dr. Young's net income for 1998 using cash-basis accounting.
2. Compute Dr. Young's net income for 1998 using accrual-basis accounting.

3 Financial Statement Analysis

The financial statements of health care institutions provide useful information to internal and external decision-makers. The primary financial statements—the balance sheet, the income statement, and the cash flow statement—present a summary of the results of operations and financial status of an organization for one or more time periods. Generally Accepted Accounting Principles (GAAP) provide a basic format for the preparation of these statements, which are required for external presentation. This basic format has already been introduced in Chapter 2. Accordingly, the material presented in this chapter will continue to follow the disclosure formats identified in the *American Institute of CPAs Audit and Accounting Guide: Health Care Organizations* (June 1, 1996). However, the reader should recognize that alternative formats and terminology may be encountered as health care managers adapt their statements to meet new organizational and other reporting requirements. The reader should become familiar with a range of terminology and, more importantly, develop a working knowledge of the components of financial reports.

The primary purpose of this chapter is to present a formalized approach to analyzing financial statements that will provide insights into the financial condition of an organization. We use hospital financial statements to illustrate the various analytic techniques. The same techniques can be applied to most health care organizations, including insurance companies, managed care organizations, and a variety of provider organizations. Before delving further into the specific analytic ratios, we first discuss some of the conceptual objectives of the income statement, balance sheet and statement of cash flows.

Role and Purposes of Financial Statements

The Income Statement

Regardless of the various titles that might be shown on an income statement, most organizations use one financial statement, or operating report, to summarize the operating results for the prior month or year. The income statement captures these operating activities in monetary terms. In other words, all of the costs and revenues associated with providing health care services during the past time period are summarized on one page in a few categories of information. Even a huge holding company, like Columbia/HCA, or Kaiser Permanente, a large health maintenance organization, can summarize its billions of dollars of revenues and associated expenses for the prior year on one sheet of paper.

One of the major purposes of a for-profit firm's income statement is to *provide indicators of profitability*. Most commercial organizations exist to make money. As we have shown earlier, not-for-profit organizations focus on increases or decreases in net assets. Health care organizations exist to improve people's wellness and cure their illness. In this text, the terms net profit, net income, and increases in net assets are generally synonymous. Negative income or a decrease in net assets is a loss ("red ink" in an earlier era).

The income statement is the primary source of information about the level of profits for the most recent time period. In addition, income statements may also contain information about operations for one or two prior periods. Profit or net income is usually indicated on the bottom line of the income statement. In fact, many readers only look at the income statement's bottom line and compare this limited view of profitability to the bottom line for other companies. Our purpose in this chapter is to ensure that you will not take a bottom line orientation and, instead, that you will look carefully at various parts of the income statement and know how profits may or may not be influenced by other indicators in the financial statements.

In order to accomplish this broader purpose, consider the *assessment of risk*. A clinic that has quite stable and acceptable levels of income or profit may be considered as low risk. On the other hand, a hospital with high profits one year and losses the next would exhibit much higher risk. Considering the variability and volatility of information in the income statement permits the reader to better understand the level of risk, uncertainty, or unpredictability that may be encountered in the future. Any organization that exhibits high levels of fluctuations in income may experience similar levels of variations in the future.

The risk assessment purpose goes hand-in-hand with the *predictability purpose*. Reading the income statement and interpreting all of its many nuances is of little value unless some predictions about the future can be made. You may call this the "fortune-telling" purpose of the income statement. By understanding prior income statements of the firm, you should be able to predict something about what future income statements may contain. By knowing if a firm was profitable in the past, you should be able to make some predictions about future profits.

Most managers make these predictions on a subjective and intuitive basis. This is an art, and requires much creative insight and many years of experience. For our purposes, just remember that an income statement is of little value unless it permits some prediction of profits that may be enjoyed or losses that may be suffered in the future.

On the other hand, many managers and analysts would like more feedback about the accuracy of prior income predictions. Unfortunately, the income statement is not designed to provide comparisons of prior predictions with actual results. However, the astute analyst will monitor his or her predictive ability by comparing prior predictions with actual results. This is just as important in an analysis of income as it is in preparing and analyzing budgets (Chapter 8).

Many of these predictions depend on how well the organization can adapt to future events. They also depend on how well the organization can sustain its current and prior levels of operations. These may be called the *adaptability and sustainability purposes* of the income statement. In order to accomplish these objectives, the income statement should provide separate information about normal operating activities. Unusual events should be separately disclosed. Income statements should reflect recurring activities in order to permit predictions about the ability to adapt in the future and in order to determine how well the firm has sustained itself in the past.

The income statement also reflects the costs necessary to maintain or sustain the organization. By looking at various categories of information on the income statement, future costs can be predicted. The costs incurred in the past that were necessary to sustain the organization's capacity to provide goods or services are shown on the income statement. By examining changes in various categories of the income statement, predictions about changes in levels of profitability may be made. Some of the ratios discussed in this chapter can help you make these predictions.

In summary, the income statement should provide information about profits or income and changes in income that affect risk and the predictability of income. It should also provide information about how well the organization has adapted to previous events and how well the organization has sustained its capacity to provide goods or services. These purposes are all related and are often based on similar ratios or similar income statement categories of information.

The Balance Sheet

One purpose of the balance sheet is to provide information about the *liquidity* of the organization. The balance sheet lists the current values of cash and other cash equivalents such as certificates of deposit and marketable securities. Comparisons of resources that can be spent versus liabilities which require future spending permit an assessment of liquidity. When your bills exceed what you have in the bank, you may be facing bankruptcy or other major changes in your lifestyle. In more elegant accounting terminology, when current liabilities are greater than current assets, an organization's liquidity is severely impaired. When liquidity suffers, the risk of bankruptcy or the need for an infusion of more funds is critical.

Another balance sheet purpose is to report the net book values of fixed and other long-term assets. This portion of the balance sheet refers to the unamortized or un-depreciated long-term assets. This balance sheet role is intended to help assess of the organization's *operating capacity* to provide future services. Since many of these values are reported at outdated or obsolete amounts, the balance sheet does not usually achieve its objective to provide useful information about the firm's operating capacity. In other words, the reader cannot determine how long the assets might continue to be used. The net book value of assets is only a proxy for their remaining useful lives. As long as assets are not fully depreciated, we assume that they will continue to provide useful, necessary and economically efficient services. This assumption is not always justified. Since current market values are not reported on the balance sheet, operating capacity cannot really be assessed.

A third balance sheet role identifies the amounts and relative timing associated with debts and other liabilities. When is the debt due? In what amounts? This balance sheet role also relates to liquidity in identifying immediate debt payments that must be made. On an overall basis, this is the balance sheet's *debt management* role. On the whole, most balance sheets provide useful information about the amounts and maturities of outstanding liabilities. An assessment of relative amounts and trends in debt provides much useful information about debt management's risks.

A fourth and final balance sheet role concerns the *residual claims* of investors and owners. As discussed in Chapter 2, one entire section of the balance sheet includes invested capital and retained earnings (net assets for not-for-profit organizations). This section may be viewed, in entirety, as a set of residual claims on the organization's net assets. Since this final section of the balance sheet role reflects residual interests, it is used primarily to analyze any *residual* difference between assets and liabilities.

This section of the balance sheet does not provide any indication of market values, nor does it indicate how much cash might be "left over" if the firm's assets were sold. It only provides an indicator of owners' relative interests. This role is often misunderstood and may be misleading because changes in this section of the balance sheet often lag far behind the real changes that occur in real estate and other external markets. This residual information is also relevant for not-for-profit and governmental organizations. As we have seen earlier, it is often called "Net Assets" or "Fund Balance." As the relative proportion of debt or equity (net assets) changes, investors or other constituencies may perceive themselves as better off or worse off relative to creditors and other constituencies. As noted before, the balance sheet does not really meet the objectives that would best reflect investors' or owners' residual interests. Using historical costs on the balance sheet distorts the assessment of these relative interests.

Four different balance sheet roles or purposes have been described as involving liquidity, operating capacity, debt management, and residual claims. Even though most balance sheets do not meet two of these objectives, managers' choices of accounting principles and methods should try to enhance the achievement of each of these four objectives. Users of balance sheets must know which sections relate to each role, and where to locate the relevant information. While reading the following sections, refer again to these four roles to see how each part of the balance sheet is linked to each purpose. When looking at actual balance sheets, think about these four roles and ask whether each has been effectively satisfied, or how each might be enhanced.

The Statement of Cash Flows

Many of balance sheet's purposes can also be extended to the cash flow statement. For example, the cash flow statement is certainly concerned with *liquidity*. Have the cash flows been managed effectively, and in such a way that the organization's bills are paid on a timely basis? The cash flow statement provides a vivid and easily understood indication of changes in cash balances. It also suggests reasons for why the cash balances have changed.

In similar fashion, the cash flow statement addresses the *operating capacity* issue as it summarizes the year's investing activities. Investing activities are usually intended to maintain or achieve shifts in the firm's operating capabilities. As a separate section of the cash flow statement, all of the investing activities are clearly disclosed, in terms of transactions that have recently occurred. Therefore, the cash flow statement is one of the best sources of *changes in operating capacity.*

Likewise, the cash flow statement has a separate section on financing activities, which relates to the *debt management* objective. Since the cash flow statement summarizes all changes in long-term debt, it is an excellent source for examining how managers might be changing their *debt management strategies* by obtaining more debt or reducing debt. While managers might not explicitly disclose such strategies, they are often apparent when cash flow statements for several periods are compared and analyzed.

Financial Analysis

The magnitude of data presented in typical financial statements makes it difficult to formulate judgments about the financial condition of an organization without further analysis. For example, Tables 3-1 and 3-2 present three years of financial statements for one not-for-profit hospital, Community General Hospital. These statements are used to illustrate the typical financial analysis techniques that can be applied to either for-profit or not-for-profit organizations. Effective analysis of these statements requires a systematic approach. One of the more useful evaluation tools is **ratio analysis**.

A ratio expresses the relationship between two numbers, such as current assets and current liabilities. Unfortunately, by itself, a single ratio calculation is difficult to evaluate, unless some standards or normative values are available for comparative purposes. As we will show, two kinds of comparisons are usually possible. Comparisons with industry norms and comparisons with prior ratio values in the same organization can provide useful insight.

Professional organizations such as the American Hospital Association, the Center for Healthcare Industry Performance Studies (CHIPS) or the Medical Group Management Association (MGMA) have been collecting data from health care providers for many years. They routinely publish median or average ratios for different types of institutions. These ratios can serve as standards for similar institutions. These standards can be useful in assessing the financial condition of a health care organization. When several years of financial data are available, a series of ratios examining the same relationships for consecutive periods of time can provide valuable information about the financial condition of an organization. Trends in a series of ratios can provide information about the direction of a change in financial condition. When we use the term "norms," we are providing our own subjective assessment of a desirable target, or acceptable range of the ratios discussed in this chapter. We have, of course, used a variety of actual data sources, which are often medians or averages, to determine our recommended "norms." We often state these "norms" in terms of ranges that would be relevant and valid over a three to five year period. Many of our illustrations and end-of-chapter materials are based on actual health care organizations' performance and achievements.

For example, the **current ratio** is commonly computed as the relationship between current assets and current liabilities (current ratio = current assets / current liabilities). This ratio is then used to make judgments about the ability of an organization to meet its short-term obligations. From the 1998 data for Community General Hospital in Table 3-1, a current ratio of 1.68 can be computed (12,890,000 / 7,655,155 = 1.68). Our norms would indicate a range of 1.2 to 2.2. The actual hospital industry performance in 1992 was 1.90.[1] Using a single data point for 1998 might indicate that Community General's ability to meet its current liabilities is somewhat problematic. However, when the ratios for the previous two years are computed, a different evaluation might be made. The ratios from 1996 to 1998 are 1.36, 1.51, and 1.68 .

Table 3-1   Community General Hospital Balance Sheet.

	12/31/96	12/31/97	12/31/98
Assets			
Current Assets:			
Cash	$50,000	$150,000	$275,000
Marketable securities	1,188,000	1,039,000	1,214,000
Accounts receivable	10,529,000	12,072,000	14,295,000
Less allowances for			
doubtful accounts	(3,488,000)	(3,899,000)	(4,529,000)
Net accounts receivable	$7,041,000	$8,173,000	$9,766,000
Supplies inventory	800,000	910,000	1,035,000
Prepaid expenses	542,000	565,000	600,000
Total current assets	9,621,000	10,837,000	12,890,000
Assets limited as to use, net of			
amounts required to meet current obligations:	0	0	0
Property and Equipment	51,763,812	57,774,950	61,013,373
Less accumulated			
depreciation	(21,521,072)	(25,550,621)	(30,243,852)
Property and equipment, net	30,242,740	32,224,329	30,769,521
Other assets	17,312,374	20,178,412	26,864,858
Total assets	$57,176,114	$63,239,741	$70,524,379
Liabilities and Net Assets			
Current Liabilities:			
Accounts payable	$2,870,000	$2,417,000	$2,275,000
Notes payable	398,000	520,000	612,000
Current portion of			
long-term debt	345,077	346,877	349,155
Accrued salaries	2,437,000	2,858,000	3,369,000
Other current liabilities	1,050,000	1,050,000	1,050,000
Total current liabilities	7,100,077	7,191,877	7,655,155
Long-Term Debt:			
Mortgage payable	5,272,114	4,927,037	4,580,160
Less current maturities	(345,077)	(346,877)	(349,155)
Net long-term debt	4,927,037	4,580,160	4,231,005
Net assets, unrestricted	45,149,000	51,467,704	58,638,219
Total liabilities and			
net assets	$57,176,114	$63,239,741	$70,524,379

Table 3-2   Community General Hospital Income Statement.

	FYE* 12/31/96	FYE 12/31/97	FYE 12/31/98
Unrestricted Revenues, Gains and Other Support:			
Net inpatient revenue	$70,140,266	$78,345,560	$92,573,914
Net outpatient revenue	6,844,450	7,843,175	9,267,576
Net patient service revenue	76,984,716	86,188,735	101,841,490
Other service revenues	1,463,280	1,609,608	1,770,569
Total revenues, gains and other support	78,447,996	87,798,343	103,612,059
Operating Expenses:			
Salaries	36,925,010	44,403,200	52,339,563
Fringe benefits	5,495,751	6,852,136	8,695,810
Fees	2,015,407	2,253,412	2,540,480
Supplies	10,838,836	12,024,161	13,974,501
Utilities	1,962,513	2,394,266	2,921,055
Provision for bad debt	8,267,318	7,422,553	9,161,125
Depreciation	3,250,178	4,029,549	4,693,531
Interest	484,208	454,003	423,721
Other expenses	3,402,125	3,776,359	4,191,758
Total expenses	72,641,346	83,609,639	98,941,544
Operating income	5,806,650	4,188,704	4,670,515
Contributions from foundation	2,939,544	2,079,000	2,427,000
Increase in unrestricted net assets	$8,746,194	$6,267,704	$7,097,515
Per diem inpatient revenue	$831.73	$905.73	$1035.07
Per diem operating income	$103.71	$72.46	$79.36
Patient days	84,331	86,500	89,437

*FYE, fiscal year ending.

This definitely represents a positive trend, and it appears that the management of Community General is making significant improvement in this area.

The use of ratio analysis as a management tool requires some caution for several reasons. First, definitions for the same ratio may vary. Thus, the analyst must document which definition is used and must interpret the results accordingly. In this chapter, we use some common definitions, but alternatives are available. Second, finding a comparison group that matches a provider in all aspects is difficult. Third, since there is some leeway allowed in preparing financial statements in accordance with GAAP, alternative methods of preparation can influence the ratios computed. Authoritative information concerning financial statement presentation in accordance with GAAP can be found in the industry audit guides published by the American Institute of Certified Public Accountants.[2] Finally, interpretation of the ratios often involves judgment. Different analysts may interpret the same results somewhat differently.

National Data Analysis Sources

It would be very difficult for an individual manager to collect the comparative data necessary to use ratio analysis effectively. However, readily available sources of such data exist. The American Hospital Association publishes annual summary data on hospitals' financial performance. This information can also be purchased in an electronic format to facilitate the analysis. The Medical Group Management Association (MGMA) conducts an annual survey of its members. This information is published in summary form each year. Other sources of comparative financial performance data would include Robert Morris Associates, Health Care Investment Analysts, the Center for Healthcare Industry Performance Studies (CHIPS), and Health Plan Employer Data and Information Source (HEDIS) data (which includes indicators of outcomes, patient satisfaction and financial performance).

Ratio Categories

Ratios can be used to facilitate evaluation of the financial condition of an organization. This evaluation is more effective if the ratios are combined into categories that reflect similar management actions or strategies.

Liquidity ratios and capitalization ratios focus primarily on the balance sheet, whereas profitability ratios generally use data from the income statement. Turnover ratios use data from both the balance sheet and the income statement. Collectively, the ratios enable management to make informed judgments about the health care organization's financial condition and performance.

Liquidity ratios enable an analyst to assess how the organization manages its short-term liquidity and its working capital. **Capitalization ratios** permit an examination of long-term financing strategies including the amount of long-term debt financing, changes in capital structure, and the ability to repay existing long-term debt. **Turnover ratios** facilitate the analysis of output ratios, using the income statement as a measure of outputs and the balance sheet as a measure of inputs. **Profitability ratios** are sometimes called performance ratios because they summarize the primary dimensions of an organization's fiscal and financial performance, generally linking the income statement and the balance sheet.

Each of the categories will be discussed in greater detail and defined specifically in Figure 3-1 as the financial statements for Community General, a not-for-profit hospital, are evaluated in the next section. One technical caveat concerning Figure 3-1 must be noted: wherever the term "cash" is indicated, we always mean to include all forms of cash and cash equivalents. Therefore, any financial instruments that the organization construes and states as cash or cash equivalents will be included in our ratio definitions.

Illustration: Community General Hospital

The financial statements of Community General, presented in Tables 3-1, 3-2 and 3-3, are similar to the financial statements issued by many not-for-profit hospitals. To illustrate the basic elements of financial analysis, ratios are computed for Community General using its financial statements. Although a hospital is used in the sample problem, the same methods could be used in analyzing the financial statements of any health care firm. The importance of different ratios will vary for different types of health care organizations. For example, turnover ratios may be less important for a managed care organization that is not as capital-intensive as a hospital because managed care organizations do not usually have as high a proportion of fixed assets as hospitals.

Liquidity Ratios

Perhaps the ratio most frequently used to reflect short-term liquidity is the **current ratio**. It relates current assets to current liabilities and is useful in identifying possible short-run financial problems. The term **current assets** is usually interpreted to mean those assets that will be converted to cash in less than one year. Similarly, **current liabilities** are those liabilities that are to be paid within one year. A current ratio greater than one (1.0) is considered a sign of prudent fiscal management, for this allows a margin of safety in the ability to meet current obligations. Based on the 1996-98 trends in its current ratios, it appears that Community General has been slowly improving its management of current assets and current liabilities as it is now at the mid-range of our suggested norms. Many firms operate successfully with current ratios that are close to 1.0. Therefore, Community General's low current ratio may reflect prudent management of current assets and could minimize the cost of holding them. However, it may also reflect a narrow margin of safety to meet current liabilities. Should cash flow be reduced for any reason, alternative sources of funds such as short-term financing may be needed on short notice to meet current obligations.

Figure 3-1   Commonly Used Ratios.

I.   **Liquidity**

$$\text{Current Ratio} = \frac{\text{Current assets}}{\text{Current liabilities}}$$

$$\text{Quick Ratio} = \frac{\text{Cash} + \text{Net accounts receivable} + \text{Marketable securities}}{\text{Current liabilities}}$$

$$\text{Acid Test Ratio} = \frac{\text{Cash} + \text{Marketable securities}}{\text{Current liabilities}}$$

$$\text{Net Working Capital Per Bed} = \frac{\text{Net working capital}}{\text{Available beds}} = \frac{\text{Current assets} - \text{Current liabilities}}{\text{Available beds}}$$

$$\text{Cushion Ratio} = \frac{\text{Cash} + \text{Marketable securities} + \text{Board - designated restricted cash}}{\text{Annual Debt Service}}$$

$$\text{Daily Cash Flow} = \frac{\text{Operating expenses} - (\text{Depreciation} + \text{Other non - cash charges})}{\text{Days in period}}$$

$$\text{Days of Cash Available} = \frac{\text{Cash}}{\text{Daily cash flow}}$$

II.   **Turnover Ratios***

$$\text{Total Asset Turnover} = \frac{\text{Total revenues}}{\text{Total assets}}$$

$$\text{Accounts Receivable Turnover} = \frac{\text{Net patient service revenue}}{\text{Net accounts receivable}}$$

$$\text{Accounts Receivable Collection Period} = \frac{365 \text{ days}}{\text{Accounts receivable turnover}}$$

$$\text{Average Accounts Payable Turnover} = \frac{\text{Cost of supplies}}{\text{Accounts payable}}$$

$$\text{Accounts Payable Payment Period} = \frac{365}{\text{Accounts payable turnover}}$$

Figure 3-1 continued

$$\text{Inventory Turnover} = \frac{\text{Cost of supplies}}{\text{Supplies inventory}}$$

$$\text{Current Asset Turnover} = \frac{\text{Total revenues}}{\text{Current assets}}$$

$$\text{Cash Asset Turnover} = \frac{\text{Total revenues}}{\text{Cash}}$$

$$\text{Average Daily Patient Revenue} = \frac{\text{Total revenues}}{\text{Days in period}}$$

$$\text{Average Daily Operating Expenses} = \frac{\text{Operating expenses}}{\text{Days in period}}$$

* (Gross or net revenue figures can be used although net revenues reflect the more conservative and useful approach. However, for external comparisons, the basis used should be made explicit.)

III.   Profitability Ratios

$$\text{Operating Margin} = \frac{\text{Operating income}}{\text{Total revenues}}$$

$$\text{Return on Assets} = \frac{\text{Increase in unrestricted net assets (or net income)}}{\text{Total assets}}$$

$$\text{Allowances Ratio} = \frac{\text{Charity care} + \text{Bad debts} + \text{Contractual allowances}}{\text{Gross patient revenues}}$$

$$\text{Return on Equity} = \frac{\text{Increase in unrestricted net assets (or net income)}}{\text{Net assets}}$$

$$\text{Prefinancing Return on Net Assets and Long-term Debt} = \frac{\text{Increase in unrestricted net assets (or net income)} + \text{Interest expense}}{\text{Net assets} + \text{Long-term debt}}$$

Figure 3-1   continued

$$\text{Bad Debt Ratio} = \frac{\text{Provision for bad debt}}{\text{Net patient service revenue}}$$

IV.   **Capitalization Ratios**

$$\text{Long-term Debt to Total Assets Ratio} = \frac{\text{Long - term debt}}{\text{Total assets}}$$

$$\text{Times Interest Earned} = \frac{\text{Operating income} * \ + \ \text{Interest expense}}{\text{Interest expense}}$$

$$\text{Fixed Charge Coverage} = \frac{\text{Operating income} * \ + \ \text{Interest expense} \ + \ \text{Lease obligations}}{\text{Interest expense} \ + \ \text{Lease obligations}}$$

Debt Service Coverage

$$= \frac{\text{Operating income} * + \ \text{Depreciation expense} + \text{Annual debt service requirements}}{\text{Annual debt service requirements}}$$

*Some analysts use increase in net assets or net income instead of operating income when the health care provider has significant income from other sources (e.g. contributions, extraordinary items, etc.) that are expected to continue.

Table 3-3   Community General Hospital Cash Flow Statement (abbreviated).

	1997	1998
Operating Activities		
Collections from patients	$85,096,735	$102,019,057
Payments to employees	(43,982,200)	(51,828,563)
Other operating activities	(36,416,021)	(44,813,701)
Cash Provided by Operating Activities	4,698,514	5,376,793
Financing Activities		
Contributions	2,079,000	2,427,000
Incur (redeem) long-term debt	(346,887)	(349,155)
Cash Provided by Financing Activities	1,732,113	2,077,845
Investing Activities		
Purchase "other assets"	(2,906,038)	(6,686,446)
Purchase land, buildings, and equipment	(1,981,589)	1,454,808
Cash Used in Investing Activities	(4,887,627)	(5,231,638)
Increase in Cash	$1,543,000	$2,223,000

1996 Computation

$$\text{Current Ratio} = \frac{\text{Current assets}}{\text{Current liabilities}} = \frac{9,621,000}{7,100,077} = 1.36$$

Community General's current ratios are:

Ratio	1996	1997	1998	Norms
Current	1.36	1.51	1.68	1.2 to 2.2

To further assess liquidity, many analysts also compute a quick ratio. The quick ratio represents a more stringent definition of current assets, as only cash, net patient accounts receivable, and marketable securities are considered available to meet current liabilities.

1996 Computation

$$\text{Quick Ratio} = \frac{\text{Cash} + \text{Net patient accounts receivable} + \text{Marketable securites}}{\text{Current liabilities}}$$

Community General's quick ratios are: $\dfrac{8,279,000}{7,100,077} = 1.17$

Ratio	1996	1996	1998	Norms	US Hospital 1992 Median
Quick	1.16	1.30	1.47	1.0 to 2.0	1.67[4]

The quick ratios for Community General also indicate an improvement in the liquidity position over the three years as noted, and that the hospital is operating at the mid-range of our suggested norms.

A more focused liquidity ratio is called the **acid test ratio**.

$$\text{Acid Test Ratio} = \frac{\text{Cash} + \text{Marketable securities}}{\text{Current liabilities}}$$

The acid test ratio looks at "spendable" resources because marketable securities can be turned into cash very quickly.

1996 Computation

Community General's acid test ratios are: $\dfrac{50,000 + 1,188,000}{7,100,077} = .17$

Ratio	1996	1997	1998	Norms	US Hospital 1992 Median
Acid Test	.17	.17	.19	.10 to .30	.54[5]

Community General's acid test results are quite stable and well within the indicated norms. One might expect more volatility in this ratio unless managers explicitly manage their cash balances in order to achieve certain targets at the end of each year. For example, one organization may try to show high cash balances at the end of the year as a safety measure or to instill confidence in potential investors, while others might try to whittle its cash balances down to almost nothing at the end of the year.

To summarize, all three liquidity ratios (current, quick, and acid test ratios) indicate that Community General is increasing current assets in relation to its current liabilities. If a firm has easy access to short-term debt or other sources of short-term funds, then a relatively low liquidity position will tend to minimize the costs associated with managing current assets. In other words, the funds that would have been used to provide liquidity can be used to provide other, perhaps more essential, patient services. If alternative short-term sources of funding are not available, and some major payers delay payment for any reason, Community General could find itself in a cash bind. The increasing trend in these ratios over the three-year period may indicate that management has been making a concerted effort to improve its liquidity position.

Some additional liquidity ratios are of particular interest to investors. The first of these is the **net working capital per bed** ratio (Figure 3-1). It normalizes net working capital by beds to facilitate comparisons across organizations. Any liquidity measure from the balance sheet could be used as the numerator of a similar ratio.

A variety of cash-based ratios might also be calculated in order to further assess the hospital's liquidity. Many cash ratios rely on data from the statement of cash flows (especially using data on cash flow from operations). While we only illustrate three cash ratios in Figure 3-1, other accounting texts illustrate a variety of useful cash-based performance ratios.[6] One of the more interesting cash ratios is used by Standard & Poor's in determining its credit ratings. Their ratio is the **cushion ratio,** which is the only cash ratio we will discuss in depth.

$$\text{Cushion Ratio} = \frac{\text{Cash} + \text{Marketable securities} + \text{Board - designated restricted cash}}{\text{Annual debt service}}$$

The cushion ratio is interesting on several counts because it includes cash and other short-term investments (marketable securities and other cash equivalents); it includes cash in board designated accounts (which may have otherwise been ignored in a liquidity analysis); and it ties the balance sheet and income statement together. The numerator emphasizes "substance over form;" it should include all forms of liquid, spendable cash or cash equivalents. In general, all ratios should emphasize and include terms that are defined on a "substance over form" basis; i.e., include all similar items that properly reflect liquidity, or profitability, etc. In many cases, it is instructive to compute the ratio first using a narrow definition of the terms, and, second, to compute the same ratio using much broader and more inclusive definitions.

To get a complete understanding of an organization's cushion ratio, one might calculate it first as indicated above, using only internally-restricted liquid assets, and then in a second calculation include all liquid assets some of which might be restricted by donors. This second calculation might also extend the entity definition to include related foundations or other closely-controlled affiliates. In other words, the substance over form question requires the analyst to look for other sources of liquidity that may be controlled by the health care organization.

In the denominator of the cushion ratio, two financial statements are tied together where the annual interest expense is added to the annual principal repayments on long-term debt. Sometimes, the annual debt service is shown in the notes to the financial statements. In other cases, the annual principal payments must be estimated. Principal payments can also sometimes be found on the cash flow statement. What is most interesting about the denominator is that there is no single source where annual debt service can always be found. The astute analyst must often piece together the various elements, or estimate them.

In order to calculate annual debt service, find the interest expense on the income statement, and the payments on long-term debt, or the current maturities of long-term debt on the balance sheet. In our example, we use the current portion of long-term debt, from the prior year's balance sheet, that is, "lagged" by one year, because the balances shown at the beginning of the year are expected to be paid during the year. We use the interest expense from the current income statement; though more correctly, we should use the actual interest paid, which is also sometimes shown on the statement of cash flows.

$$\text{Annual Debt Service} = \text{Interest expense} + \text{Annual principal payments}$$

$$\text{Community General's 1997 Cushion Ratio} = \frac{150,000 + 1,039,000 + 0}{454,003 + 345,077} = \frac{1,189,000}{799,080} = 1.49$$

Using our "lagged" approach, we cannot calculate the cushion ratio for 1996. Its cushion ratios for two years are:

Ratio	1997	1998	Norms
Cushion	1.49	1.93	1.0 to 3.0

While Community's cushion ratios have improved, they are still not at the level required for investment grade bonds or other investments. It has increased, slightly, but not to the level expected by Standard & Poor's, which expects a cushion ratio greater than 6.0.

Turnover Ratios

One of management's primary responsibilities is the efficient use of assets. **Turnover** or **activity ratios** can provide useful information in this area. Data from both the balance sheet and the income statement are needed to compute turnover ratios.

The **total asset turnover ratio** is a key indicator of how efficiently assets are being used to generate revenues. This ratio shows the amount of revenue obtained from each dollar of assets.

1996 Computation

$$\text{Total Asset Turnover (TAT) ratio} = \frac{\text{Total revenues, gains and other support}}{\text{Total assets}}$$

$$\text{TAT} = \frac{78,447,996}{57,176,114} = 1.37$$

Community General's total asset turnover ratios are:

Ratio	1996	1997	1998	Norms	US Hospital 1992 Median
TAT	1.37	1.38	1.47	1.0 to 1.1	.91[7]

Community General appears to be making excellent use of its assets to create revenue. Any result greater than 1.0 for this ratio implies that management is monitoring investments in assets relatively closely and maximizing the assets' ability to generate revenues.

Another highly informative turnover ratio is the **accounts receivable turnover ratio** and its related statistic, the **average collection period**. These ratios are the primary ones tracked by experienced health care managers in provider firms, mainly because of the size of the investment in receivables at most hospitals and the often lengthy collection periods from third-party payers. Managed care organizations and other payers would not be as concerned about accounts receivable because they receive their funds regularly each month in the form of premiums or other contractual payments.

1996 Computation

$$\text{Accounts Receivable Turnover (ART)} = \frac{\text{Net patient service revenue}}{\text{Net accounts receivable}}$$

$$= \frac{76,984,716}{7,041,000} = 10.93$$

$$\text{Average Collection Period (ACP) (in days)} = \frac{365 \text{ days}}{\text{Accounts receivable turnover}}$$

$$= \frac{365 \text{ days}}{10.9} = 33.49 \text{ days}$$

Community General's ratios are:

Ratio	1996	1997	1998	Norms	US Hospital 1992 Median
ART	10.93	10.54	10.43	4.0 to 12.0	5.37 [8]
ACP	33.49	34.63	35.00	30.0 to 75.0	72.0 [9]

Overall, Community General's average collection period is excellent; however, the decreasing trend in accounts receivable turnover, which results in a slight increasing trend in the average collection period, might be of slight concern to management. It may mean that collection procedures are becoming lax, a different type of patient is being served, or the major third-party purchasers (payers) are changing their payment policies.

A similar approach to the accounts receivable computations can be used for accounts payable, inventory and current assets. The number of days' usage in each category and the length of the payment period can identify potential problems before they become serious and result in poor vendor relationships. For example, with respect to accounts payable the **accounts payable turnover** and **accounts payable payment period** are:

<u>1996 Computation</u>

$$\text{Accounts Payable Turnover (APT)} = \frac{\text{Cost of supplies}}{\text{Accounts payable}} = \frac{10,838,836}{2,870,000} = 3.78$$

$$\text{Accounts Payable Payment Period (APPP)} = \frac{365 \text{ days}}{\text{Accounts payable turnover}} = \frac{365 \text{ days}}{3.78}$$
(payment period in days)

$$= 96.56 \text{ days}$$

For Community General, the turnover ratios are:

Ratio	1996	1997	1998	Norms
APT	3.78	4.97	6.14	5.00 to 8.00
APPP	96.56	73.44	59.45	45.00 to 70.00

Community General seems to be doing an excellent job of utilizing its assets. Its total asset turnover ratio is on the high side (of our norms), and its average collection period for accounts receivable is very good. However, two possible areas of concern include the slight change in the average collection period and the slow payment to vendors for supplies. The long accounts payable cycle is in keeping with Community General's low current ratio and helps the cash flow by delaying payment as much as possible. However, the slow payment for supplies could strain vendor relationships since most vendors allow only 30 days before payment is due. If Community General were to run into liquidity problems in the future and need additional time to make payment, its creditors may not be very receptive. However, note that each of these ratios improve significantly in 1997 and 1998, as APT almost doubled and the length of the payment period (APPP) was reduced by more than 33%.

Several other turnover ratios are also illustrated in Figure 3-1. One shows how an **inventory turnover ratio** is analogous to both accounts receivable and accounts payable turnover ratios. Note that each has an income statement element in the numerator and a balance sheet element in the denominator. Similarly, **current asset and cash turnover ratios** are also illustrated in Figure 3-1. The final set of turnover ratios is used to express average daily flows. We illustrate **average daily revenue and expense ratios** because many planning models require daily estimates of such income statement elements. Similarly, any income statement element can be defined on a daily basis. What we have left unstated is how to calculate the number of days in the period. The two options here are: calendar days or business days. Our only advice is to be consistent in your choice of one or the other. A hospital may use calendar days, on the basis of its round-the-clock operations, while a managed care organization might use business days.

Profitability Ratios

Profitability ratios provide a more global perspective to performance evaluation of health care organizations. They indicate how much better off the organization is as a result of profits or changes in net assets. Two ratios that are closely related are the operating margin and the return on assets.

The **operating margin ratio** expresses the difference between the revenues received from providing services and the expenses required to support these revenues as a percentage of total revenues. We use operating income, or excess of revenues over expenses, in the numerator of this ratio because it most clearly expresses the financial impact of "core business" operations, as compared to other sub-totals that may be shown elsewhere on the income statement. However, some analysts may prefer to use net income (or change in net assets) as the numerator in this ratio. When net income is used, the ratio is called the total margin ratio.

The **return on assets ratio** expresses the net income (increase in unrestricted net assets) as a percentage of the assets employed to provide services or products. This is an overall profitability ratio because it uses the "bottom line" on the income statement. Both operating margin and return on assets ratios provide managers with a perspective on how revenues, expenses, and assets were used to provide health care services or products. If the operating margin is too low, management has the option of raising prices or reducing expenses. Either alternative would result in an increase in the operating margin. If the return on assets is low, management can either increase the operating margin as indicated above or reduce the amount of assets utilized.

<u>1996 Computations</u>

$$\text{Operating Margin (OM)} = \frac{\text{Operating income}}{\text{Total revenues}} = \frac{5,806,650}{78,447,996} = 0.074$$

$$\text{Return On Assets (ROA)} = \frac{\text{Increase in unrestricted net assets (or net income)}}{\text{Total assets}} = \frac{8,746,194}{57,176,114} = 0.153$$

Community General's ratios are:

Ratio	1996	1997	1998	Norms	US Hospital 1992 Median
OM	0.083	0.048	0.045	0.03 to 0.06	.029 [10]
ROA	0.153	0.099	0.101	0.03 to 0.06	.045 [11]

The return on assets for Community General is very good, but the declining trend in operating margin and return on assets may indicate a potential problem. The declining operating margin may be due to a number of factors, including an increase in government-sponsored or managed care patients for whom the hospital is paid at discounted rates. The decline in **operating margin** may also indicate that management is not raising rates at a fast enough rate. Another possible explanation might include inefficient or costly operations. Many factors contribute to positive and negative operating margins. These profitability ratios are just summary measures of many inter-related factors.

Another ratio commonly used to diagnose profitability is the **bad debt ratio**. This ratio measures the amount of patient service revenues that are lost to uncollected accounts receivable. In our example we compare bad debt expenses to net patient service revenue as opposed to calculating a bad debt ratio against only inpatient or outpatient revenues.

<u>1996 Computations</u>

$$\text{Bad debt ratio} = \frac{\text{Provision for bad debts}}{\text{Net patient service revenue}} = \frac{8,267,318}{76,984,716} = 0.11$$

Community General's bad debt ratios are:

Ratio	1996	1997	1998	Norms
Bad Debt	0.110	0.086	0.090	0.05 to 0.15

This fairly stable ratio indicates that the collection procedures used to manage bad debts over these three years, have been effective.

The **allowances ratio** may be used to determine the amounts of allowances deducted from gross patient revenue for charity care, courtesy allowances, and contractual discounts. This ratio is less important now that allowances and discounts are not shown on the income statement. Under managed care, a variety of ratios involving discounts will be helpful. To evaluate such issues, the appropriate data will have to be obtained from the notes or some other less convenient source. Since the allowances ratio has been de-emphasized, we do not illustrate its calculation for Community General Hospital.

Two other profitability ratios are also shown in Figure 3-1. These include the **return on equity ratio** and the **prefinancing return on net assets and long-term debt**. These show the returns to residual claimants and the returns to all suppliers of long-term capital, respectively. We do not illustrate their calculation for Community General Hospital.

Capitalization Ratios

The final group of ratios to be analyzed concentrates on capital structure and ability to pay existing long-term debt issues. These ratios help evaluate the firm's financial flexibility and the amount of potential risk in the financing of assets. Another commonly used term for this group of ratios is **leverage ratios**. Basically, financial leverage refers to the substitution of debt for equity financing with the goal of increasing return on equity. Leverage usually assumes that debt is less costly than equity, such that having more debt will reduce the firm's financing costs relative to the costs of obtaining equity financing. Increasing proportions of debt usually mean reduced flexibility in obtaining future financing (further lending may not be available) and increased risks (due to increased variability in net income). When the proportion of debt in the firm's capital structure becomes too high, lenders may also increase the cost of debt (interest expense) for the firm.

The **long-term debt to total assets ratio** is just one component of determining the relative composition of debt and equity financing. This same information could be obtained from a vertical analysis, or percentage composition ratio, described elsewhere.[12] The long-term debt to total assets ratio contains the most important component of a complete vertical analysis. The second major indicator of financial risk associated with capitalization is the **times-interest-earned ratio**, which evaluates the ability to pay existing debt payments. We use operating income, or excess of revenues over expenses, in the numerator of this ratio, because it most closely approximates the sustainable, or long-term, income flows that can be expected in the future. Since the times-interest-earned ratio is a proxy for risk, we are most interested in how this ratio is likely to evolve in the future. The major capitalization ratios for Community General are:

1996 Computations

$$\text{Long - term Debt to Total Assets (LTD) ratio} = \frac{\text{Long - term debt}}{\text{Total assets}} = \frac{4,927,037}{57,176,114} = 0.09$$

$$\text{Times - Interest - Earned (TIE) ratio} = \frac{\text{Operating income} + \text{Interest expense}}{\text{Interest expense}} = \frac{5,806,650}{484,208} = 11.99$$

Ratio	1996	1997	1998	Norms	US Hospital 1992 Median
LTD	0.09	0.07	0.06	0.30 to 0.60	.34 [13]
TIE	11.99	9.23	11.02	2.50 to 7.50	2.47 [14]

The long-term financial structure of Community General indicates that considerable **debt capacity** exists. If Community General sets a maximum debt capacity of 50% of total assets, then its long-term debt capacity in 1997 is $31,619,857 [=.5(63,239,714)]. With only $4,580,160 in long-term debt currently outstanding, Community General has $27,039,697 in additional debt capacity. This estimate of additional long-term debt capacity is reinforced by the times-interest-earned ratio of 9.23, which is much higher than the industry norms. It appears that Community General has considerable flexibility in its financial structure to meet future requirements and can borrow as needed on a long-term or a short-term basis.

Two other capitalization ratios are also described in Figure 3-1. These include the **fixed charge coverage ratio** and the **debt service coverage ratio**. Neither ratio is calculated for Community General Hospital, given its already healthy times-interest-earned ratio and its large amount of additional debt capacity. No new insights would be gained by making these calculations.

Overall Assessment

The financial ratios computed for Community General indicate a healthy overall financial condition with flexibility in financing for the future. The minimal use of debt indicates that the approximately $20 million increase in the land, building, and equipment account from 1996 to 1998 has been financed through either internally generated funds or donations. The low level of long-term debt provides the borrowing capacity that will permit Community General to take advantage of opportunities such as joint ventures, mergers, and the like. In addition, more information on the $41.5 million held in other investments would be helpful in assessing the hospital's overall financial condition. The hospital also has used its assets well to generate revenues as well as profits. Although its short-term liquidity has been improving, Community General's management should evaluate why it remains low. It should pay special attention to the slow payment of accounts payable. Improvements in short liquidity will also make the hospital more able to obtain long-term debt at reasonable rates.

This analysis of Community General Hospital has used only the more commonly recognized relationships. The number of ratios that can actually be computed is constrained only by the imagination of the analyst. Figure 3-1 provides a variety of ratios that can be used in financial analysis. The ratios that we have illustrated are usually computed first; if questions arise, then additional ratios may be necessary. We have barely scratched the surface in terms of illustrating how financial analysis can be conducted. These techniques may be compared to "peeling an onion" in that the analyst is always trying to gain better understanding and more insight into the financial performance of a health care organization. By calculating a few ratios, the analyst may just uncover more questions that may require additional insight and ratio calculations tailored to the specific institution.

The Return on Assets Approach

Health care firms must manage their resources in such a manner as to enable the organization to provide needed health services in the future. To meet community health care needs, an organization must be financially healthy as well as have the right personnel and equipment. It must have the operating capacity to provide the necessary services. One way to accomplish this goal is to determine a **required return on assets**. The required return must, at a minimum, match current inflation effects, provide for new technologies (either replacement or new equipment needs), provide new services demanded by customers or clients, and deal with political and environmental risks (such as recessions or economic controls, taxes, etc.). The exact required return that will meet these needs is unknown, but subjective estimates can be made. For example, Table 3-4 illustrates one approach to estimating the required return: the basic factor approach.

This approach is especially valuable for not-for-profit organizations, where a market price for equity securities cannot be used to establish the required returns. The manager of such an organization will have to use its strategic plan to identify the most crucial threats and opportunities. Each of these can be ranked in terms of expected future costs. The most important factors can then be expressed in terms of the return on assets necessary to achieve each objective. The basic technique is based on the concept that a firm's goals can be expressed in terms of future returns and that these goals can be summed to obtain an estimate of a future required return on assets. Table 3-4 indicates that an 8% goal might be sufficient for a hypothetical organization. Each organization must conduct its own analysis and determine its own required future rate of return.

It is possible to meet the required return on assets either by increasing the total margin ratio or by increasing the asset turnover ratio. This relationship can be developed in the following manner:

$$\text{Total Margin Ratio} = \frac{\text{Net income}}{\text{Total revenues}} \quad \text{multiplied by}$$

Table 3-4   Estimated Total Required Return on Assets.*

Basic Factors	Estimated Average Annual Rate of Return Required (%)
Inflation	3.0 %
Technology	2.0
Expansion of Existing Services	1.0
New Services	1.0
Risk of Recession, Economic Controls, etc.	<u>1.0</u>
Required Return on Assets	8.0%

* Long, H.W. "Valuation as a Criterion in Not-for-Profit Decision-Making" *Health Care Management Review* 1(Summer): 34-46, 1976.

$$\text{Asset Turnover Ratio} \quad = \quad \frac{\text{Total revenues}}{\text{Total assets}} \quad \text{equals}$$

$$\text{Return On Assets} \quad = \quad \frac{\text{Net income}}{\text{Total assets}} \quad .$$

Understanding these relationships is important to the health care decision-maker. For example, if net income cannot be increased to meet required returns because of payor constraints on payments or other competitive conditions, increasing the utilization of assets may be the only way to increase the firm's return on assets. In today's health care environment, managers must consider these alternatives to meet the desired goals.

Using this approach, the following ratios can be calculated for Community General Hospital:

	1996	1997	1998
Total Margin Ratio	11.1%	7.1%	6.85%
Asset turnover ratio	1.37	1.39	1.47
Return on assets ratio	15.3%	9.9%	10.1%

Clearly, Community General's return on assets has decreased after 1996. It is approaching the point of jeopardizing its required return objective of 8% as identified in Table 3-4. However, it is important to note that a large proportion of Community General's change in unrestricted net assets is due to contributions from a foundation. If these relationships are recalculated without reference to those contributions, then the return on assets for 1998 is only 6.6%. Such a result is clearly below the 8% target.

This example illustrates the necessity for looking at ratios from several perspectives and perhaps calculating the same ratio using alternative elements from the financial statements. In order to estimate future relationships, then only the sustainable components of income should be included. If Community General's contribution from the foundation will continue, then "no worries, mate." If the contribution is suspect, or if the amount may decrease significantly, then the achievement of historical rates of return may be in jeopardy.

Note how Community General's increase in its asset turnover ratio helped, to some extent, offset the decline in operating margin (from 1996 to 1998). In other words, more effective and efficient use of operating rooms, laboratories, radiology, computer systems, and dietary equipment offset a lower margin between net charges and expenses. If the prevailing practice in health care organizations of having a dollar in assets create only a dollar in patient revenues could be significantly improved (a ratio of seven or eight is typically expected in non-health care organizations), health care providers would be using their assets more effectively and may not need a massive capital base. Such a change might even lower the cost of providing health care to the community. In Community General, increasing the asset turnover ratio to 3.0 would increase the return on assets to 0.132, which is much closer to the required total return. The other choice is to continue to seek donations and grants, or to reduce the level of services offered.

Economic Consequences and Managerial Incentives

Many managers, especially in for-profit firms, are generally motivated to achieve and report the highest net income possible. Managers in not-for-profit firms might have similar objectives where promotions, prestige, and other perquisites are at stake. Readers of financial statements must understand this inherent bias. Even accountants are motivated to cooperate with management in reporting the highest incomes possible—to keep managers happy and to increase their chances of being rehired next year! As you will learn in further study of financial accounting, there are limits to how high net earnings can be under GAAP and as to how cooperative accountants can be in maximizing earnings.

The economic consequences of increasing earnings by virtue of accounting adjustments do not generally result in any increase in cash flows or other tangible, spendable resources. The accounting devices by which earnings can be increased usually affect some element of the balance sheet which may be unlikely to have a long-term benefit for the firm. Adjustments or manipulations of earnings are the subject of many of the notes to the financial statements. As such, the notes must be studied carefully, along with the financial analysis ratios discussed earlier. The simple equations presented in this chapter can be used to interpret changes in revenues, expenses, and earnings that are often discussed in the notes. The analyst can also focus on how these changes affect the balance sheet. The knowledgeable analyst will understand, after further study of financial accounting, which changes that increase net income are really improvements for the firm and which are merely a sham. Of course, many possible accounting adjustments and re-valuations are somewhere in between, neither a sham nor a blessing. In many cases, it will take a number of years before the final realization will be known.

As to managerial incentives, income statement users must be aware of how managers might inflate revenues and earnings, or how expenses might be deferred or reduced, which will also increase net income. It is through these kinds of manipulations that managers might try to achieve an early, or unwarranted, promotion. Or, they might be trying to gain a salary increase or reach a threshold level of performance where a bonus would be earned. While managers are known to be responsive to these types of incentives, the linkage between their actions and any manipulation of earnings is not as clear. There is much ambiguity between actions that might increase cash flow versus actions that would have no effect on cash flow. In fact, some instances have been reported where managers have increased earnings, increased taxes, and decreased cash flows to the firm. This would be an extreme case of "perverse incentives" where managers thought that higher earnings were better than higher cash flows.

These issues can be explored through further study of financial accounting. Specific examples may be encountered in the end-of-chapter materials or in projects assigned by your instructor. For now, readers may start to think about how the data in financial statements might reflect manager's ambitions and aspirations, along with the economic reality that must be analyzed in each decision situation. Users of financial statements must be alert to issues where "form over substance" prevails, where the reporting choices are not consistent with economic reality and where the firm is worse off under the accounting choices that were made. In most cases, managers and other constituencies will prefer "substance over form," and financial statements that clarify the substance will always be preferred over those that obscure and confuse the reader.

Summary

Ratio analysis is an effective management tool to pinpoint possible problem areas before they can become serious. It allows managers to concentrate their efforts on the more pressing problem areas. It helps identify areas for further attention. The routine calculation of these ratios can be done on a pocket calculator or personal computer, using a spreadsheet or using data base program. The availability of comparative data from national services will also make ratio analysis techniques accessible to managers in a variety of health care settings.

The examples in this chapter have illustrated these ratio techniques in the context of a not-for-profit hospital. Similar analyses can be applied to other health care providers, as well as to payer organizations such as insurance companies or managed care organizations. In all cases, the reader of financial statements must be careful to understand the underlying motivations and incentives facing the provider or the payer. Do not be confused by a mechanical application of these techniques; instead, use them to understand the meaning and implications of the decisions made by managers in these organizations.

Appendix Chapter 3A
Expanded Balance Sheet & Income Statement Equations For NFP Firms

Financial statements are not stand-alone, independent documents. They must relate to each other; they must be internally consistent. A balance sheet cannot indicate that the firm is extremely healthy, while the income statement shows that it has suffered three years of huge losses. Conversely, three years of high profits would generally result in a fairly sound balance sheet. In the rare event that these generalizations do not hold, then the analyst's first question is to find out why the statements are inconsistent.

In order to provide more formality to these relationships, income statements and balance sheets must *articulate*. That is, when some positive event occurs on the income statement, there must be a corresponding positive effect on the balance sheet. When losses or expenses are recorded on the income statement, there is a corresponding negative effect on the balance sheet. Accountants have a formal, ritualized procedure for transferring or closing all of the income statement effects onto the balance sheet. While we are not going to discuss these procedures in detail, we are going to use the accounting equation as an interpretative device to understand and show how transactions affect both the income statement and the balance sheet. Once this equation is understood, it will help the analyst interpret ratio relationships that depend on both balance sheet and income statement data. An expanded equation can be used to help interpret such difficult issues as decreases in asset values or as extraordinary losses.

This new equation can be quite simple, or it can build on the complex equations presented in the Appendix to Chapter 2. For starters, we will use the simple version to review how the income statement and balance sheet relate or articulate with each other. The purpose of this appendix is to:

1. Expand the relationships first introduced in the Appendix to Chapter 2.
2. Show how these equations can be used to examine the interface and articulation between the income statement and balance sheet.
3. Give the analyst a tool that can be used to make predictions about future balance sheet relationships, once the income forecasts have been made.

At the beginning of the year, the familiar expression must hold:

$$\text{ASSETS} = \text{LIABILITIES} + \text{NET ASSETS}$$

As revenues are earned, and as expenses are matched with revenues the income statement may also be shown in equation form:

$$\text{REVENUES} - \text{EXPENSES} = \text{OPERATING INCOME}$$

$$\text{OPERATING INCOME} + \text{CONTRIBUTIONS} = \text{INCREASE IN NET ASSETS}$$

At the end of the period, the accounting equation must also be in balance as the change in net assets will also impact the balance sheet equation. On the other hand, losses would result in decreases in net assets. At the end of the period, the accounting equation could be stated in the following form:

$$\text{ASSETS} = \text{LIABILITIES} + \text{NET ASSETS (beginning)} + \text{INCREASE IN NET ASSETS}$$
$$[\text{or}, - \text{DECREASES}]$$

which can then be summarized in the ending balance sheet as:

$$\text{ASSETS} = \text{LIABILITIES} + \text{NET ASSETS (ending)}$$

where:

$$\text{NET ASSETS (beginning)} + \text{INCREASE IN NET ASSETS} = \text{NET ASSETS (ending)}$$
$$[\text{or}, - \text{DECREASES}]$$

The final equation at the end of the period will be just as at the beginning:

$$\text{ASSETS} = \text{LIABILITIES} + \text{NET ASSETS}$$

To show these effects in numerical terms, consider a company with the following balance sheet equation at the beginning of the period:

$$\$100,000 = \$40,000 + \$60,000$$

Now, assume that this company has an income statement equation as follows:

$$\text{REVENUES} - \text{EXPENSES} = \text{OPERATING INCOME}$$

$$\$165,000 - \$95,000 = \$70,000$$

If we assume that all of these income effects have resulted in increases in net assets (that is, operating income equals the increase in net assets), then the new balance sheet equation at the end of the period must be:

$$\$170,000 = \$40,000 + (\$60,000 + \$70,000)$$

$$\$170,000 = \$40,000 + \$130,000$$

In other words, the new balance sheet has $70,000 in additional assets and $70,000 in additional net assets. This short-hand version of the combined balance sheet and income statement equation is very important to a complete understanding of financial statement relationships.

The next step is to include revenues and expenses in the basic equation, without showing operating income at all. Now, we combine the basic balance sheet equation with the income statement equation such that operating income is not shown at all, because algebraically it would be redundant to do so. This new summary equation can form the basis for subsequent analyses.

$$\text{ASSETS} = \text{LIABILITIES} + \text{NET ASSETS (beginning)} + \text{REVENUES} - \text{EXPENSES} + \text{CONTRIBUTIONS}$$

This equation indicates the complete articulation of the balance sheet and the income statement. The first two terms are familiar balance sheet items. The last three terms show how the beginning balances in net assets are combined with revenues and expenses to arrive at the ending balances in net assets. To verify this relationship, it can be expressed algebraically in a more complete form as:

$$\text{ASSETS} = \text{LIABILITIES} + \text{NET ASSETS (beginning)} + \text{REVENUES} - \text{EXPENSES} + \text{CONTRIBUTIONS}$$

$$\text{NET ASSETS (beginning)} + \text{REVENUES} - \text{EXPENSES} + \text{CONTRIBUTIONS} = \text{NET ASSETS (ending)}$$

Note that these equations ignore any new investments or withdrawals or distributions. They ignore dividends and other changes in capital accounts. Next we show how the example data just presented applies to these equations at the beginning and end of the period:

$$\text{ASSETS} = \text{LIABILITIES} + \text{NET ASSETS}$$

$$\$100,000 = \$40,000 + \$60,000$$

$$\text{ASSETS} = \text{LIABILITIES} + \text{NET ASSETS (beginning)} + \text{REVENUES} - \text{EXPENSES} + \text{CONTRIBUTIONS}$$

$$\$170,000 = \$40,000 + \$60,000 + \$165,000 - \$95,000 + 0$$

$$\text{ASSETS} = \text{LIABILITIES} + \text{NET ASSETS}$$

$$\$170,000 = \$40,000 + \$130,000$$

Finally to show how the ending balance in net assets is computed using the net assets equation:

$$\text{NET ASSETS (beginning)} + \text{REVENUES} - \text{EXPENSES} + \text{CONTRIBUTIONS} = \text{NET ASSETS (ending)}$$

$$\$60,000 + \$165,000 - \$95,000 = \$130,000$$

These equations are very powerful and can be used to capture every conceivable accounting transaction, except new investments or dividends or withdrawals. This additional nuance is not covered in this text. The net assets equation is simply a reconciliation or a transition between the beginning balance in net assets and the ending balance in net assets. At this point, the whole series of equations should be reviewed to verify that each equation is clear and to see how they differ. Note the similarities in two equations, where one equation includes Operating Income as an explicit term, while the other includes its determinants (Revenues and Expenses). While these equations are not illustrated in the end-of-chapter material, your instructor may provide further examples.

Notes

1. Cleverley, W.O., "Trends in the Hospital Financial Picture" *Healthcare Financial Management* (February): 57, 1994.
2. American Institute of Certified Public Accountants (AIPCA), *Audit and Accounting Guide: Health Care Organizations.* New York, 1996.
3. Contact W.O. Cleverley at the Center for Healthcare Performance Studies (CHIPS), Columbus, Ohio, or see their annual report titled, *The (1995) Almanac of Hospital Financial & Operating Statistics.*
4. Cleverly, *op. cit.*
5. *Ibid.*
6. Suver, J., B. Neumann, and K. Boles. *Management Accounting for Healthcare Organizations, 3rd Edition.* Healthcare Financial Management Association and Pluribus Press, Chicago, IL, 1992.

Murray, D., B. Neumann, and P. Elgers. *Using Financial Accounting: An Introduction*, West Publishing Co. St. Paul, 1996.
Granof, M., P. Bell, and B. Neumann. *Accounting for Managers and Investors, 2nd Edition.* Prentice Hall, Englewood Cliffs, NJ, 1993.

7. Cleverley, *op. cit.*
8. *Ibid.*, p. 62.
9. *Ibid.*, p. 57.
10. *Ibid.*, p. 59.
11. *Ibid.*, p. 57.
12. Suver, Neumann, and Boles, *op. cit.*
    Murray, Neumann and Elgers, *op. cit.*
    Granof, Bell and Neumann, *op. cit.*
13. Cleverley, *op. cit.*
14. *Ibid.*

Bibliography

Cleverley, W.O. "Trends in the Hospital Financial Picture" *Healthcare Financial Management* (February): 57, 1994.

Granof, M., P. Bell, and B. Neumann. *Accounting for Managers and Investors, 2nd Edition.* Englewood Cliffs, NJ: Prentice Hall, 1993.

Health Care Committee and Health Care Audit Guide Task Force. Federal Government Division of the AICPA. *AICPA Audit and Accounting Guide: Health Care Organizations.* Washington, D.C.: AICPA, June 1, 1996.

Long, H.W. "Valuation as a Criterion in Not-for-Profit Decision-Making" *Health Care Management Review* 1(Summer): 34-46, 1976.

Murray, D., B. Neumann, and P. Elgers. *Using Financial Accounting: An Introduction.* St. Paul: West Publishing Co., 1996.

Suver, J., B. Neumann, and K. Boles. *Management Accounting for Healthcare Organizations, 3rd Edition.* Chicago, IL: Healthcare Financial Management Association and Pluribus Press, 1992.

Terms and Concepts

accounts payable payment period
accounts payable turnover
accounts receivable turnover
acid test ratio
activity ratios
allowances ratio
average collection period
average daily patient revenue
bad debt ratio
capitalization ratio
cash turnover ratio
cushion ratio
current assets
current asset turnover ratio
current liabilities
current ratio
debt capacity
debt service coverage ratio

fixed charge coverage ratio
inventory turnover ratio
leverage ratio
liquidity ratio
long-term debt to total assets ratio
net operating margin
operating margin ratio
prefinancing return on net assets and long-term debt
profitability ratio
quick ratio
ratio analysis
required return on assets
return on assets ratio
return on equity ratio
times-interest earned ratio
total asset turnover ratio
turnover ratios
working capital per bed ratio

Questions and Problems _____

3-1 Explain the relationship among the primary financial statements of a health care provider.

3-2 Explain why financial ratios are more meaningful than simply the entry for a single account or a group of accounts. Why must one be cautious when analyzing and interpreting a single ratio?

3-3 Why would liquidity ratios be valuable in determining whether a health care provider could use cash to pay for a long-term asset (e.g., a CT scanner)?

3-4 What are the distinctions between turnover and profitability ratios? What are capitalization ratios and why are they useful? What types of third parties would be most interested in them?

3-5 Why do you think that not-for-profit as well as proprietary institutions must earn a "profit" or return on equity?

3-6 Why should administrators in not-for-profit health care organizations be concerned about meeting a required return on assets?

3-7 Explain asset turnover, net operating margin, and return on assets in your own words. What is the relationship between asset turnover and net operating margin in achieving a required return on assets?

3-8 Why is the availability of national data analysis sources useful to health care financial managers? What precautions must be taken with the use of data from such sources?

3-9 Why do you think it imperative to separate operating from nonoperating revenues and expenses when calculating ratios or analyzing the financial condition of an organization?

3-10 Should depreciation or interest expense be included in the figure for net operating income? Why?

For the following problems, use the associated financial statements.

3-11 A. From the accompanying financial statements of St. Ann's Hospital, compute the following ratios.
1. Current ratio
2. Operating margin
3. Return on assets
4. Long-term debt ratio

B. What is your assessment of the financial condition of St. Ann's Hospital?

3-12 A. Compute the following ratios for Hot Springs Community Hospital:
   1. Current ratio
   2. Operating margin
   3. Return on assets
   4. Long-term debt to total assets ratio

B. Analyze the financial statements for Hot Springs Community Hospital. What recommendations would you make to the managers of the hospital?

3-13 A. Compute the following ratios for PacifiCare Health Systems:
   1. Liquidity ratios
   2. Turnover ratios
   3. Performance ratios
   4. Capitalization ratios

You should only compute the ratios that you think are important in each category.

B. Analyze the financial performance of PacifiCare Health Systems.

Problem 3-11
St. Ann's Hospital
Consolidated Financial Reports

Assets	1992	1991	Revenues	1992	1991
Current assets	$2,685,733	$2,510,773			
Fixed assets	3,871,521	3,899,044			
Other assets	53,095	58,939	Net patient service revenue	$10,045,961	$8,842,617
Total assets	$6,610,349	$6,468,756	Other operating revenue	170,608	138,763
			Total operating revenue	$10,216,569	$8,981,380

Liabilities and Net Assets:			Expenses:		
Current liabilities	$ 810,171	$ 842,937	Nursing services	$ 3,816,836	$ 3,248,137
Long-term			Other professional	1,651,426	1,470,261
liabilities	1,623,318	1,728,341	General services	1,559,889	1,415,699
Total liabilities	$2,433,489	$2,571,278	Fiscal services	387,518	321,333
			Administrative services	1,790,919	1,678,675
			Provision for bad debts	813,058	458,852
			Total expenses	$10,019,646	$ 8,592,957
			Operating income	$ 196,923	$ 388,423
Net assets	$4,176,860	$3,897,478	Contributions	82,460	15,745
Total liabilities and net assets	$6,610,349	$6,468,756	Increase in un-restricted net assets	$ 279,383	$ 404,168

Problem 3-12
Hot Springs Community Hospital
Unaudited Detailed Statement of Revenue and Expenses
For the Twelve Months Ended June 30, 1997

Operating Revenues	July-December 1996	January-June 1997	Total
Patient Service Revenue (net)	$ 663,738	$ 774,547	$ 1,438,285
Ancillary Service Revenue (net)			
Surgery Recovery Room/ Anesthesiology	104,349	152,002	256,351
Central Supply/IV	223,192	242,018	465,210
Emergency Room	73,108	107,284	180,392
Cardio-Pulmonary/EKG/Respiratory Therapy	100,441	115,499	215,940
Laboratory/Blood Bank	214,416	322,516	536,932
Radiology/Nuclear Medicine/ Ultrasound	121,902	123,136	245,038
Pharmacy	170,471	231,303	401,774
Physical Therapy	39,666	51,001	90,667
Total Ancillary Service Revenue (net)	$1,047,545	$1,344,759	$2,392,304
Other Revenue	22,650	28,229	50,879
Total Revenue	$1,733,933	$2,147,535	$3,881,468
Expenses			
Nursing Services	273,227	287,884	561,111
Ancillary Services	552,422	657,562	1,209,984
General Services	263,500	268,082	531,582
Administrative/Fiscal	349,917	373,741	723,658
Provision for Bad Debt	85,681	77,412	163,093
Total Operating Expenses Before Rent, Interest, Depreciation and Amortization	$1,524,747	$1,664,681	$3,189,428
Income Available for Rent, Interest Depreciation, and Amortization	$ 209,186	$ 482,854	$ 692,040
Rent, Interest, Depreciation, and Amortization	772,924	796,519	1,569,443
Total Expenses (memo total)	$2,297,671	$2,461,200	$4,758,871
Increase (decrease) in Unrestricted Net Assets	($563,738)	($313,665)	($877,403)

Problem 3-12
Hot Springs Community Hospital
Pro Forma Unaudited Balance Sheet

Assets		June 30, 1997
Cash		$34,231
Patient Accounts Receivable	$1,192,444	
Less Allowance for Doubtful Accounts	(123,532)	1,068,912
Inventory		93,018
Prepaid expenses		4,617
Pre-Opening expenses		115,804
Total assets		$ 1,316,582

Liabilities and net assets		
Accounts payable		$121,008
Accrued salary/payroll tax		26,673
Accrued property taxes		40,667
Accrued audit fees		5,500
Accrued expenses		56,083
Blue Cross financing		29,493
CSNB Note	$480,518	
Plus accrued interest	9,884	490,402
Total liabilities		$ 769,826
Net assets		$ 546,756
Total Liabilities and Net Assets		$ 1,316,582

Problem 3-13
PacifiCare Health Systems, Inc.
Statement of Income

	Year Ended September 30 1997
Revenues	
Group premiums	$87,162,983
Interest and other income	2,736,268
Total revenues	$89,899,251
Expenses	
Health care services	
Medical services	$34,376,519
Hospital services	26,246,979
Other	6,473,636
Total health care services	$67,097,134
Marketing, general, and administrative	11,297,602
Interest	384,296
Total expenses	$78,779,032
Income before taxes	$11,120,219
Provision for taxes	5,435,000
Net income	$ 5,685,219
Earnings per share	$1.06

Problem 3-13
PacifiCare Health Systems, Inc.
Balance Sheet

Assets	September 30, 1997
Current assets	
Cash and equivalents	$ 4,151,180
Short-term interest-bearing investments	33,231,680
Receivables, net	2,043,913
Prepaid expenses and taxes	1,021,360
Total current assets	$40,448,133
Equipment and leasehold improvements, at cost, net	
of accumulated depreciation and amortization	
(1997: $701,367; 1996: $343,184)	1,546,501
Interest-bearing investments (restricted)	742,108
Other assets	2,563,763
Total assets	$45,300,505
Liabilities and stockholders' equity	
Current liabilities	
Medical claims and accruals	
Hospitals	$ 8,610,000
Incentives and other amounts payable to	
participating medical groups	2,490,000
Total medical claims and accruals	$11,100,000
Accounts payable	1,473,302
Accrued liabilities	1,173,713
Unearned premium revenues	698,651
Long-term debt due within one year	332,949
Total current liabilities	$14,778,615
Long-term debt due after one year	2,392,783
Total liabilities	$17,171,398
Stockholders' equity	
Preferred shares, par value $1.00 per share;	
10,000,000 shares authorized; none outstanding	
Common shares, par value $.50 per share; 20,000,000	
shares authorized, 5,893,600 shares issued and	
outstanding	2,946,800
Additional paid-in capital	17,152,225
Retained earnings	8,030,082
Total stockholders' equity	$28,129,107
Total liabilities and stockholders' equity	$45,300,505

3-14 A. Compute the following ratios for Triangle Hospice:
1. Liquidity ratios
2. Performance ratios

B. Analyze the financial statements of Triangle Hospice. Why are two columns used to report the financial information? Should this approach be used? Why or why not?

3-15 A. From the following financial statements of Adams Cooperative Health Enterprise (ACHE), compute the listed ratios for 1996 and 1995, its first two years of operation:
1. Current ratio
2. Fixed asset turnover
3. Return on assets
4. Long-term debt to total asset ratios

B. What events could account for the changes in the net assets and operating income from 1995 to 1996?

C. How would you assess ACHE's current financial situation based on the information given?

D. What recommendations, if any, would you make for future financial administration of ACHE?

3-16 Jefferson-Madison Ambulatory Center (J-MAC) is the product of a recent merger of Jefferson Ambulatory Care (JAC) and Madison Outpatient Service Center, Inc. (MOSCI). The center operates weekdays. The organizations' financial statements follow.

A. Calculate the following ratios for the two agencies for 1996.
1. Quick ratio
2. Accounts receivable turnover
3. Average collection period
4. Long-term debt to total assets ratio

B. Which agency seemed less financially stable before the merger? Will the combined agency's financial condition be better or worse than the two independent agencies separately? Why?

C. What course of action would you suggest to further improve J-MAC's situation?

Problem 3-14
Triangle Hospice, Inc.
Statements of Support, Revenue, and Expenses and Changes in Fund Balances
Year Ended December 31, 1997

	Current Funds Unrestricted	Furniture and Equipment Funds	Total 1997
Public Support and Revenue			
Public Support			
Contributions	$ 39,306	$ 185	$ 39,491
Grants	7,500		7,500
Total public support	$ 46,806	$ 185	$ 46,991
Revenue			
Investment income	3,116		3,116
Miscellaneous			
Total revenue	$ 3,116		$ 3,116
Total public support and revenue	$ 49,922	$ 185	$ 50,107
Expenses			
Program Services			
Patient care	35,727	60	35,787
Training & staff development	12,945	22	12,967
Public and professional education	3,885	6	3,891
Total program services	$ 52,557	$ 88	$ 52,645
Supporting Services			
Management and general	27,468	178	27,646
Fund raising	3,171	29	3,200
Total supporting services	$ 30,639	$ 207	$ 30,846
Total expenses	$ 83,196	$ 295	$ 83,491
Decrease in net assets	($33,274)	($ 110)	($ 33,384)
Net assets, beginning of year	$56,624	$ 1,832	
Net assets, end of year	$23,350	$ 1,722	

Problem 3-14
Triangle Hospice, Inc.
Balance Sheet

December 31, 1997

Assets	Current Funds Unrestricted	Furniture and Equipment Funds	Total 1997
Cash	$21,812		$21,812
Certificates of deposit			
U.S. government securities			
Marketable securities: corporate stock (market value $1,392 in 1997 and $580 in 1996)	1,306		1,306
Contributions and accounts receivable	561		561
Prepaid expenses	551		551
Furniture and equipment, at cost, less accumulated depreciation of $561	____	1,722	1,722
Total assets	$ 24,230	$ 1,722	$25,952

Liabilities and Net Assets

Liabilities:			
Accounts payable	$ 880		$ 880
Accrued payroll taxes			
Total liabilities	$ 880		$ 880
Net Assets:			
Unrestricted, available for general activities	$ 23,350		$23,350
Restricted for furniture and equipment fund	____	$ 1,722	1,722
Total liabilities & net assets	$ 24,230	$ 1,722	$25,952

Problem 3-15
Adams Cooperative Health Enterprise
Balance Sheets: General Funds
12/31/95 and 12/31/96

Assets	1996	1995
Current assets	$ 3,042,159	$ 2,438,776
Fixed assets	7,101,233	5,874,231
Other assets	387,184	558,432
Total assets	$10,530,576	$ 8,871,439

Liabilities and Net Assets		
Current liabilities:		
Accounts and notes payable	$ 514,503	$ 345,798
Staffing and payroll-related	1,043,720	841,621
Other short-term payables	8,765	10,102
Total current liabilities	$1,566,988	$ 1,197,521
Long-term liabilities		
Long-term debt	$ 6,500,772	$ 5,950,728
Note payable to		
development fund	2,000,000	2,000,000
Total long-term liabilities	$ 8,500,772	$ 7,950,728
Total liabilities	$10,067,760	$ 9,148,249
Net assets	$ 462,816	$ (276,810)
Total liabilities and net assets	$10,530,576	$ 8,871,439

Problem 3-15
Adams Cooperative Health Enterprise
Income Statements
1/1/95 to 12/31/95 and 1/1/96 to 12/31/96

Revenues	1996	1995
Net enrollee revenue	$4,875,990	$2,830,865
Other operating revenue	581,282	123,744
Total revenues	$5,457,272	$2,954,609
Expenses		
Physician salaries and expenses	$1,227,850	$1,124,818
Nursing salaries and expenses	594,243	305,720
Other salaries and expenses	305,986	213,412
Supplies	914,361	486,257
Utilities	45,764	38,110
Depreciation	613,228	542,333
Bad Debt Expense	21,260	24,645
Interest and other	205,521	280,479
Total	$3,928,213	$3,015,774
Operating income from operations ($1,005,008 paid in dividends to owners in 1996).	$1,529,059	$ (61,165)

Problem 3-16
Jefferson-Madison Ambulatory Center
Balance Sheets
10/31/96

	JAC	MOSCI
Current assets		
Cash	$ 1,420,214	$ 6,987
Accounts receivable	613,285	2,271,569
Less allowance for		
doubtful accounts	(100,496)	(97,820)
Inventory	2,584,333	616,312
Prepaid and deferred expenses	291,408	915,485
Total current assets	$ 4,808,744	$3,712,533
Fixed assets:		
Property and buildings	4,681,246	1,427,648
Equipment	3,926,817	2,637,904
Less accum. depreciation	(2,342,789)	(554,137)
Net fixed assets	$ 6,265,274	$3,511,415
Total assets	$11,074,018	$7,223,948
Current liabilities		
Accounts and rates payable	$1,562,043	$2,128,784
Accrued expenses	500,285	724,833
Total current liabilities	$2,062,328	$2,853,617
Long-term liabilities:		
Long-term property debt	1,893,427	1,118,423
Long-term debt, other	2,724,630	3,693,807
Total long-term debt	$4,618,057	$4,812,230
Total liabilities	$6,680,385	$7,665,847
Net assets	$4,393,633	$ (441,899)
Total liabilities and net assets	$11,074,018	$7,223,948

Problem 3-16
Income Statements
11/1/95 to 10/31/96

	JAC	MOSCI
Revenues		
Net patient charges	$1,945,843	$1,455,418
Other operating revenue	241,650	85,840
Total revenues	$2,187,493	$1,541,258
Expenses		
Payroll-related expenses	$1,089,135	$ 891,245
Supplies and utilities	546,808	288,117
Depreciation	500,850	62,255
Interest	256,380	210,335
Other (including bad debts)	97,415	15,063
Total operating expenses	$2,490,588	$1,467,015
Increase (decrease) in net assets	$ (303,095)	$ 74,243

3-17 A. Analyze the financial statements for Global Medical Center. Compute any ratios you consider necessary to complete your analysis.

   B. Why are unamortized bond issue costs listed as other assets?

3-18 A. Analyze the financial statements of Multi Hospital Systems.

   B. Explain the goodwill accounts on the balance sheets.

3-19 A. Analyze the Financial Statements of the Aspen Clinic. As a minimum, the current ratio and the relevant turnover ratios and performance ratios should be calculated.

   B. What does the "Assets Limited as to Use" account classification represent?

3-20 A. Analyze the financial condition of University Hospital.

   B. University Hospital uses a modified cash basis of accounting. What difficulties does this create?

3-21 A. Analyze the liquidity position of Community Hospital. What recommendations would you make to the hospital administrators?

   B. What is the meaning of the specific-purpose funds entry "Due from general fund"?

   C. Analyze the capitalization ratios for Community Hospital. If you were a banker, would you feel secure in making a long-term loan to this institution? Explain your decision.

   D. Analyze the financial performance of Community Hospital. What recommendations would you make to the board of trustees?

   E. If you had to quickly assess one of the following, what ratios might you use?
      1. a hospital's overall financial position
      2. a health administrator's performance
      3. a patient accounts collection department's performance

3-22 As a consultant, write a letter to the board of Rocky Mountain Hospice explaining your assessment of their financial condition on December 31, 1997.

Problem 3-17
Global Medical Center
Statement of Revenues and Expenses

For the Six Months Ended June 30	1997	1996
Net inpatient services revenue	$6,963,645	$6,101,084
Net outpatient services revenue	1,080,441	894,041
Total patient service revenue	$8,044,086	$6,995,125
Other operating revenues	111,568	92,992
Total revenues	$8,155,654	$7,088,117
Operating expenses		
Salaries and employee benefits	3,886,011	3,443,833
Professional fees	340,067	273,291
Provision for bad debts	949,479	558,439
Supplies and other expenses	2,395,362	2,044,713
Operating expenses	$7,570,919	$6,320,276
Revenue before capital expenses	$ 584,735	$ 767,841
Capital Expenses:		
Interest	211,038	215,600
Depreciation	229,028	224,952
Capital expenses	$ 440,066	$ 440,552
Operating income	$ 144,669	$ 327,289
Contributions	68,544	64,557
Increase in net assets	$ 213,213	$ 391,846

Problem 3-17
Global Medical Center
Balance Sheet

As of June 30	1997	1996
Assets		
Current assets:		
Cash	$ 189,817	$ 2,121
Net patient receivables	3,030,972	3,134,429
Inventories	434,656	415,061
Prepaid expenses and other	127,644	65,465
Total current assets	$3,783,089	$ 3,617,076
Other assets:		
Investments	562,000	310,000
Unamortized bond issue costs	98,072	103,703
Property, plant, and equipment		
Less accumulated depreciation	5,151,719	5,203,611
Total other assets	$5,811,791	$5,617,314
Total assets	$9,594,880	$9,234,390
Liabilities and Net Assets		
Current liabilities:		
Current installments of long-term debt	$170,806	$146,000
Accounts payable	509,811	471,266
Accrued expenses	319,390	192,166
Total current liabilities	$1,000,007	$ 809,432
Deferred revenue	137,660	119,660
Long-term debt		
Bonds	$4,389,692	$4,560,355
Capitalized lease obligation	69,850	
Total liabilities	$5,597,209	$5,489,447
Net assets	$3,997,671	$3,744,943
Total liabilities and net assets	$9,594,880	$9,234,390

Problem 3-18
Multi Hospital Systems
Income Statement

	Year Ended December 31, 1995
Revenues (net)	
Services	$24,962,677
Systems sales	23,121,366
Interest and dividends	340,576
Other income	261,809
Total revenues	$48,686,428
Costs and expenses	
Costs of services	$13,619,276
Costs of systems sold	11,778,087
Research and development costs	1,818,631
Selling and administrative expenses	15,844,112
Provision for bad debts	101,360
Interest	94,502
Total expenses	$43,255,968
Income before taxes	$ 5,430,460
Income taxes	2,314,000
Net income	$ 3,116,460
Earnings per share	$1.35
Weighted average of shares outstanding	2,316,797

Problem 3-18
Multi Hospital Systems
Consolidated Balance Sheets

As of December 31	1995	1994
Assets		
Current assets		
Cash	$ 824,270	$ 2,520,291
Marketable securities, at cost, less $206,000 allowance for decline in market value in 1995, plus accrued interest	9,650,307	2,325,189
Accounts receivable, less $126,000 allowance for doubtful accounts in 1995, $101,000 in 1994	14,225,113	12,247,918
Unbilled work at estimated realizable value	1,584,197	1,106,176
Supply and equipment inventories	3,610,914	2,375,915
Prepaid expenses and other assets	1,276,512	1,159,980
Total current assets	$31,171,313	$21,735,469
Property and equipment, at cost less accumulated depreciation and amortization	12,912,996	9,007,226
Software products, less $691,239 accumulated amortization in 1995, $396,000 in 1994	3,302,227	527,123
Goodwill, less $226,316 accumulated amortization in 1995, $154,318 in 1994	2,495,937	2,567,935
Other intangibles, less $598,296 accumulated amortization in 1995, $153,500 in 1994	2,386,325	544,703
Other assets	1,004,695	931,892
Total assets	$53,273,493	$35,314,348

Problem 3-18
Multi Hospital Systems
Consolidated Balance Sheets, continued

As of December 31	1995	1994
Liabilities and Stockholders' Equity		
Current liabilities		
Current portion of long-term debt	$ 790,579	$ 248,833
Acquisition payment due	1,550,000	
Accounts payable	4,578,592	4,267,574
Accrued expenses	1,070,473	743,827
Accrued payroll	713,637	581,892
Client deposits and unearned income	1,243,774	684,530
Deferred income taxes	4,773,611	3,947,907
Total current liabilities	$14,720,666	$10,474,563
Long-term debt, less current portion	1,014,488	263,317
Deferred income taxes	2,418,408	954,408
Total liabilities	$18,153,562	$11,692,288
Stockholders' equity:		
Preferred stock, par value $1.00, 1,000,000 shares authorized, none issued		
Common stock, par value $.01, 10,000,000 shares authorized, 2,611,656 issued in 1995	26,117	22,368
Capital in excess of par value	23,881,060	15,487,566
Retained earnings	11,212,754	8,112,126
Total stockholders' equity	$35,119,931	$23,622,060
Total liabilities and stockholders' equity	$53,273,493	$35,314,348

Problem 3-19
Aspen Clinic, Inc.
Statements of Revenues and Expenses
for the Years Ended October 31, 1997 and 1996

	1997	1996
Operating Revenues (net)		
Daily patient services	$1,001,352	$ 971,213
Ancillary services	3,459,613	2,943,119
Other	73,257	33,427
Net operating revenues	$4,534,222	$ 3,947,759
Operating Expenses		
Salaries, wages, and employee benefits	1,679,484	1,754,943
Supplies and other expenses	1,278,711	1,155,557
Specialists' fees	530,036	354,883
Depreciation	203,033	202,028
Provision for bad debts	203,173	224,423
Contract expenses	62,119	32,365
Interest and amortization expense	160,070	194,527
Other	19,787	21,996
Operating expenses	$4,136,413	$3,940,722
Operating income	$ 397,809	$ 7,037
Nonoperating Revenues (Expenses):		
Contributions, net	105,947	144,382
Investment income	92,993	55,848
Rental income, net	81,106	73,683
Gain (loss) on disposal of equipment	5,703	(37,587)
Total nonoperating revenues	$ 285,749	$ 236,326
Increase in net assets	$ 683,558	$ 243,363

Problem 3-19
Aspen Clinic, Inc.
Balance Sheets
October 31, 1997 and 1996

Assets	1997	1996
Current assets:		
Cash	$ 64,325	$ 166,353
Accounts receivable from patient services, net of allowances for uncollectible accounts of $275,000 in 1997 and $175,000 in 1996	332,260	421,511
Supplies inventory	190,568	166,860
Assets limited as to use required for current liabilities	151,522	117,683
Pledges receivable, net of allowances for uncollectible pledges of $67,000 in 1987 and $63,000 in 1996	8,620	33,120
Other current assets	55,725	34,322
Total current assets	$ 803,020	$ 939,849
Land, buildings, and equipment, net	$3,521,774	$3,476,966
Assets limited as to use:		
Board-designated funded depreciation	897,243	300,000
Funds required by Series 1987 Revenue Bonds	351,032	353,058
	$1,248,275	$ 653,058
Less: required for current liabilities	(151,522)	(117,683)
Total assets limited as to use	$1,096,753	$ 535,375
Other assets:		
Unamortized bond issuance costs	101,525	113,290
Note receivable	6,600	7,495
Total assets	$5,529,672	$5,072,975

Liabilities and Fund Balances		
Current liabilities:		
Accounts payable	$ 148,039	$ 85,108
Payable to an affiliate	10,242	246,728
Estimated payable to third-party agencies	120,000	105,000
Current maturities of long-term debt	80,000	79,316
Accrued interest payable	71,522	73,735
Other liabilities and accrued expenses	142,086	150,215
Total current liabilities	$ 571,889	$ 740,102
Long-term debt, net of current maturities	1,935,000	2,015,000
Total liabilities	$2,506,889	$2,755,102
Net Assets:		
Unrestricted	2,998,562	2,315,004
Restricted	24,221	2,869
Total net assets	$3,022,783	$2,317,873
Total liabilities and net assets	$5,529,672	$5,072,975

Problem 3-20
University Hospital
Summary of Revenues and Expenses
as of July 31, 1997

Patient Revenues:	
Inpatient Services	$ 8,385,303
Outpatient Services	1,427,635
Emergency Services	1,096,729
Per Diem Ancillary Services	9,135,010
Itemized Ancillary Services	6,003,787
Patient Revenues	$26,048,464
Nonpatient Revenue	448,205
State Appropriation	13,315,368
Pay Plan Appropriation	901,749
Total revenue	$40,713,786
Operating Expenses:	
Academic Salaries	889,323
Classified and Other Wages	18,485,992
Resident and Intern Salaries	2,196,238
Other Payroll Expenses	3,118,100
Services and Supplies	12,232,103
Bad Debt Expense	3,057,807
Depreciation	1,304,761
Interest	187,000
Operating expenses	$41,471,324
Operating income (loss)	($ 757,538)

Problem 3-20
University Hospital
Balance Sheet
July 31, 1997

<u>Current General Fund</u>

Current assets:		
Cash		$ 8,797,497
Marketable securities		750,693
Cash & cash equivalents		$ 9,548,190
Investments		1
Patient and contract receivables	$11,869,985	
Less: Allowance for doubtful accounts	(5,222,839)	$ 6,647,146
Medicare/Medicaid Payments		
Receivables	$ 229,416	
Less: Allowance for doubtful accounts	(107,479)	$ 121,937
Inventories		1,103,192
Total current assets		$17,420,466
Net assets		$17,420,466

Problem 3-21
Community Hospital
Statement of Revenue and Expenses

| | Year Ended June 30 | |
	1997	1996
Net patient service revenue	$21,187,739	$18,583,344
Other operating revenue	499,680	493,665
Total revenues	$21,687,419	$19,077,009
Operating expenses		
Professional care of patients	11,649,229	10,141,372
Dietary	1,165,543	1,100,139
Household and property	1,626,921	1,461,717
Administrative and general	1,836,102	2,232,979
Bad debt expense	2,551,538	1,994,393
Interest	127,502	198,059
Depreciation	1,030,606	978,589
	$19,987,441	$18,107,248
Operating income	$ 1,699,978	$ 969,761
Unrestricted contributions	155,715	121,801
Gain (loss) on disposition of assets	10,388	(19,301)
Subtotal	$ 166,103	$ 102,500
Increase in net assets	$ 1,866,081	$ 1,072,261

Problem 3-21
Community Hospital
Consolidated Balance Sheet
Unrestricted Funds

	June 30	
Assets	1997	1996
General fund		
Current assets		
Cash in bank and on hand	$ 116,620	$ 181,045
Certificate of deposit	420,777	300,938
Investment: at cost (which		
approximates market)	124,635	
Receivables		
Patients' charges (net of allowance		
for doubtful accounts and		
contractual adjustments of		
$633,074 in 1997 and $511,833		
in 1996)	2,822,021	2,241,197
Estimated contractual adjustments, net	75,898	282,356
Other	14,289	5,851
Inventories	526,096	482,025
Prepaid and deferred expenses	238,647	33,930
Total current assets	$ 4,338,983	$ 3,527,342
Property, plant, and equipment		
Land and land improvements	961,330	481,626
Buildings and improvements	13,893,623	14,090,895
Equipment	10,135,961	8,553,794
Total property, plant, and equipment	$24,990,914	$23,126,315
Less accumulated depreciation	8,879,729	7,955,372
Net property, plant, and equipment	$16,111,185	$15,170,943
Other assets	54,965	12,701
Total general fund assets	$20,505,133	$18,710,986
Specific-purpose funds		
Cash	$ 11,320	$ 11,705
Certificate of deposit		100,000
Due from general fund	59,030	50,036
Total specific-purpose funds	$ 70,350	$ 161,741
Development fund		
Cash	$ 150,905	$ 9,578
Certificates of deposit	179,918	169,260
Pledges receivable	58,707	656,874
Interest receivable	29,701	1,169
Investments	110,320	83,423
Note receivable from operating fund	284,468	
Due from specific purpose fund	10,666	16,666
Total development fund assets	$ 824,685	$ 936,970

Problem 3-21
Community Hospital
Consolidated Balance Sheet
Unrestricted Funds, continued

	June 30	
	1997	1996
Liabilities and Net Assets		
Current liabilities		
7.5% unsecured note payable to bank	$	$ 164,318
Accounts payable: trade	956,399	677,396
Salaries, wages, and fees payable	639,882	520,873
Advances: intermediary	220,050	196,740
Payroll taxes and withholdings	136,866	63,866
Other accrued expenses	93,757	61,468
Current maturities of long-term debt	419,855	112,358
Total current liabilities	$ 2,466,809	$ 1,797,019
Long-term debt	859,467	817,682
Due to specific purpose fund	59,030	50,036
Note payable to development fund	284,468	
Total liabilities	$ 3,669,774	$ 2,664,737
Net assets	$ 16,835,359	$16,046,249
Total liabilities and net assets	$ 20,505,133	$18,710,986
Specific-purpose fund		
Due to development fund	$ 10,666	$ 16,666
Specific-purpose fund balance	59,684	145,075
Total liabilities and net assets	$ 70,350	$ 161,741
Development fund		
Accounts payable		$ 106,414
Interest payable		1,498
Building loan payable		455,500
Development fund balance	$ 824,685	373,558
Total liabilities and net assets	$ 824,685	$ 936,970

Problem 3-22
Rocky Mountain Hospice, Inc.
Balance Sheet
December 31, 1997

Assets	Total All Funds	Operating Funds	Equipment Funds
Cash	$11,473	$11,473	
Certificates of deposit	20,000	20,000	
U.S. government securities	26,838	26,838	
Marketable securities: corporate stock (market value $580)	505	505	
Contributions and accounts receivable	3,817	3,817	
Accounts receivable: employees	582	582	
Prepaid expenses	1,303	1,303	
Furniture and equipment	1,832		$ 1,832
Total Assets	$66,350	$64,518	$ 1,832
Liabilities and net assets			
Liabilities			
Accounts payable	$ 1,158	$ 1,158	
Accrued payroll taxes	6,736	6,736	
Total Liabilities	$ 7,894	$ 7,894	
Net assets	$58,456	$56,624	$ 1,832
Total Liabilities and Net Assets	$66,350	$64,518	$ 1,832

Problem 3-22
Rocky Mountain Hospice, Inc.
Statement of Support, Revenue, and Expenses
and Changes in Fund Balances
Year Ended December 31, 1997

	Total All Funds	Operating Funds	Equipment Funds
Support and Revenue			
Grant income	$ 6,587	$ 6,587	
Contributions	7,662	7,662	
Interest income	6,616	6,616	
Miscellaneous income	806	186	$ 620
Total support and revenue	$ 21,671	$ 21,051	$ 620
Expenses			
Program services			
Patient care	8,098	8,098	
Training and staff development	11,037	11,037	
Public and professional education	6,848	6,848	
Total program services expenses	$ 25,983	$ 25,983	
Supporting services			
General and administrative	16,463	16,233	230
Fund raising	235	235	
Total supporting services expenses	$ 16,698	$ 16,468	$ 230
Total expenses	$ 42,681	$ 42,451	$ 230
Increase (decrease) in net assets	($21,010)	($21,400)	$ 390

3-23 A. Evaluate the financial performance of Investor Owned Systems.
   B. What trends are important in your analysis?
   C. What major problem areas would you report to the board of directors?

3-24 A. Compute the following ratios for United Health Plan, Inc.:
   1. Liquidity ratios
   2. Turnover ratios
   3. Profitability ratios
   4. Capitalization ratios

   B. Evaluate the financial performance of United Health Plan, Inc.
   C. In what areas would you like more information?

3-25 A. Assess the financial performance of United Hospitals.
   B. What ratios do you think are crucial to your analysis?

3-26 A. Assess the financial condition of the United Hospital Fund of New York.
   B. Are ratios for the individual funds important to your analysis?

3-27 A. Analyze the financial statements of Holderness and Company. What ratios do you think are important in this type of organization? (Hint: Holderness and Company is primarily an investment company.) What key assumptions did you make in computing your ratios?
   B. Explain the deferred income tax and deferred compensation accounts.

Page intentionally left blank.

Problem 3-23
Investor Owned Systems
Consolidated Statements of Income

(dollars in millions, except per share amounts)	1996	1995	1994
Net revenues	$9,362.1	$9,021.1	$8,346.8
Costs and expenses			
Maintenance	1,656.1	1,646.9	1,587.9
Depreciation	1,664.5	1,602.7	1,347.3
Other operating expenses	2,811.4	2,656.0	2,450.0
Bad debt expense	111.0	107.0	96.5
Taxes other than income taxes	694.2	719.5	714.0
Total costs and expenses	$6,937.2	$6,732.1	$6,195.7
Other income:	33.3	30.3	61.5
Income before interest expense and income taxes	$2,458.2	$2,319.3	$2,212.6
Interest expense	390.4	421.9	436.6
Income before income taxes	$2,067.8	$1,897.4	$1,776.0
Income taxes	929.4	819.7	785.4
Net income	$1,138.4	$1,077.7	$ 990.6
Earnings per share*	$ 7.87	$ 7.35	$ 6.78
Dividends per share*	$ 4.79	$ 4.40	$ 4.00
Average common shares outstanding (millions)*	144.6	146.7	146.1

*Share and per share data have been restated to reflect three-for-two stock split effective December 31, 1996.

Problem 3-23
Investor Owned Systems
Consolidated Balance Sheets, continued

	Dec. 31, 1996	Dec. 31, 1995
Liabilities and Shareowners' Equity		
Current liabilities:		
Debt maturing within one year	$ 227.7	$ 227.6
Accounts payable	1,304.2	1,244.0
Accrued payroll	93.1	102.7
Accrued taxes	505.7	395.7
Income taxes deferred for one year	185.9	141.4
Advance billing and customers' deposits	204.5	192.3
Dividend payable	178.8	160.7
Accrued interest	96.4	115.2
Total current liabilities	$ 2,796.3	$ 2,579.6
Long and intermediate-term debt	4,496.6	4,517.6
Deferred credits:		
Accumulated deferred income taxes	2,805.3	2,572.4
Unamortized investment tax credits	921.4	935.9
Other	110.8	93.8
Total deferred credits	$ 3,837.5	$ 3,602.1
Shareowners' equity:		
Common stock (at par value)	146.9	98.1
Proceeds in excess of par value	5,855.5	5,616.5
Reinvested earnings	2,250.0	1,802.9
Treasury stock, at cost	(643.4)	(68.0)
Total shareowners' equity	$ 7,609.0	$ 7,449.5
Total liabilities and shareowners' equity	$ 18,739.4	$18,148.8

Page intentionally left blank.

Problem 3-24
United Health Plan, Inc.
Combined Statements of Net Income

	Year Ended December 31, 1995
Revenues	
Members' dues	$3,309,453
Supplemental charges to members	138,923
Medicare, Health Plan members	496,309
Nonplan and industrial	81,402
Other	48,816
Total revenues	$4,074,903
Expenses	
Medical services	1,830,100
Hospital services	1,312,268
Outpatient pharmacy and optical services	242,605
Other benefit costs	196,927
Bad debt expense	145,060
Community service programs, less $10,329 from research grants and contracts	36,645
Total medical and hospital services	$3,763,605
Health Plan administration	117,362
Total expenses	$3,880,967
Operating income	$ 193,936

Problem 3-24
United Health Plan, Inc.
Statement of Cash Flows (Abbreviated)

	Year Ended December 31, 1995
Cash Provided by Operations	$ 350,254
Other sources of cash:	
Working capital loans	121,995
Investments designated for facilities expenditures	(353,086)
Liability for physicians' retirement plan benefits	56,134
Other long-term liabilities	(17,620)
Proceeds from long-term borrowings	484,119
Bond funds held by trustees and deferred	
debt issuance expenses	(44,330)
Total sources of cash	$ 597,466
Uses of Cash:	
Land, buildings, and equipment, net	$ 487,474
Principal payments on long-term debt	36,256
Securities segregated for physicians'	
retirement plan obligation	56,134
Acquisitions	1,227
Other	16,375
Total uses of cash	$ 597,466

Problem 3-24
United Health Plan, Inc.
Balance Sheet

	December 31, 1995
Assets	
Current assets:	
Cash, including interest-bearing deposits and short-term investments	$ 206,154
Accounts receivable	
Members' dues	90,003
Medicare	53,863
Patients, less allowance for uncollectible accounts of $21,972	62,417
Other	11,636
	$ 217,919
Inventories	47,330
Prepaid expenses	38,428
Total current assets	$ 509,831
Cash and Securities Segregated for Physicians' Retirement Plan Obligation	383,769
Investments Designated for Facilities Expenditures	389,966
Bonds Funds Held by Trustees and Deferred Debt Issuance Expenses	76,106
Land, Buildings, and Equipment	
Land	229,348
Buildings and improvements	1,630,040
Equipment	526,426
Construction in progress	306,802
	$2,692,616
Less accumulated depreciation	857,367
	$1,835,249
Other assets	19,798
Total assets	$3,214,719

Problem 3-24
United Health Plan, Inc.
Balance Sheet, continued

	December 31, 1995
Liabilities and Net Worth	
Current liabilities:	
Notes payable	$ 44,975
Accounts payable and accrued expenses	224,570
Due to associated medical groups	123,164
Payroll and related charges	132,165
Liability for self-insured losses	70,745
Dues collected in advance	65,401
Revenue deferred to reduce dues rates	44,145
Other liabilities	66,447
Current installments on long-term debt	42,145
Total current liabilities	$ 813,757
Long-Term Liabilities, less current portion:	
Debt	877,969
Liability for physicians' retirement plan benefits	383,769
Liability for self-insured losses	133,403
Revenue deferred to reduce dues rates	28,047
Liability for postretirement benefits	38,439
Total liabilities	$1,461,627
Net worth	$ 939,335
Total liabilities and net worth	$3,214,719

Problem 3-25
United Hospitals,
Balance Sheet

Amounts in Thousands	December 31, 1996

Assets

Current assets:

Cash, including interest-bearing deposits and short-term investments	$	85,526
Accounts receivable		
Members' dues		93,810
Patients, less allowance for uncollectible accounts of $13,454		68,460
Medicare		40,689
Other		14,262
		217,221
		57,328
Prepaid expenses		50,873
Total current assets	$	410,948
Land, buildings, and equipment:		
Land		270,860
Buildings and improvements		1,938,417
Equipment		624,330
Construction in progress		284,286
Total land, buildings, and equipment	$	3,117,893
Less accumulated depreciation		745,860
	$	2,372,033
Other assets		789,374
Total assets	$	3,572,355

Problem 3-25
United Hospitals
Statement of Net Income

Amounts in Thousands	Year Ended December 31, 1996	
Revenues:		
Members' dues	$3,645,196	81.4%
Supplemental charges to members	151,058	3.4
Medicare, Health Plan members	531,872	11.9
Nonplan and industrial	82,958	1.8
Other	65,838	1.5
Total revenues	$4,476,922	100.0
Expenses:		
Medical services	1,994,810	44.6
Hospital services	1,438,688	32.1
Outpatient pharmacy and optical services	281,942	6.3
Other benefit costs	233,378	5.2
Bad debt expense	179,077	4.0
Community service programs, less $10,329 from research grants and contracts	39,733	.9
Total Medical and Hospital Services	$4,167,628	93.1
Health Plan administration	126,830	2.8
Total Expenses	$4,294,458	95.9
Operating Income	$ 182,464	4.1

Problem 3-26

United Hospital Fund of New York
Statement of Income, Expenses, and Changes in Fund Balances

Year ended February 28, 1996

| | Unrestricted funds | | | | Year ended February 28, 1995 |
	General	Board Designated Endowment	Restricted Endowment	Total	Total
Income					
Public Support:					
The Greater New York/ United Way	$ 5,835,271			$ 5,835,271	$5,314,771
Contributions	1,328,472			1,328,472	1,328,941
Grants	290,976			290,976	319,395
Legacies		$ 223,282		223,282	349,486
Total public support	$ 7,454,719	$ 223,282		$ 7,678,001	$ 7,312,593
Other Income:					
Income from services to hospitals	195,112			195,112	158,578
Investment income	2,608,893			2,608,893	2,427,164
Other	277,077			277,077	58,221
Total other income	$ 3,081,082			$ 3,081,082	$ 2,643,963
Total income	$10,535,801	$ 223,282		$10,759,083	$ 9,956,556

Problem 3-26

United Hospital Fund of New York
Statement of Income, Expenses, and Changes in Fund Balances (cont.)
Year ended February 28, 1996

	Unrestricted funds		Restricted Endowment	Total	Year ended February 28, 1995 Total
	General	Board Designated Endowment			
Expenses					
Program Services:					
Allocation to hospitals and affiliated org'ns	$ 6,347,872			$ 6,347,872	$6,004,110
health care programs	1,893,787			1,893,787	1,391,248
Patient Origin Information Systems					225,132
Support Services:					
Administrative and general	1,806,318			1,806,318	1,269,081
Fund raising	605,934			605,934	680,202
Total Expenses	$10,653,911			$10,653,911	$ 9,569,773
Excess of Income (Expenses) before Appreciation on Investments	(118,110)	223,282		105,172	386,783
Appreciation on investments		6,261,452	1,527,360	7,788,812	2,224,725
Increase (decrease) in net assets	(118,110)	$6,484,734	$ 1,527,360	$ 7,893,984	$ 2,611,508
Net assets; beginning of year	$ 1,462,152	23,843,474	5,894,741	$31,200,367	$28,588,859
Interfund Transfers	1,269		(1,269)		
Net assets: end of year	$ 1,345,311	$30,328,208	$ 7,420,832	$39,094,351	$31,200,367

Problem 3-26

United Hospital Fund of New York
Statement of Assets, Liabilities, and Fund Balances
Year ended February 28, 1996

| | Unrestricted funds | | | | Year ended February 28, 1995 |
	General	Board Designated Endowment	Restricted Endowment	Total	Total
Assets					
Cash and cash equivalents:					
Checking accounts	$ 145,546	$ 327,654	$ 144	$ 473,344	$ 396,364
Interest-bearing accounts and demand notes	2,227,062			2,227,062	3,806,096
Receivable from Greater New York/ United Way	2,025,271			2,025,271	1,354,771
Investments in marketable securities, at fair market value (cost $29,332,152 - 1986 and $26,458,841 -1985)		29,682,854	7,320,688	37,003,542	29,047,535
Other assets	342,931	317,700	100,000	760,631	639,400
Office furniture, equipment and leasehold improvements, at cost, less accumulated depreciation and amortization of $170,802 - 1986 and $418,037, - 1985	742,370			742,370	229,042
Total assets	$ 5,483,180	$30,328,208	$ 7,420,832	$43,232,220	$35,473,208

Problem 3-26

United Hospital Fund of New York
Statement of Assets, Liabilities, and Fund Balances (cont.)
Year ended February 28, 1996

| | | Unrestricted funds | | | Year ended February 28, 1995 |
	General	Board Designated Endowment	Restricted Endowment	Total	Total
Liabilities					
Accounts payable and other liabilities	789,223			789,223	597,715
Designated allocations payable	2,782,285			2,782,285	3,138,421
Undesignated allocations payable	566,361			566,361	536,705
Total liabilities	$4,137,869			$ 4,137,869	$4,272,841
Net Assets					
Board or donor designated	313,440	30,328,208	7,420,832	38,062,480	29,986,903
Unrestricted	1,031,871			1,031,871	1,213,464
Total net assets	$1,345,311	$30,328,208	$7,420,832	$39,094,351	$31,200,367
Total liabilities and net assets	$5,483,180	$30,328,208	$7,420,832	$43,232,220	$35,473,208

Problem 3-27

Holderness and Company
Statement of Income and Retained Earnings
Year Ended December 31, 1991

Income:		
Dividends on stocks		$ 224,331
Interest		60,501
Gain on sale of securities		600,322
Total income		$ 885,154
Expenses:		
Salaries	$34,801	
Deferred officer compensation	5,000	
Taxes other than income	12,176	
Office rent	1,318	
Telephone and telegraph	783	
Professional services	7,525	
Office supplies and expense	171	
Miscellaneous	1,212	
Total expenses		$ 62,986
Income before income taxes		$ 822,168
Income taxes		
Current	208,662	
Deferred	(850)	$ 207,812
Net income		$ 614,356
Retained earnings at beginning of year		1,296,809
Retained earnings at end		
of Year, before dividends		$1,911,165
Cash dividends @ $2.80 per share		(173,243)
Retained earnings, at end of year		$1,737,922
Earnings Per Common Share		$9.92

Problem 3-27
Holderness and Company
Balance Sheet
December 31, 1991

<u>Assets</u>
Current assets:
Cash $ 63,848
Marketable securities (at cost)
  Stocks (market
  $2,864,862.00) $ 1,468,394
  Bonds (market
  $779,311.00)
  (maturity $945,000.00) $ 841,019
  Accrued interest 16,193 857,212 $ 2,325,606

  Accounts receivable: brokers 56

  Total current assets $ 2,389,510

Deferred income taxes 2,700

Total assets $ 2,392,210

<u>Liabilities and Stockholders' Equity</u>

Current liabilities:
  Accounts payable $ 3,823
  Accrued taxes, other than income 6,352
  Income taxes 193,062

  Total current liabilities $ 203,237

Deferred Compensation 15,000

Total liabilities $ 218,237

Stockholders' equity:
  Common stock, par value
  $10.00 per share; authorized
  150,000 shares; issued 86,050
  shares $ 860,500
  Retained earnings 1,737,921
  $2,598,421

Less: common stock in treasury,
  24,338 shares at cost 424,448.00 $ 2,173,973

Total liabilities and stockholders' equity $ 2,392,210

4 Cost Definitions and Cost Behavior

While the previous chapters introduced financial statements that may have used terms involving costs, we have not been very specific about how to define costs. Recall that financial statements are usually prepared for external users, like bankers, other creditors, investors, etc. These external users are usually "outside" the organization and they have diverse backgrounds and needs. They usually do not have a "real-time" need for the information and often they can rely on last year's or last quarter's data. Consequently, financial statements prepared for external users are almost always based on Generally Accepted Accounting Principles (GAAP).

On the other hand, detailed costing data are usually prepared for and used by managers within a health care organization. These "internal" managers have more immediate access to detailed data within the organization. They have an even greater variety of needs because their possible decisions are almost infinite. We are, thus, moving from financial accounting to focus, instead, on managerial accounting. The purpose of management accounting is to provide information for decision making. The decision makers can specify the kinds of information they find most relevant. Managers and financial managers define costs in a way that is most helpful for the decision at hand.

Cost analysis is an important part of most decisions made by health care managers. Whether one is a manager or clinician in a health care organization, terms such as cost per unit, cost management, and cost-benefit are continually used. This chapter provides an overview of the most common cost-related concepts and terms and then relates those concepts to the variability or "behavior" of costs. You will find, in this chapter and thereafter, a variety of costs. You will also find that costs should be defined according to the decision or purpose for which they will be used. Chapter 5 applies some of these cost concepts to short-term decision-making in the context of cost-volume-profit and differential analysis.

This chapter presents the internal role of accounting information next, followed by some basic premises supporting managerial accounting information. Several categories of cost classifications are defined and discussed. Finally, a method of estimating total costs is demonstrated.

Internal Role of Accounting Information

In order to understand managers' needs for different types of information, the management control process must first be described. There are five activities in this process. They are data collection, planning, implementing, controlling and evaluating. All of these activities are performed in light of the organization's objectives and goals. Figure 4-1 describes the management control process, assuming the collection of appropriate data. This **data collection** activity often involves both internal and external data. Relevant data can include information about competitors, social and economic policies, payment rules and practices, demographics, and the health needs of the community. Much of this relevant information is not found in the firm's ongoing, routine information systems. Our focus, however, is on cost information that generally should be available in the firm's information system; or, at least, on costs that can be constructed and re-arranged on the basis of information found within the firm's information system.

The second activity in which managers engage, **planning**, is often episodic and non-routine, based on reactions to competitors or other environmental changes. Again, we focus more on routine parts of the planning process, such as budgeting. In such cases, the information requirements can be more precisely anticipated. They can be more often generalized or extrapolated from one planning scenario to the next. Chapter 8 deals more fully with these planning and budgeting issues. In any event, managers will want detailed information about various kinds of costs, in order to plan more effectively. While we cannot provide a complete inventory of these kinds of costs and the decisions to which they might relate, one of the purposes of this chapter, and following chapters, is to illustrate some of these costs in typical decision contexts. Other, more advanced courses in cost accounting can provide broader coverage of these issues.

Figure 4-1 Management Control Cycle.

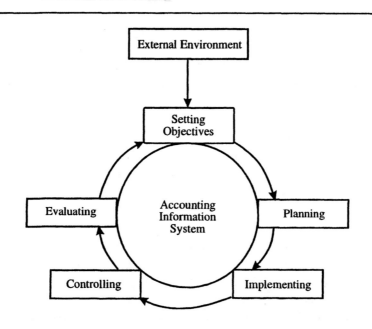

The third activity in the management control process is to implement decisions. Financial managers are less involved in **implementation**. Managers have the authority to implement decisions and they are held responsible for their decisions.

It is in the final part of the management control process where managers obtain the most useful information for **controlling** and **evaluating** their performance. This last activity could also be called **performance assessment**. The control phase involves many different kinds of costing information as managers try to assess how well their plans are being implemented. Control processes are complex. They involve important behavioral reactions because they often affect people's performance. The impact of management accounting information on people's behavior is often subtle, but with long-term consequences. Because of this important link to human behavior, it is crucial that financial managers be concerned with the most accurate, the most relevant, and the most well-understood costing concepts.

There is often a "veil" or barrier between the manager or clinician and the financial manager. Our goal is to pierce that veil and make some of these costing concepts more understandable and more useful to managers. Consequently, many of the subsequent chapters will rely on the costing concepts and definitions that are introduced in this chapter. As you proceed through this text, you may find it helpful to review this chapter in conjunction with subsequent chapters that examine various phases of the management control process. At this point, remember that management accounting occurs simultaneously with management decision-making. Management accounting is intertwined throughout Figure 4-1, as information about costs and cost behavior is used by managers in many different ways, as they make both short and long-term decisions.

Basic Premises of Managerial Accounting Information

A thorough understanding of management accounting rests on ten basic premises. These premises affect the determination of costs, and they affect many of the activities in the management control process.

Premise One

Management account information must *serve a purpose*. It must provide information about some **cost object** or objective. Once the objective is known, then the information most suitable for that purpose can be specified.

Premise Two

Management accounting information must be *relevant* to the decision at hand. In order to facilitate and improve manager's decisions, information must be relevant and useful. Costing information, especially, must rest on this premise. Costing algorithms or definitions used in one organization, or in one set of computer software, may be irrelevant and counter-productive in another health care organization. Chapter 5 emphasizes this relevance factor.

Premise Three

Management accounting information is often *future-oriented,* which means it is based on estimates and forecasts. It does not depend on the same level of precision and verifiability often found in financial accounting. Uncertainty, which is inherent in predicting the future, is often a factor that must be included in the manager's decision processes. While formal ways to deal with uncertainty are not presented in this text, the subjective nature of costs must be considered. The most useful method of dealing with uncertainty, in terms of this text, will be to test alternative scenarios to determine whether the recommended decision might change under any of the possible alternative scenarios.

Premise Four

Management accounting often focuses on *incremental costs* (and incremental revenues). Costs that differ between two alternatives will often be the deciding factor in making a decision. By separating the incremental, or differential costs, the financial manager can greatly assist the manager in making the proper choice. We will show how using certain types of costs may actually mislead the decision maker when incremental costs are not separately disclosed. Incremental costs are discussed in Chapter 5.

Premise Five

Financial managers must often emphasize *cash flows* as compared to accrual accounting numbers. Differential cash flows associated with each decision are often the most important decision factors. To the extent that cost information mirrors these cash flows, then managers will make better decisions. In other words, accrual-based costs may not always reflect cash flows. Managers who want to improve the firm's cash flows need to look at both factors.

Premise Six

Managers must also consider the *time value of money.* A dollar today is worth more than a dollar next year, or ten years later. This factor affects long-range decisions, primarily those that involve purchasing or selling fixed assets. We will take up this concept in more detail in Chapter 13.

Premise Seven

Managers must consider the *behavioral impact* of their decisions. Similarly, financial managers must consider the impact of their information on the managers, and on the managers' decisions. Numbers are affected by the people who provide them; people are influenced by numbers. We cannot stress too much the importance of these behavioral factors. Further study of management processes will increase your understanding of these behavioral factors. These issues are most important in the context of budgeting and performance reporting.

Premise Eight

A particular behavioral impact concerns the issue of *responsibility* or *accountability*. Managers should only be evaluated in areas where they can exercise control. *Controllability* is a necessary corollary to accountability. Managers should be accountable for processes and decisions which they can affect or control. This criterion of ability to change, or impact, will be used to define certain kinds of costs later in this chapter. At a minimum, managerial performance reports should distinguish between controllable and noncontrollable costs. Controllable costs should not be intermingled with other costs.

Premise Nine

Timely information is also essential. Managerial accounting information that is too late to help the decision process is almost worthless. In many cases, estimates must be used because the actual data will not be known until after the decision needs to be made. For example, for evaluating payer-provider contracts, estimates may be necessary because the actual data will not be available for several months, or it may be too expensive to achieve higher levels of precision.

Premise Ten

The final premise relates to the value of information versus the cost to provide it, which can be called the *cost versus benefit* of information. In many cases, this benefit/cost criterion might be applied to the decision regarding whether to gather additional information; i.e. are the benefits of more precise information worth the cost of the getting the additional information?

The ten premises provide a foundation for understanding managerial cost accounting data. These premises are referenced throughout this text. Depending on the decision setting, some premises may be linked. In this situation, they need to be considered simultaneously.

Cost Concepts

Unfortunately for the manager, the term cost has come to have numerous meanings in today's health care environment. This ambiguity requires that managers be aware of the many different ways the term is used and where each is relevant to decision-making. Exhibit 4-1 presents many different cost-related terms, classified into several categories. A discussion of each term follows.

Asset Valuation

Accountants are very concerned about asset valuation because assets are transformed into expenses when resources are used. Expenses are just expired assets. Costs are recognized as assets are used. For example, as a computer is used by a physician or by a managed care organization, its periodic amortization is shown on the income statement as an expense. There is a causal link between assets, their valuation, and the costs that ultimately are used for

Exhibit 4-1 Types of Cost by Category.

Asset Valuation

> Cash basis of accounting
> Accrual basis of accounting
> Historical costs
> Replacement costs

Responsibility Accounting

> Controllable costs
> Noncontrollable costs

Traceability

> Direct costs
> Indirect costs
> Full costs

Commitment

> Committed costs
> Non-committed costs

Actual and Budgeted

> Budgeted costs
> Actual costs

Relevance

> Incremental (differential) costs
> Sunk costs
> Opportunity costs

Cost Behavior

> Fixed costs
> Variable costs
> Total costs
> Mixed costs
> Semi-fixed costs
> Semi-variable costs

performance reports and the related expenses that appear in income statements. For short-term assets, the asset and the expense are recognized in the same accounting period. An example is salary or wage expense. Because these two events happen so close together, valuation is not an issue. For long-term assets, the asset is on the balance sheet for more than one year, and the expense is recognized over the course of this time frame. An example is depreciation of equipment. The concern in this section is with long-term assets.

Part of the accountant's concern for asset valuation was discussed in Chapter 2, in the context of cash versus accrual accounting. The concern regarding how much to value an asset stems from the ambiguity of the word value. For instance, value can mean: (1) how much something means to us; (2) how much we could sell an item for (market value); (3) how much it would cost to replace an asset (replacement cost); (4) the benefit we think we will receive as a result of owning an item; and (4) how much we paid for it.

For balance sheet presentation purposes, under GAAP long-lived (fixed) assets are valued at their **historical cost** (the actual purchase price plus related costs necessary to put the assets into service). Valuing assets at historical costs standardizes how assets are reported on the balance sheet. However, if not interpreted carefully, it can be quite misleading in times of inflation. For instance, in Exhibit 4-2, the value that would be reported on the balance sheet for the old gastroscope is $2,271. This amount represents the **net book value** of the gastroscope, which is equal to the historical cost of $5,300 less accumulated depreciation of $3,029.

It should be apparent, though, that it would cost considerably more than $2,271 to replace the equipment today. The **replacement cost** is $8,200, which is comprised of the $7,800 cost of a new machine and the $400 it would take to bring the new asset into working condition. Replacement cost is only one of several ways to determine the current value of an asset.

The second concern in asset valuation is when to recognize on the income statement the expenses associated with an asset which has already been purchased. As discussed in Chapter 2, under the *cash basis* of accounting, costs are recognized when cash is paid out; that is, when an expenditure occurs. In Exhibit 4-2, the expenditure for the new gastroscope would be $2,000, the amount of the down payment. Using the *accrual basis* of accounting recognizes expenses as the asset produces benefits, that is, as it is used in producing goods or services. When the accrual basis of accounting is used, a portion of the historical cost, called depreciation, is recognized on the income statement during each period of the useful life of the asset. Depreciation is classified as an expense. The annual expense associated with the new gastroscope is the annual depreciation expense of $1,171.

Responsibility Accounting

The second category of cost terms relates to **managerial control** and holding managers responsible for their actions and decisions. The first classification of cost terms, **controllable** versus **noncontrollable,** refers to the ability of management to influence the amount of expense associated with delivering a service or a product. Those costs over which managers have major discretion are called controllable costs, whereas those over which a manager can exercise little discretion are considered noncontrollable costs by that manager. For instance, if a department head can control the number and salary of the employees needed to run the new equipment, then these labor costs are deemed to be controllable. On the other hand, if the number of persons hired and their salaries are beyond the department head's decision-making domain, then these costs are considered noncontrollable with regard to this department manager. Two additional points should be noted: (1) most costs are controllable somewhere in the organization, and (2) employees should only be held accountable for those costs over which they have control. The controllability concept is important for many planning decisions, for performance evaluation, and for cost control.

Exhibit 4-2 Data Concerning the Purchase of a New Gastroscope.

Tertiary Hospital is considering replacing, in January 19X5, the fiberoptic gastroscope it purchased in 19X1. Below are some data concerning the old (19X1) and the replacement (19X5) gastroscopes.

		19X1	19X5
(1)	Purchase price of fiberoptic gastroscope and related equipment (light source, accessories, etc.)	$5,300	$7,800
(2)	Associated set-up costs (room renovations, wiring, etc.)	$500	$400
(3)	Estimated useful life	7 years	7 years
(4)	Actual technological life	5 years	4 years
(5)	Depreciation method	Straight line	Straight line
(6)	Depreciation expense per year	$829	$1,171
(7)	Accumulated depreciation 12/31/X4	$3,029	0
(8)	Number of tests per year	30	30
(9)	Cost per year	$40	$65
(10)	Expected increase in revenues	0	0
(11)	Terms on new gastroscope: $2,000 down, net 24 months @ 17% interest		

Traceability

This concept refers to whether or not a cost can be traced to a cost object. **Direct costs** are those costs that can be traced to a **cost object**—specific units of activity, outputs such as visits, or organizational units such as departments—in an economically feasible manner; costs that cannot be specifically traced are called **indirect costs**. For instance, in Exhibit 4-2, it is likely that certain labor and supply costs can be directly traced to procedures using gastroscopes, but various other items, such as the portion of overall clinic administration associated with such procedures will probably have to be estimated. They are considered indirect costs. When combined, direct costs and indirect costs comprise **full costs**. Full costing calculations will add direct costs to some share of indirect costs (to equal the full costs of some particular cost object).

Often, whether a cost is considered direct or indirect depends on the ability of the accounting system to track the cost. The rule of thumb for managerial control is to try and make as many costs as possible direct costs. The methods for handling indirect costs, called cost allocation, is covered in Chapter 6.

Commitment

Another set of managerial control-related cost terms is committed versus non-committed costs. Returning to Exhibit 4-2, assume that the organization has a budget of $100,000 for fixed expenses during the next budget period. If all of this amount is obligated, for instance to make payments on leases, loans, and insurance, all $100,000 is considered a **committed cost**, or money that management really cannot reallocate to purchase a new gastroscope. On the other hand, if management has complete discretion over whether the money is spent, the cost is considered to be **non-committed**. Committed costs usually arise in relation to fixed assets where management is obligated to pay certain expenditures, such as mortgage payments, over a period of time. The distinction between committed and non-committed costs is often used for budgeting and planning decisions, particularly under responsibility accounting schemes.

Actual and Budgeted

The final set of costs associated with managerial control is budgeted versus actual costs. In fact, for the mid-level manager, this set of costs may be the most important. **Budgeted costs** are those costs that the organization plans to incur during a budget period. **Actual costs** are the expenses actually incurred during a budget period. Managerial uses of budgeted and actual costs are discussed in more detail in Chapter 9. These categories are useful for evaluating performance of managers.

Relevance

Another category of costs relates to providing **relevant** information for managerial decision making, known as **incremental** or **differential costs**. These are the additional costs of one alternative over another. In Exhibit 4-3, Smertha Clinic is deciding between two programs; an incremental cost analysis would focus on the fact that alternative A provides $3,000 more in net income per month over the useful life of the two projects than does alternative B. This method can be compared to a total cost analysis, which would compare the total costs of each program. The incremental cost analysis ignores the sunk costs that are equal under each alternative. It asks the crucial question: "how much better off will we be under one alternative than the others?" Wherever costs or revenues are equal or common, or sunk, relative to several alternatives, they can be ignored in the numerical analysis of each alternative.

Exhibit 4-3 shows how the incremental cost analysis of two alternatives is easier to understand and present than is a total cost analysis (in the bottom section of Exhibit 4-3). The incremental difference is the essential item of interest to most managers and most decision-makers. Exhibit 4-3 shows how the expansion of the Stop Smoking Clinic will generate $3,000

Exhibit 4-3 An Illustration of Incremental Cost Analysis vs. Total Cost Analysis.

Smertha Clinic is considering whether to expand its stop-smoking clinic or keep the clinic as is and open a new weight-loss program using presently unused space and labor. The stop-smoking program already earns $5,000 per month. The data the clinic has compiled regarding the smoking clinic are as follows:

	Current	**Expansion Proposed**
Revenue	$15,000	$25,000
Expenses	10,000	12,000
Net Income	$5,000	$13,000

The weight-loss program is expected to cost an additional $7,000 a month, but bring in an additional $12,000 in revenues a month.

Incremental Cost Analysis:

	(A) Stop Smoking	**(B) Weight Loss**	**Incremental (Decremental) Difference (A vs. B)**
Incremental Revenues	$10,000	$12,000	$(2,000)
Incremental Expenses	2,000	7,000	(5,000)
Incremental Net Income	$ 8,000	$ 5,000	$ 3,000

Explanation: If the clinic has definitely decided to offer one or the other of these two alternatives, then the *incremental difference* is more important than the total cost. It is important to focus on the $3,000 increase in net income produced by the stop-smoking clinic expansion over the weight-loss alternative. A total cost analysis gives the same answer, but includes information not needed for analysis:

Total Cost Analysis:

	(A) Stop Smoking	**(B) Weight Loss**	**Incremental (Decremental) Difference (A vs. B)**
Revenues			
Current	15,000	15,000	—
Incremental	10,000	12,000	(2,000)
Net	25,000	27,000	(2,000)
Expenses			
Current	10,000	10,000	—
Incremental	2,000	7,000	(5,000)
	12,000	17,000	(5,000)
Net Income	$13,000	$10,000	$3,000

in additional net income, as compared to the new Weight Loss Program. The bottom section of the exhibit shows how the same results are obtained under an analysis of total costs.

The term **sunk costs** refers to costs that have already been incurred or that will *not* change as part of a particular decision. From a strictly financial point of view, sunk costs should be omitted from any financial analysis. That is, financial decision-making should be concerned with additional costs to be incurred in the future. Money that has already been spent cannot be differential since the cash flow has already occurred.

There are two sayings in common parlance that describe the concept of sunk costs: "Don't cry over spilt milk," and "Don't throw good money after bad." As an example, the authors are familiar with a state that spent almost $14 million trying to improve a poorly planned, state-wide health care management information system. After five years and numerous attempts to improve the system, the state again faced the decision: should it abandon the system, attempt to upgrade the system, or design a cheaper alternative?

From a purely financial point of view, the $14 million should have been considered a sunk cost. Each alternative should have been considered on its own merits and on the basis of future costs. However, this decision, like most decisions in the health care field, also had to consider political realities. The state's decision-makers had to be willing to face the political consequences of being accused of "throwing away" $14 million of the taxpayers' money. After considerable time and politics, the state finally abandoned the old system in favor of a simpler and less costly alternative—but not without some political repercussions for the responsible officials.

A concept related to incremental cost analysis is that of opportunity cost. **Opportunity cost** refers to the benefits (or income) foregone when choosing one option over the next best alternative. In Exhibit 4-4, if Smertha Clinic were to use the same money that it was going to spend on program A and invest it in program B (the next best alternative), we can see that the clinic is foregoing $5,000 in incremental income by not investing in program B. Thus, the opportunity cost associated with choosing program A and not choosing program B is $5,000.

Cost Behavior

The final category of cost terms is related to the volume of services or products provided. In management accounting, costs are often classified into two basic components: fixed costs and variable costs. Cost prediction is often enhanced using these two cost categories. These predicted costs are often used in planning and budgeting; therefore, by improving the quality of predicted costs, managers will also improve their planning and budgeting decisions.

Total fixed costs are those costs that do not vary in total with changes in volume. They remain the same over fairly broad ranges of volume. For instance, regardless of how many patients are seen, within a relevant range, costs such as rent, insurance, or taxes will not change. Similarly, the salaries of certain personnel, such as the basic nursing staff and top-level managers, will not change with volume. Salaries are not usually computed on the basis of volume (although commissions and bonuses may be).

Of course, any of these fixed costs may change as a result of changes in rental rates, insurance premiums, or tax rates. Changes in the number of personnel, or their salaries will

Exhibit 4-4   An Example of Opportunity Cost Analysis.

Using the data in Exhibit 7-3, Smertha Clinic compiles the following information about the two programs:

	(A) Stop Smoking	(B) Weight Loss
Incremental Revenues	$10,000	$12,000
Incremental Expenses	2,000	7,000
Incremental Income	$ 8,000	$ 5,000
Less: Opportunity Cost (B)	$ 5,000	
Incremental Income (A)	$ 3,000	

Explanation: Without considering alternative B, alternative A looks as if it will bring in an extra $8,000. However, given that alternative B will be provided if alternative A is not, then A can be seen as having not an $8,000 advantage, but only a $3,000 advantage over the next best alternative. The *opportunity cost* is therefore $5,000. Incidentally, the next best alternative may not be another capital project, but investing the money in interest-bearing accounts.

also change fixed costs. However, they do not directly change in total as a result of changes in volume (Figure 4-2). Fixed costs do vary with changes in other factors, such as the number of physicians or the number of hours that the clinic is open. Fixed costs of an insurance company may change when the number of insured changes drastically. In other words, fixed costs may be "lumpy" and may not change unless the underlying **cost driver**, that factor that causes the cost to change, is significantly different. Uncertainty may affect fixed costs as unexpected breakdowns and repairs occur. Fixed costs are also subject to immediate management control (or manipulation) as travel budgets are cut or marketing programs are expanded.

On the other hand, **variable costs** are those costs that change in a linear fashion with a change in volume. Variable costs change directly and proportionately with changes in volume. For instance, if performing a certain examination costs $10, then each time another examination is given, variable costs (and total costs) go up by $10. This cost is variable since it changes directly with a change in the number of examinations given. In this instance, the cost to examine 100 patients is $1,000. This is $990 more than the cost of examining one patient ($10 x 99 additional patients = $990).

Other examples of costs that are usually variable in health care settings include the costs of materials associated with x-rays, dietary service, and medications. Variable costs under a managed care plan would usually be described on a "per member per month (pmpm)" basis. Similarly, the costs of reinsuring major medical risks under managed care might also fluctuate according to changes in the enrolled membership base.

The above definitions focused on *total* fixed and variable costs. We now turn to a discussion of *per unit* fixed and variable costs. Whereas fixed costs do not change in total with a change in volume, they do change per unit with changes in volume (Figure 4-2). For instance, assume nursing salaries equal $10,000 per month. If one patient is seen, then nursing costs $10,000 per patient. However, if 100 patients are seen, then per patient nursing costs decrease to $100. Finally, if 500 patients are seen during a month, then nursing costs decrease to $20 per patient.

Per-unit variable costs behave in just the opposite manner. If it costs $10 in supplies per patient to administer a certain medication, then over the relevant range the per-unit variable cost, $10, will not change (although the total variable cost will). The behavior of fixed and variable total and per-unit costs in relation to changes in volume is illustrated in Figure 4-2 and Exhibit 4-5.

Figure 4-2 illustrates how fixed and variable costs can be translated into per-unit costs. As fixed costs are translated into per-unit costs, a downwards sloping curve results. These declining costs are the result of economies of scale as the fixed costs are "spread over larger volumes." On the other hand, variable costs per unit can generally be shown as a horizontal line. They will only decline outside the relevant range as economies of scale take effect. But, as long as the variable costs are constant, on a per-unit basis, then the translation of total variable costs into per-unit costs must result in a horizontal graph. These various cost behavior patterns are summarized in Table 4-1 which shows how fixed and variable costs normally react to changes in volume. Table 4-1 summarizes the graphical concepts shown in Figure 4-2.

Figure 4-2   Graphic Representation of the Behavior of Fixed and Variable Costs in Relation to Volume.

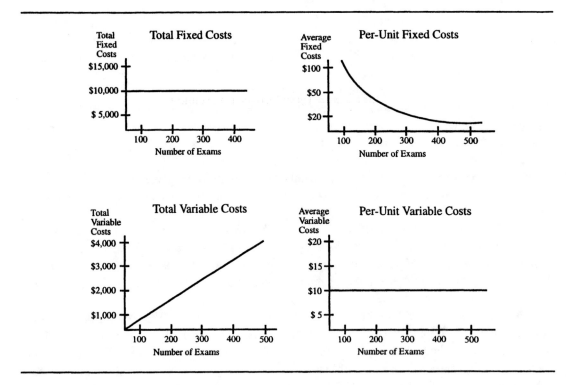

Table 4-1   Fixed and Variable Costs: Total and Per-Unit Costs in Relation to Change in Volume.

	TOTAL COSTS	PER-UNIT COSTS
Fixed	Do not change	Change
Variable	Change	Do not change

Total variable costs are depicted graphically as an upward sloping line (Figure 4-2). In more complex cases, this function may have a bend, like an "elbow" where a change in slope represents a change in the variable cost per unit. As variable costs per unit increase, the line will bend upward. As variable costs per unit decrease, the total variable cost line will bend downward. Imagine, if you will, a variable cost (per-unit) line that slopes downward to the right. What does that imply? Would you expect to find such a relationship in any health care organization? If you did, what would you do as a manager? [Answer: a downwards sloping variable cost per unit graph would indicate economies of scale. A manager who encounters such efficiencies would reward the people involved and would try to extend those economies of scale to other parts of the organization.]

The fixed vs. variable cost dichotomy is a relatively simple view of the world. It forces all costs into one category or the other. Mathematically, fixed costs plus variable costs equals total costs:

Total Costs = Fixed Costs + Variable Costs.

In reality, there are many types of costs. We use the fixed and variable cost dichotomy as a simple way of describing two typical ways that costs behave. If we understand fixed and variable costs, then other more complex variations can be dealt with using variations of the fixed-variable dichotomy.

The term **relevant range** refers to the stability of the cost relationships described above. They pertain only within certain time periods and specified volumes—those time frames and volumes pertinent to the decision being made. For instance, we can assume that rent, a fixed cost, will be constant during the budget period if there is no dramatic increase in volume. However, should volume increase beyond a realistic maximum capacity, then we may have to increase space, and thus rent or depreciation will also increase.

There are additional categories of cost behavior. **Mixed costs** are costs that contain both a variable and a fixed component. **Semi-fixed** or **semi-variable** costs vary, but not directly with changes in volume. An example of a semi-fixed cost, corresponding to the data shown in Figure 4-3, would be additional equipment rental costs that increase by $1,500 with each 100,000 increase in the number of laboratory tests.

This idea gives rise to the concept of step-fixed costs. **Step fixed costs** stay the same in total until a certain volume is reached and then increase another "step" at that point. For instance, assume that the cost of a laboratory technician is $1,500 per month. Further assume that the lab technician can handle 100,000 tests per month. For any volume greater than 100,000 tests and up to 200,000 lab tests, the total fixed cost steps up to $3,000, assuming that a second lab technician also is paid $1,500 per month. This concept is depicted in the top part of Figure 4-3.

Total Cost Equation

As indicated earlier, total costs can be viewed as the sum of fixed and variable costs. In this section, we expand these concepts, graphically and in equation form. Both the graphs and the equations will be used in the next chapter as we use these concepts to enhance managers' decision-making.

Exhibit 4-5 contains basic fixed and variable cost data for a particular service (physical exams). Notice the assumptions at the bottom of Exhibit 4-5 which are general assumptions under the fixed and variable cost formulations discussed in this chapter. Notice also the differences between total costs and per-unit costs and how these relationships fit the basic patterns graphed in Figure 4-2. Using the data in Exhibit 4-5, we can plot the number of exams (volume) on the horizontal axis, and we can plot dollars on the vertical axis. This graph is shown in Figure 4-4. We can then plot the fixed costs as a horizontal line at $10,000. We can also plot the variable costs, at $10 per exam, as a straight line, sloping upwards to the right, from the origin (0,0 point).

By next taking the variable cost line and adding it to the fixed cost line, we can get the total cost line (Figure 4-4). This total cost function simply uses the fixed costs as the "bottom layer" of the graph, with the variable costs superimposed as the "upper layer" of the graph. The new line, sloping upwards to right, which looks exactly like the total variable cost line in Figure 4-2, can now be called the total cost line. Note that variable costs are then depicted as the difference between total costs and fixed costs. Furthermore, the three points identified in Exhibit 4-5 as total costs ($10,010, $12,000, and $15,000) can be specifically identified on this new graph (Figure 4-4). As a further check of your understanding of the graph, see if you can identify the total costs associated with 400 exams [answer = $14,000].

The underlying computations necessary to complete, or extend, Exhibit 4-5 are based on our basic total cost equation. One of these is the variable cost component which suggests that total variable costs are computed by multiplying the variable cost per unit by the volume (or other cost driver). In this case the volume measure is number of exams:

Total Variable Cost = (Variable Cost per Exam) x (Number of Exams)

Figure 4-3 Illustration of Semi-fixed and Semi-variable Costs.

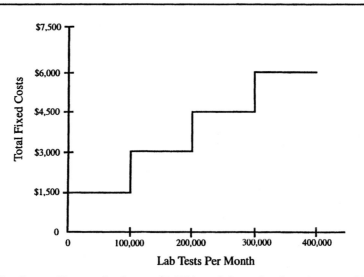

Semi-fixed (Step-fixed) costs (Assume fixed cost = $1,500/month for each volume increase of 100,000 tests)

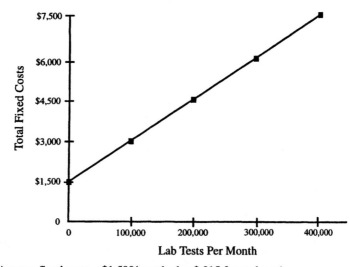

Semi-variable costs (Assume fixed costs = $1,500/month plus $.015 for each test)

Exhibit 4-5   A Comparison of the Use of Fixed and Variable Costs.

The following information is available regarding the administration of the physical exams:

Fixed Costs = $10,000
Variable Costs = $10/exam

What are the required total and per-exam costs if 200 or 500 exams are conducted?

Number of Exams	Total Fixed Cost	Fixed Cost Per Exam	Variable Cost Per Exam	Total Variable Cost	Total Cost	Total Per-unit Costs
1	$10,000	$10,000	$10	$10	$10,010	$10,010
200	$10,000	$50	$10	$2,000	$12,000	$60
500	$10,000	$20	$10	$5,000	$15,000	$30

As the number of exams increases:

A)   The total fixed costs remain the same.
B)   The per-unit fixed costs decrease.
C)   The per-unit variable cost remains the same.
D)   The total variable cost increases.
E)   The total cost increases by the amount of the increase in variable cost.
F)   The per-unit costs decreases as the number of exams increases because there are more exams over which to spread the fixed costs.

Figure 4-4   Total Costs, Including Fixed and Variable Costs, Using Data from Exhibit 4-5.

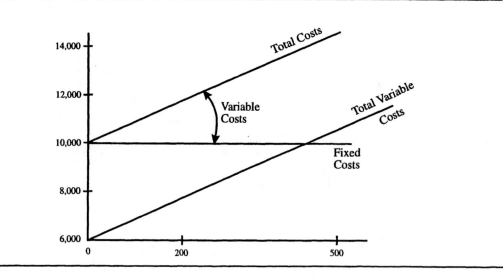

Using 400 exams as our predicted level of activity, variable costs would be predicted at $4,000:

Total Variable Cost = ($10 per exam) x (400 exams) = $4,000.

As identified in Exhibit 4-5, fixed costs are constant at $10,000. Also, as shown earlier, total cost is the sum of fixed and variable costs:

Total Cost = Fixed Cost + Variable Cost

Again, at 400 exams, total cost would be predicted at $14,000:

Total Cost = $10,000 + $4,000 = $14,000.

Simplifying the above expressions into one longer equation results in the following general expression for total cost:

Total Cost = Fixed Cost + (Variable Cost per Exam) x (Number of Exams)

Total Cost = $10,000 + ($10 per Exam) x (400 Exams)

= $10,000 + $4,000 = $14,000.

As a general form, we will always list fixed costs first, with any variable costs shown next in the total cost equation. This general expression, showing total costs, fixed costs, and variable costs (as calculated using the cost per unit and the predicted volume) is a fundamental equation that will be used through the remainder of our discussion of management accounting. The most general form of this equation, using units as the volume measure, can be shown as:

Total Cost = Fixed Cost + (Variable Cost per Unit) x (Number of Units)

Again, to check your understanding, determine the total costs that would be expected for 300 exams. Use the graph and the equation to check your result [answer = $13,000]. You should always get the same answer using either the total costs graph or the total costs equation. You may find the equation to be more precise, as it may be difficult to read exact results from a graph.

Estimating Fixed and Variable Costs Using the High-Low Method

While there are several different approaches to determining fixed and variable costs, we will only present the most basic approach in this chapter. This approach is often called the **High-Low Method**. It rests on a basic algebraic technique to determine the slope of a line, which is often called "rise over run" or "change in dollars divided by the change in activities." In algebra or economics, this technique is also known as "finding the equation for a straight line." As such, we are assuming linear relationships and we are assuming that two points will adequately represent the cost relationships in a department or health care provider.

The High-Low Method in Nine Easy Steps

This technique can be summarized as follows:

Step 1. Select two representative historical observations of costs and activities. While these observations should not be unusually high or low, one should be relatively high and the other should be relatively low. In other words, they should be some distance apart. If possible, they should be the highest cost month and the lowest cost month.

Step 2. Identify the costs and activity levels at each of these two points.

Step 3. Divide the difference in costs by the difference in activity levels, being sure to subtract both the numerator and denominator in the same order. Another check, at this stage, is to make sure that neither the numerator or denominator is negative.

Step 4. The result of Step 3 can be viewed as the slope of the line connecting the two representative observations. It can also be used as the variable cost per unit in the cost relationships and equations discussed above.

Step 5. Using one of the two representative points, substitute the total costs and the number of units, at that point, and the variable cost per unit, from Step 3, into the total cost equation:

Total Cost = Fixed Cost + (Variable Cost per Unit) x (Number of Units)

Step 6. Having made these substitutions, the only unknown in the total cost equation will be the Fixed Cost. Solve this equation for the unknown Fixed Cost.

Step 7. Prepare a new total cost equation using the calculated level of fixed costs, along with the variable cost per unit as calculated in Step 3.

Step 8. Check the accuracy of the total cost equation using the other representative point; that is, the observation that was not used in Step 5. If the same fixed costs cannot be verified using this point, or if the total costs do not agree, then you have made some mathematical error.

Step 9. Use the total cost equation to predict costs at the level of activity expected in the future. This predictive application will be expanded during our discussion of budgeting and flexible budgeting in later chapters.

Illustration of High-Low Method in Nine Easy Steps

Given the following representative observations:

Month	Costs	Activity Level
March	$50,000	2,000 visits
April	$60,000	2,300 visits
May	$67,500	2,600 visits
June	$72,000	3,100 visits
July	$80,000	3,500 visits

The following nine steps utilize the above two observations:

Step 1. March and July are selected as the months most representative of high and low costs and activities; they are not outliers and no unusual activities or events occurred in either month. They also are the highest and lowest cost months in this sample.

Step 2. The costs and activities are shown above. The costs and activity levels were both extracted from the monthly operating reports; other source documents could have been used.

Step 3. Subtract the costs, $80,000 - $50,000, to get a difference in costs of $30,000. Subtract the visits, 3,500 - 2,000, to obtain a difference in visits of 1,500. Divide the difference in costs by the difference in activities, $30,000 / 1,500 visits = $20.00.

Step 4. This result can be viewed as the slope of the line connecting the two representative points. It can also be used as the estimated variable cost ($20.00) per visit.

Step 5. Using the data from March, construct a total cost equation using all the known data:

$$\text{Total Cost} = \text{Fixed Cost} + (\text{Variable Cost per Unit}) \times (\text{Number of Units})$$
$$= \text{Fixed Cost} + (\$20.00 \text{ per Visit}) \times (2000 \text{ Visits})$$

Step 6. Solve the total cost equation for the unknown amount of Fixed Costs.

$$\$50,000 = \text{Fixed Cost} + \$40,000$$
$$\$10,000 = \text{Fixed Cost}$$

Step 7. Prepare a new total cost equation:

Total Cost = $10,000 + ($20.00 per Visit) x (Number of Visits)

Step 8. Check the total cost equation using the second representative observation (July):

$80,000 = $10,000 + ($20.00 per Visit) x (3,500 Visits)
$80,000 = $10,000 + $70,000
$80,000 = $80,000

This equality proves the mathematical accuracy of our earlier calculations.

Step 9. The total cost equation, as determined in Step 7, can now be used in other applications as a way of predicting costs in some future month.

The terms that we solved for in the total cost equation are known as estimated **coefficients** or **cost factors**. In our example above, the $10,000 is a fixed cost coefficient and the $20.00 is the variable cost per visit coefficient. These coefficients or cost factors will be used in later applications of budgeting and cost analysis. For now, concentrate on how these coefficients are calculated, and on how they are used in the total cost equation. Be sure that you fully understand the total cost equation and that you can use the High-Low Method to determine either of its two cost coefficients.

The determination of the fixed and variable components of cost is often quite difficult in the delivery of health services. Their determination is greatly enhanced through the use of regression analysis, a statistical technique. The availability of calculators and computers that can perform regression analysis has greatly facilitated this process.

Summary

An understanding of costs and cost behavior is fundamental to good financial management. This is true for any organization whether it is part of the health care sector or not. Unfortunately, the term "cost" has many different meanings in everyday usage and among managers. This chapter reviewed many of the most common cost terms using the following broad categories of costs: asset valuation, responsibility accounting, traceability, commitment, actual and budgeted numbers, relevance, and cost behavior. We discussed the key point regarding how the appropriate cost definitions should be matched with the decisions that managers are making.

We identified how fixed and variable costs are combined to form total costs, using both a graph of total costs and a total cost equation. A fundamental equation was developed using the following general expression: Total Cost = Fixed Cost + (Variable Costs per Unit) x (Number of Units). This expression will be used in subsequent chapters to improve managers' cost predictions. We showed how the High-Low Method can be used to calculate the fixed cost coefficient and the variable cost per unit coefficient in this equation.

Bibliography

Kolb, D.S. and J.L. Horowitz. "Managing the Transition to Capitation" *Healthcare Financial Management* (February): 64-69, 1995.

Krueger, D. and T. Davidson. "Alternative Approaches to Cost Accounting" *Topics in Health Care Financing* 13(4): 1-9, 1987.

Orloff, T.M., et al. "Hospital Cost Accounting: Who's Doing What and Why" *Health Care Management Review* 15(4): 73-78, 1990.

Ryan, J. B. and S.B. Clay. "Understanding the Law of Large Numbers" *Healthcare Financial Management* (October): 22-24, 1995.

Terms and Concepts

actual costs
budgeted costs
coefficient cost factor
committed costs
controllable costs
controlling
cost driver
cost object
data collection
differential costs
direct costs
evaluating
fixed costs
full costs
high low method
historical costs
implementation

incremental costs
indirect costs
managerial control
mixed costs
net book value
non-committed costs
non-controllable costs
opportunity costs
performance assessment
planning
relevant
relevant range
replacement costs
semi-fixed costs
semi-variable costs
step fixed costs
sunk costs
variable costs

Questions and Problems _____

4-1 Explain the relationship between historical cost, book value, and replacement cost of assets.

4-2 Why is asset valuation problematic?

4-3 Give an example in which each of the following expenses would be classified as controllable—and as noncontrollable.
   -fire insurance
   -supplies cost
   -overtime laboratory technician wages

4-4 The expenses listed in question 4-3 could also be direct or indirect. Give examples of situations in which they would be indirect.

4-5 Why is it a good idea to make as many costs as possible direct costs?

4-6 Would the monies in a funded depreciation account be used for committed or non-committed costs?

4-7 Why is there more than one opportunity cost that must be accounted for when deciding to build a psychiatric wing instead of a new ICU?

4-8 Draw a graph that shows the following:
   a. Fixed costs at $20,000.
   b. Variable costs at $20.00 per visit.
   c. Total costs at 1000, 2000, 3000 and 4000 visits.
   d. Calculate cost per unit at 1000, 2000, 3000, and 4000 visits.

4-9 Prepare equations for fixed, variable and total costs, using the data in the preceding problem.

4-10 Draw a graph that shows the following:
   a. Fixed costs at $45,000.
   b. Variable costs at $12.00 per visit.
   c. Total costs at 1500, 2500, 3500 and 4500 visits.
   d. Calculate cost per unit at 1500, 2500, 3500, and 4500 visits.

4-11 Prepare equations for fixed, variable and total costs, using the data in the preceding problem.

4-12 Draw a graph that shows variable costs that change under the following conditions:
    a. Variable costs at $15.00 per visit for 0-2000 visits.
    b. Variable costs at $12.00 per visit for 2001-5000 visits.

4-13 Prepare equations for variable costs, using the data in the preceding problem.

4-14 Draw a graph that shows variable costs that change under the following conditions:
    a. Variable costs at $22.00 per visit for 0-3000 visits.
    b. Variable costs at $13.00 per visit for 3001-6000 visits.

4-15 Prepare equations for variable costs, using the data in the preceding problem.

4-16 Draw a graph that shows fixed costs that change under the following conditions:
    a. Fixed costs of $300,000 for 0-3000 visits.
    b. Fixed costs of $450,000 for 3001-6000 visits.
    c. Fixed costs of $550,000 for more than 6000 visits.
    d. Calculate cost per unit at 1000, 2000, 3000, 4000, 5000, 6000 and 7000 visits.

4-17 Prepare equations for fixed costs, using the data in the preceding problem.

4-18 Draw a graph that shows fixed costs that change under the following conditions:
    a. Fixed costs of $115,000 for 0-2000 visits.
    b. Fixed costs of $210,000 for 2001-4500 visits.
    c. Fixed costs of $350,000 for more than 4500 visits.
    d. Calculate cost per unit at 1000, 2000, 3000, 4000, and 5000 visits.

4-19 Prepare equations for fixed costs, using the data in the preceding problem.

4-20 Given the following data, use the High-Low Method in Nine Easy Steps to develop a Total Costs Equation:

Month	Costs	Activity Level
March	$80,000	3,400 visits
April	$60,000	2,300 visits
May	$67,500	2,600 visits
June	$72,000	3,100 visits
July	$80,000	3,500 visits

4-21 With regard to the preceding problem:

    a. Draw a graph of the data.
    b. Show your Total Costs Equation on the same graph.

   c. Comment on how well the equation "fits" the data.
   d. How would you explain the non-representative points to other managers?
   e. Calculate the average activity level over the five months.
   f. Predict the total costs at this level of activity.
   g. Enter this prediction on your graph and comment on how well the Total Costs Equation "fits" with your prediction.
   h. Comment on how well the average activity level represents the entire data set.

4-22 Given the following data, use the High-Low Method in Nine Easy Steps to develop a Total Costs Equation:

Month	Costs	Activity Level
March	$85,000	3,600 visits
April	$62,000	2,400 visits
May	$69,500	2,750 visits
June	$73,500	3,200 visits
July	$82,000	3,400 visits

4-23 With regard to the preceding problem:

   a. Draw a graph of the data.
   b. Show your Total Costs Equation on the same graph.
   c. Comment on how well the equation "fits" the data.
   d. How would you explain the non-representative points to other managers?
   e. Calculate the average activity level over the five months.
   f. Predict the total costs at this level of activity.
   g. Enter this prediction on your graph and comment on how well the Total Costs Equation "fits" with your prediction.
   h. Comment on how well the average activity level represents the entire data set.

4-24 Given the following data, use the High-Low Method in Nine Easy Steps to develop a Total Costs Equation:

Month	Costs	Activity Level
March	$99,000	1,200 visits
April	$60,000	2,300 visits
May	$67,500	2,600 visits
June	$72,000	3,100 visits
July	$80,000	3,500 visits

Note: It is not obvious which months are the most representative.

4-25 With regard to the preceding problem:

    a. Draw a graph of the data.
    b. Show your Total Costs Equation on the same graph.
    c. Comment on how well the equation "fits" the data.
    d. How would you explain the non-representative points to other managers?
    e. Calculate the average activity level over the five months.
    f. Predict the total costs at this level of activity.
    g. Enter this prediction on your graph and comment on how well the Total Costs Equation "fits" with your prediction.
    h. Comment on how well the average activity level represents the entire data set.

4-26 Given the following data, use the High-Low Method in Nine Easy Steps to develop a Total Costs Equation:

Month	Costs	Activity Level
March	$85,000	3,600 visits
April	$22,000	3,400 visits
May	$69,500	2,750 visits
June	$73,500	3,200 visits
July	$62,000	2,400 visits

Note: It is not obvious which months are the most representative.

4-27 With regard to the preceding problem:

    a. Draw a graph of the data.
    b. Show your Total Costs Equation on the same graph.
    c. Comment on how well the equation "fits" the data.
    d. How would you explain the non-representative points to other managers?
    e. Calculate the average activity level over the five months.
    f. Predict the total costs at this level of activity.
    g. Enter this prediction on your graph and comment on how well the Total Costs Equation "fits" with your prediction.
    h. Comment on how well the average activity level represents the entire data set.

4-28 Data for the Radiology Department at Palm Springs Hospital are as follows:

Month	Number of X-rays	Department Costs
January	6,150	280,000
February	7,100	290,000
March	5,200	230,000

April	4,150	200,000
May	4,400	220,000
June	3,100	170,000
July	3,800	180,000
August	5,650	240,000
September	5,850	260,000
October	6,200	270,000
November	6,450	285,000
December	6,300	280,000

a. Draw a graph of the data.
b. Use the High-Low Method in Nine Easy Steps to develop a Total Costs Equation.
c. Show your Total Costs Equation on the same graph.
d. Comment on how well the equation "fits" the data.
e. How would you explain the non-representative points to other managers?
f. Calculate the average activity level over the twelve months.
g. Predict the total costs at this level of activity.
h. Enter this prediction on your graph and comment on how well the Total Costs Equation "fits" with your prediction.
i. Comment on how well the average activity level represents the entire data set.
j. Assume a 10% growth factor from December of the current year to January of the following year. Predict the total costs using your Total Costs Equation.
k. Enter this prediction on your graph and comment on how well the Total Costs Equation "fits" with your prediction.
l. Write a short memo to your superior explaining how this prediction might be used, and identify any reservations you may have regarding this prediction.

4-29 Data for the Pathology Department at Palm Desert Hospital are as follows:

Month	Number of Tests	Department Costs
January	4,150	285,000
February	5,100	295,000
March	3,200	235,000
April	2,150	210,000
May	2,400	225,000
June	1,900	175,000
July	2,100	195,000
August	3,950	245,000
September	3,850	265,000
October	4,200	275,000
November	4,450	295,000
December	4,300	285,000

a. Draw a graph of the data.
b. Use the High-Low Method in Nine Easy Steps to develop a Total Costs Equation.
c. Show your Total Costs Equation on the same graph.
d. Comment on how well the equation "fits" the data.
e. How would you explain the non-representative points to other managers?
f. Calculate the average activity level over the twelve months.
g. Predict the total costs at this level of activity.
h. Enter this prediction on your graph and comment on how well the Total Costs Equation "fits" with your prediction.
i. Comment on how well the average activity level represents the entire data set.
j. Assume a 10% growth factor from December of the current year to January of the following year. Predict the total costs using your Total Costs Equation.
k. Enter this prediction on your graph and comment on how well the Total Costs Equation "fits" with your prediction.
l. Write a short memo to your superior explaining how this prediction might be used, and identify any reservations you may have regarding this prediction.

4-30 Data for the Laundry Department at Palm Vista Hospital are as follows:

Month	Pounds of Laundry	Department Costs
January	206,000	280,000
February	208,100	290,000
March	205,500	230,000
April	204,300	200,000
May	204,800	220,000
June	203,500	170,000
July	203,950	180,000
August	205,650	240,000
September	205,890	260,000
October	205,600	270,000
November	206,450	285,000
December	206,750	280,000

a. Draw a graph of the data.
b. Use the High-Low Method in Nine Easy Steps to develop a Total Costs Equation.
c. Show your Total Costs Equation on the same graph.
d. Comment on how well the equation "fits" the data.
e. How would you explain the non-representative points to other managers?
f. Calculate the average activity level over the twelve months.
g. Predict the total costs at this level of activity.
h. Enter this prediction on your graph and comment on how well the Total Costs Equation "fits" with your prediction.

i.   Comment on how well the average activity level represents the entire data set.
j.   Assume a 1% growth factor from December of the current year to January of the following year. Predict the total costs using your Total Costs Equation.
k.   Enter this prediction on your graph and comment on how well the Total Costs Equation "fits" with your prediction.
l.   Write a short memo to your superior explaining how this prediction might be used, and identify any reservations you may have regarding this prediction.

4-31 Data for the Medical Records Department at Palm Date Hospital are as follows:

Month	Number of Records	Department Costs
January	24,250	285,000
February	25,100	295,000
March	23,400	235,000
April	22,350	210,000
May	22,450	225,000
June	21,980	175,000
July	22,345	195,000
August	23,950	245,000
September	23,876	265,000
October	24,345	275,000
November	24,567	295,000
December	24,300	285,000

a.   Draw a graph of the data.
b.   Use the High-Low Method in Nine Easy Steps to develop a Total Costs Equation.
c.   Show your Total Costs Equation on the same graph.
d.   Comment on how well the equation "fits" the data.
e.   How would you explain the non-representative points to other managers?
f.   Calculate the average activity level over the twelve months.
g.   Predict the total costs at this level of activity.
h.   Enter this prediction on your graph and comment on how well the Total Costs Equation "fits" with your prediction.
i.   Comment on how well the average activity level represents the entire data set.
j.   Assume a 2% growth factor from December of the current year to January of the following year. Predict the total costs using your Total Costs Equation.
k.   Enter this prediction on your graph and comment on how well the Total Costs Equation "fits" with your prediction.
l.   Write a short memo to your superior explaining how this prediction might be used, and identify any reservations you may have regarding this prediction.

4-32 Data for the Pathology Department at Palm Desert Hospital have become somewhat "scrambled" as a new computer system was installed.

Month	Number of Tests	Department Costs
January	1,150	285,000
February	5,100	595,000
March	1,200	735,000
April	4,150	110,000
May	2,400	225,000
June	1,900	175,000
July	2,100	195,000
August	3,950	245,000
September	3,850	265,000
October	4,200	275,000
November	4,450	295,000
December	4,300	285,000

a. Draw a graph of the data.
b. Use the High-Low Method in Nine Easy Steps to develop a Total Costs Equation.
c. Show your Total Costs Equation on the same graph.
d. Comment on how well the equation "fits" the data.
e. How would you explain the non-representative points to other managers?
f. Calculate the average activity level over the most representative months.
g. Predict the total costs at this level of activity.
h. Enter this prediction on your graph and comment on how well the Total Costs Equation "fits" with your prediction.
i. Comment on how well the average activity level represents the entire data set.
j. Assume a 10% growth factor from December of the current year to January of the following year. Predict the total costs using your Total Costs Equation.
k. Enter this prediction on your graph and comment on how well the Total Costs Equation "fits" with your prediction.
l. Write a short memo to your superior explaining how this prediction might be used, and identify any reservations you may have regarding this prediction.

4-33 Data for the Laundry Department at Palm Vista Hospital have been lost due to a fire:

Month	Pounds of Laundry	Department Costs
January	205,600	290,000
February	206,200	298,000
March	204,400	232,000
April	203,400	204,000
May	206,600	224,000

June	206,500	175,000
July	209,950	186,000
August	208,650	247,000
September	206,890	265,000
October	207,600	279,000
November	—	—
December	—	—

a. Draw a graph of the data.
b. Use the High-Low Method in Nine Easy Steps to develop a Total Costs Equation.
c. Write a short memo to your superior explaining how this prediction might be used, and identify any reservations you may have regarding this prediction.

4-34 Data for the Medical Records Department at Palm Date Hospital has become unreliable as new personnel were trained:

Month	Number of Records	Department Costs
January	24,250	285,000
February	25,100	295,000
March	23,400	235,000
April	22,350	210,000
May	22,450	225,000
June	21,980	175,000
July	22,345	195,000
August	23,950	245,000
September	33,987	265,000
October	14,345	275,000
November	34,678	295,000
December	14,300	285,000

a. Draw a graph of the data.
b. Use the High-Low Method in Nine Easy Steps to develop a Total Costs Equation.
c. Write a short memo to your superior explaining how this prediction might be used, and identify any reservations you may have regarding this prediction.

5 Short-Term Decision-Making

This chapter provides information that is useful for making short-term decisions. These decisions usually last a year or less and involve no new long-lived assets. Long-term decisions, in which the analyst must consider the time value of money, are discussed in Chapter 13.

Cost-volume-profit analysis (CVP analysis), often called **break even analysis,** is discussed in the first part of the chapter. It is often used when making routine planning decisions that are related to output volume and pricing. The most relevant types of costs for these decisions are fixed and variable costs.

The second part of the chapter discusses short-term non-routine decisions. These decisions involve choosing between alternative sets of actions or accepting a minimum price for an output. They are made on the basis of incremental or differential costs (or revenues).

Cost-Volume-Profit Analysis

There are three main purposes for cost-volume-profit analysis: (1) to determine the volume of output necessary to achieve a financial goal such as break even (zero profit); (2) to determine a price to cover fixed and variable, thus, full costs of outputs; and (3) to evaluate different environmental scenarios and managerial actions. We begin with a discussion of break even analysis and proceed to discussions of achieving profit goals for both tax-exempt and taxable firms. For these analyses, we start with the case in which the organization or organizational subunit produces a single output and payment is for each individual unit of output (fee-for-service). Other analyses show additional uses of CVP analyses. Later we expand to the more realistic situation in which the organization produces multiple outputs or where there may be multiple payers for its outputs. Finally, we demonstrate how CVP analysis differs for providers of health care services not paid on a fee-for-service basis.

The Break Even Equation

Break even analysis incorporates the following basic cost equation presented in the previous chapter:

$$\text{Total Costs} = \text{Total Fixed Costs} + \text{Total Variable Costs, or}$$

$$TC = TFC + TVC.$$

As noted in Chapter 4, although fixed costs do not vary directly and proportionately with respect to the volume of output, variable costs do. Total variable costs are equal to the **variable cost per unit (VCU)** multiplied by the number of units of products or services provided, or

$$TVC = (VCU) \times Q$$

where Q stands for quantity of services or products. Therefore, the total cost equation can be expanded as

$$TC = TFC + (VCU \times Q).$$

Exhibit 5-1 illustrates how the basic cost equation can be used to project total costs for three different levels of service (2500, 3000 and 3500 examinations). Since it is difficult to predict actual volumes of output precisely, using this cost equation may increase the likelihood that actual costs are more likely to correspond to the estimated costs.

The total cost equation is combined with a revenue equation for cost-volume-profit analysis. Just as variable costs are comprised of the cost per unit times the number of units, when clients pay for each output, total revenue equals the price per unit times the number of units of output provided. In equation form:

$$\text{Total Revenue} = \text{Revenue Per Unit} \times \text{Quantity, or}$$

$$TR = RU \times Q.$$

In economics, this is simply known as "price times quantity." This relationship holds whether we are considering full charges, discounted rates, or flat fees (per patient) or whether the output is a service or a product. For a fee-for-service provider, revenues are the clinic prices per visit, or hospital prices per day or per stay multiplied by the number of clinic visits or hospital days or hospital patients. For a health service payer or managed care plan, revenues are the monthly premiums multiplied by the number of enrolled members. As with the total cost equation, the revenue equation can be used to prepare revenue budgets for alternative volumes of output.

Break even means that the revenue generated from providing health care services or products just equals the costs of those services or products. This can be expressed most clearly by an equation that sets revenues equal to costs:

$$\text{Total Revenue} = \text{Total Costs, or}$$

$$TR = TC.$$

Substituting the simple "price times quantity" revenue relationship into this equation gives us

$$RU \times Q = TC.$$

Exhibit 5-1   Use of the Cost-Volume-Profit Formula to Calculate Total Projected Costs.

A. A community health care organization (CHO) projects the following costs and volume for an annual well-baby check-up program for next year:

> Total Fixed Costs = $25,000
> Variable Costs = $5 per examination
> Number of Examinations = 3,000

Determine the total projected cost of these exams.

Solution: TC = TFC + (VCU x Q)
            TC = $25,000 + ($5 x 3,000)
            TC = $25,000 + $15,000
            TC = $40,000

B. The CHO is not quite sure how many patients there will be. Therefore, it wants to make both a conservative and liberal estimate of total costs using the information in part A.

Calculate total projected cost based on volume estimates of (a) 2,500 and (b) 3,500 examinations.

Solution: (a) TC = FC + (VCU x Q)   (b) TC = FC + (VCU x Q)
                TC = $25,000 + ($5 x 2,500)   TC = $25,000 + ($5 x 3,500)
                TC = $25,000 + $12,500   TC = $25,000 + $17,500
                TC = $37,500   TC = $42,500

C. Summary: The total cost will always equal the sum of the fixed and variable costs. In this example, total costs increase by $5 per patient examined because of the cost of supplies used in each visit.

This formula treats total costs as a single, lump-sum amount that might be relevant in some contractual settings. It can be applied as a simplified break even model in a health care setting as shown in Exhibit 5-2. This exhibit illustrates how one of the elements in this equation can be treated as an "unknown" and the equation can then be "solved" for the missing element. In the first part of Exhibit 5-2, we solve for the revenue or price per unit (RU) that would have to be charged within the specified cost and volume limits. In the second part, we determine the quantity of patients necessary to break even, given the specified cost and a specified limit on the $8.00 price. In each case, by setting revenues equal to costs, we are achieving break even when we solve for a missing term in the equation. As in any linear algebraic problem, we can only solve for one unknown. Therefore, we must manipulate these relationships in such a way that only one element is not known.

We can also expand the cost side of the equation to include fixed and variable costs. This results in the following **break even equation** or **break even formula**:

Exhibit 5-2   Determining Prices and Quantities Necessary to Break Even when Costs are Pre-Set.

A.   A health department (HD) projects the following (costs and volume) for the administration of screening tests next year:

> Total Cost = $25,540 (all fixed)
> Number of Screening Tests = 3,000

Determine the rate that would have to be charged per test to break even.

Solution: RU x Q = TC
RU x 3,000 = $25,540 (all fixed)
RU = $25,540/3,000
RU = $8.51

B.   Another health department normally charges $8.00 per client and cannot change its rates.

Determine the number of clients which must be screened to break even if the total cost remains at $25,540.

Solution: RU x Q = TC
$8.00 x Q = $25,540
Q = 25,540/$8.00
Q = 3,193

C.   Summary: At the break even point, total revenues equal total costs. The total revenue is comprised of two components: revenue per unit (RU) and the number of units. This information may be used to calculate prices, number of service, or total cost if two of the three items in the equation, RU x Q = TC, are known.

$$TR = TC$$

$$RU \times Q = TFC + (VCU \times Q).$$

Figure 5-1 illustrates the relationship between revenues and costs. This graph contains the same cost lines as shown in the previous chapter. Note how fixed costs are described by the horizontal line at the bottom of the graph. Then, variable costs are added to the fixed costs. The sum of fixed costs plus variable costs equals total costs.

The total revenue line in Figure 5-1 is the diagonal line from the origin. This is simply the "price times quantity" equation drawn on a graph. It must start from the origin because a zero quantity of services will result in zero revenues. It must increase positively and proportionately because each unit of service is assumed to be charged the same price. If that assumption is incorrect, then we would have a non-linear relationship, or perhaps a "kinked" relationship if prices are "discounted" after a certain quantity level is reached. These non-linearities are beyond the scope of this text.

The point of intersection of the Total Revenue line with the Total Cost line, where total revenues equal total costs, is the break even point.

Be sure you fully understand each line on this graph and how a change in one factor will change the graph. For example, how will an increase in fixed costs be shown? How will it affect break even? [Answer: The fixed costs line will move up, and the break even point will increase.] Furthermore, how will an increase in revenue per unit (price) change the total revenue line? How will it affect break even? [Answer: The total revenue line will have a steeper slope and the break even point will decrease.]

Figure 5-1   Cost-Volume-Profit Graph Using the Numbers Calculated in Exhibit 5-1.

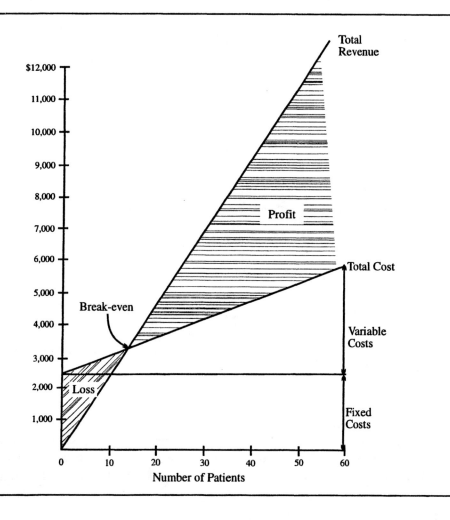

Exhibit 5-3   Determining the Number of Clients and Rates for an Alcoholism Treatment Center.

A. An alcoholism treatment center (ATC) projects the following costs and rates:

Total Fixed Costs = $25,000
Variable Costs = $.15
Rate Per Unit of Service = $10

Determine how many clients must be seen to break even.

Solution: RU x Q = TFC + (VCU x Q)
                         $10Q = $25,000 + $.15Q
                         Q = $25,000/$9.85
                         Q = $2,538

B. If another ATC projects the following information:

Total Fixed Costs = $25,000
Variable Costs Per Unit = $.15
Clients = 3,000

Determine the price or rate the ATC must charge each client to break even.

Solution: RU x Q = FC + (VCU x Q)
                     RU x 3,000 = $25,000 + .15(3,000)
                             RU = (25,000 + $450)/3,000
                             RU = $8.48

C. Summary: The break even formula can be used to calculate rates, number of units of service, and fixed and variable costs using the equation RU x Q = FC + (VCU x Q) if no more than one of the variables in the equation is unknown.

Exhibit 5-3 illustrates how the revenue and cost equation can be combined to calculate break even in a health care organization. It shows how the break even equation can be used to determine the quantity of clients necessary to break even under certain price and cost constraints. It later shows how the revenue per unit (RU) can be determined under different cost and volume projections.

Contribution Margin

The break even point can also be found by using the contribution margin. The **contribution margin** is the difference between revenues and variable costs. It is the amount that outputs contribute to covering fixed costs. Under fee-for-service (FFS) payment plans, contribution margin can be calculated on a per-unit basis as the difference between the unit sales

Exhibit 5-4   Calculations Using Contribution Margins.

To Determine Break Even Point (in units)

Item	Amount	Ratios
Revenues	$221.88/unit =	100.00%
Variable Cost	$ 50.00/unit =	22.53%
Contribution Margin	$171.88/unit =	77.47%

Total Fixed Costs to be covered = $2,500

Thus, BEQ = $2,500/$171.88 = approx. 15 units to break even

To Determine the Break Even Point (in dollars)

Contribution ratio: 77.47% or .7747 (see above)

Total Fixed Costs to be covered: $2,500

Thus, BE$ = $2,500/.7747 = $3,227 to break even in dollars (or 15 units x $221.88)

---

price (revenue per unit) and the unit variable cost (VCU),

$$CMU = RU - VCU.$$

The **contribution margin per unit (CMU),** is generally constant for all volumes within the relevant range.

Using the data from Exhibit 5-4, Figure 5-1 indicates that total revenues increase more rapidly than do total costs. This phenomenon happens because each unit of service yields $221.88 of revenue (RU), but only costs $50 per unit (VCU). The contribution margin per unit (CMU) in this example is $171.88 (RU – VCU = $221.88 – $50.00).

If one knows the total fixed costs, the number of unit sales needed to break even can be calculated by dividing the fixed costs by the contribution margin per unit.

$$BEQ = \frac{\text{Total Fixed Costs}}{\text{Contribution Margin per Unit}}$$

$$BEQ = \frac{TFC}{CMU}$$

Using the data in the example in Exhibit 5-4, the break even quantity can be calculated as:

$$BEQ = \frac{\$2,500}{\$171.88} = 14.54$$

BEQ = 15 patients (rounded upwards).

Contribution Margin Ratio

It is also possible to calculate the break even point in terms of revenue dollars. First, it is necessary to determine the proportion of each revenue dollar that is available to meet fixed costs after covering variable costs. This proportion is called the **contribution margin ratio**. It is equal to the contribution margin per unit divided by revenue per unit:

$$\text{Contribution Margin Ratio (CMR)} = \frac{\text{Contribution Margin per Unit}}{\text{Revenue per Unit}} = \frac{\text{CMU}}{\text{RU}}$$

Without showing the exact derivation, the contribution margin ratio can also be obtained from an entirely different, but related calculation. This alternative calculation does not require per unit data. Instead, it divides the contribution margin (in dollars) by the total revenue (in dollars):

$$\text{Contribution Margin Ratio} = \frac{\text{Contribution Margin (dollars)}}{\text{Total Revenue (dollars)}} = \frac{\text{CM}}{\text{TR}}$$

Be careful not to confuse the two alternative calculations of the contribution margin ratio. Even though the contribution margin ratio (CMR) can be calculated under either alternative, with the same answer, the terms in each equation cannot be interchanged.

In order to calculate break even in dollar terms, total fixed costs are divided by the contribution margin ratio:

$$\text{Break Even Level (in dollars)} = \frac{\text{Total Fixed Costs}}{\text{Contribution Margin Ratio}} \quad \text{or}$$

$$BE\$ = \frac{\text{TFC}}{\text{CMR}}$$

An example of using the contribution margin ratio to determine BE\$ is shown in Exhibit 5-4. Note that once you have calculated the break even quantity, you can simply multiply your answer by the price (RU) to obtain the point of equality shown in dollars. Incidentally, some organizations expand the format shown in the top half of Exhibit 5-4 as a way of recasting their income statements for internal reporting. In other words, the contribution margin ratio and its related terms are so useful and so insightful that monthly operating reports can be designed to emphasize these relationships.

Exhibit 5-4 also shows that revenue ratios can be calculated by dividing revenue, variable cost and contribution margin by revenue. The resulting ratio for revenues (revenues/ revenues) must be 100%. The whole is always equal to the sum of its parts. At least in accounting, this dictum usually holds. If so, there is an interesting complementary relationship involving the contribution margin ratio. A **variable cost ratio** can also be constructed by dividing by revenues:

$$\text{Variable Cost Ratio} = \frac{\text{Total Variable Costs}}{\text{Total Revenues}} = \frac{TVC}{TR} = VCR$$

Alternatively, using per unit data:

$$\text{Variable Cost Ratio} = \frac{\text{Variable Cost per Unit}}{\text{Revenue per Unit}} = \frac{VCU}{RU} = VCR$$

Again, the careful analyst must not interchange the terms in each of these equations, even though the resulting ratios should be the same. Now we show how the whole is equal to the sum of its parts, using a slight variation of the income statement equation:

Revenue – Total Variable Costs = Contribution to Fixed Costs

TR – TVC = Contribution Margin (in dollars)

Now, divide this equation by total revenue (in dollars) to obtain the related percentages:

$$\frac{TR}{TR} - \frac{TVC}{TR} = \frac{\text{Contribution Margin}}{\text{Total Revenue}} = CMR$$

$$100\% - VCR = CMR.$$

Alternatively, VCR + CMR = 100%. Once you know either the VCR or the CMR, you automatically know the other. This is known as a complementary relationship. If someone asserts that variable costs are 60% of revenues, then you will immediately recognize that the contribution margin ratio is 40%.

Cost-Volume-Profit Analysis and Profits

The break even equation is applicable where zero profits are acceptable. However, in many cases, a health care organization, whether for-profit or not-for-profit, must plan to earn a profit on a particular service, group of services or products. If this is the case, then the revenues generated must not only cover costs, but must be sufficient to provide some margin, or profit, as well. The break even equation can be expanded to include various other financial objectives. In this section, we illustrate how profits can be included in the equation by including profits as a new fixed cost. The cost-volume-profit equation becomes:

Total Revenue = Fixed Costs + Variable Costs + Profit   or

$$RU \times Q = TFC + (VCU \times Q) + P.$$

Note that the cost-volume-profit equation can be easily restated into a form that is similar to the categories found on many income statements:

Total Revenue – Variable Costs – Fixed Costs = Profit.

Figure 5-2 illustrates the revenue and cost relationships including a profit goal. This graph contains the same cost lines as shown in Figure 5-1. Note how total fixed costs continue to be described by the horizontal line at the bottom of the graph. Desired profits are now shown as a separate horizontal "layer" on top of the fixed costs. As before, variable costs are drawn in as a diagonal line above profits and fixed costs. The sum of fixed costs plus desired profits plus variable costs represents the manager's total financial objectives.

The revenue line is also shown in Figure 5-2, which is the same revenue line shown in Figure 5-1 as the diagonal line from the origin. The point of intersection of the Total Revenue line with the Total Cost plus Profit line is the point where the profit goal is achieved. To the left of that point, the profit goal has not been met. To the right, the profit goal has been exceeded. The point at which total revenues exactly equal total costs plus profit is analogous to the break even point discussed above. Operating at this point will permit the organization to achieve its desired goal. The cost-volume-profit equation is, thus, to be more useful than the more limited break even equation.

Be sure you fully understand each line on this graph and how a change in profits will change the graph. For example, how will an increase in desired profits be shown? How will it affect the point of equality? [Answer: The desired profit line will move up, and the point where the profit goal is achieved will shift to the right (increase).] Furthermore, how will a decrease in desired profits change these relationships? How will it affect the point of equality (the break even point)? [Answer: The desired profit line will shift downwards and the point of equality (break even) will shift to the left (decrease).]

Exhibit 5-5 illustrates how the cost-volume-profit equation can be applied in a health care setting to determine the price per output or the quantity of output to produce given a price.

Profit and Taxes

The above discussion of desired profits ignores income taxes. To incorporate income taxes for the taxable firm, the cost-volume-profit equation can be further modified, as follows:

Total Revenue = Total Costs + Taxes + Profit After Taxes

Taxes usually vary as a percentage of "profits before taxes." They are not usually constant, nor do they vary directly and proportionately with respect to the quantity of services provided. Even though taxes do vary with both revenues and costs, we shall generally treat

Figure 5-2   Cost-Volume-Profit Graph Using the Numbers Calculated in Exhibit 5-5, Example B.

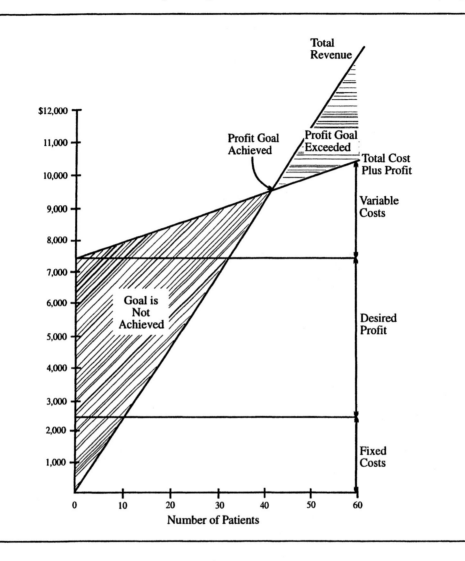

them as a constant amount. Again, this latest equation has some similarity with an income statement and can be further modified into close conformity with an income statement:

Total Revenue – Variable Costs – Fixed Costs – Taxes = Profit After Taxes

This relationship can be further simplified, even though we don't show the precise derivation, to show that the tax rate (in percentage terms) can be used along with the desired amount of profit after taxes, instead of including any specific tax amount:

Exhibit 5-5   Considering Profit in Cost-Volume-Profit Analysis.

A. A community mental health center (CMHC) desired to make a profit of $3,000 on a weight-loss clinic. Other information:

> Total Fixed Costs = $2,500
> Variable Costs = 50
> Number of Patients = 32

Determine the charge per patient necessary to achieve the desired $3,000 profit.

Solution: RU x Q = TFC + (VCU x Q) + P
RU x 32 = $2,500 + ($50 x 32) + $3,000
RU x 32 = $2,500 + $1,600 + $3,000
RU = $7,100/32
RU = $221.88

B. The CMHC desired to make a profit of $5,000 on a weight-loss clinic. Other information:

> Total Fixed Costs = $2,500
> Variable Costs Per Unit = $50
> Charge Per Patient = $250

Determine the number of patients that will have to enroll for the CMHC to break even.

Solution: RU x Q = TFC + (VCU x Q) + P
250 x Q = $2,500 + ($50 x Q) + $5,000
200 x Q = $7,500
Q = 37.5

C. Summary: The break even formula can be used to calculate rates, units of service, fixed or variable costs, and profit using the equation: RU x Q = FC + (VCU x Q) + P, if no more than one of the variables in the equation is unknown.

$$\text{Total Revenue} = \text{Fixed Costs} + \text{Variable Costs} + \frac{\text{Profit After Taxes}}{1 - \text{Tax Rate}}$$

This relationship can also be expressed in an income statement format, where the last term in the right-hand side of this equation can be viewed as "profit before taxes." In other words, dividing any after-tax amount by the complement of the tax rate (1– tax rate) will convert that number into a before-tax amount. The following income statement formula reflects taxes using this conversion:

$$\text{Total Revenue} - \text{Fixed Costs} - \text{Variable Costs} = \frac{\text{Profit After Taxes}}{1 - \text{Tax Rate}}$$

Using the data in part B of Exhibit 5-5, the quantity of output that must be produced to achieve a $5,000 after tax profit goal when the firm's marginal tax rate is 34 percent can be determined as follows:

$$\$250 \times Q = \$2,500 + (\$50 \times Q) + \frac{\$5,000}{1 - .34}$$

$$Q = 50.38.$$

Not surprisingly, as we have added more fixed costs in the form of profits and taxes, the quantity of output required to meet the financial goals has increased. Without taxes, the organization required only 37.5 patients to achieve its profit goal but required at least 50 patients to achieve the same goal with taxes on its profits.

Cost-Volume-Profit Under Cost-Based Reimbursement

As an example of how to adjust these equations, we show a modified version that reflects the impact of cost-based reimbursement. Similar adjustments can be used to show the effects of other payment plans. While cost-based payment schemes are only used by a few payers, this new formulation shows that only charge-based patients will yield any positive impact on profit. In effect, the percentage of cost-based patients could be considered equivalent to a tax on the not-for-profit organization.[1]

$$\text{Recoverable Charge} = \frac{\text{Total Fixed Costs}}{\text{VCU} \times Q} + \frac{\text{Profit}}{(Q \times \text{Proportion of Charge - Based Patients})}$$

While the derivation of this new relationship is beyond the scope of this text, the modified formula does show how the cost-volume-profit equation can be adjusted to reflect various payment conditions. The astute manager will be creative in developing pertinent relationships that reflect the payment terms appropriate to various managerial decisions.

Multiple Product or Payer Cost-Volume-Profit Analysis

The cost-volume-profit analyses in this chapter so far are relevant where the organization produces a single output or whenever prices are constant. We have assumed that the revenue per unit (RU) is the same for all payers and that there is only one product or service being provided. Most health care organizations actually produce a variety of services or products. In addition, in the health care sector, health care organizations may receive a different rate for the same output from different payers or clients. For example, for the same visit for which a physician charges $150, Medicare may pay a set fee of $100, a health maintenance organization may pay a discounted charge of $125, and Medicaid may pay $60.

Given this multi-payer, multi-product scenario, the cost-volume-profit equation can be modified to reflect a weighted average across all payers or products. Where the price for the same output differs, or where there are multiple products, the cost-volume-profit equation is:

$$(P_1 RU_1 + P_2 RU_2 + P_3 RU_3)Q = TFC + (VCU \times Q) + Profit$$

where

P_1 = proportion of payer or product type 1
P_2 = proportion of payer or product type 2
P_3 = proportion of payer or product type 3
RU_1 = Revenue per unit from payer or product 1
RU_2 = Revenue per unit from payer or product 2
RU_3 = Revenue per unit from payer or product 3.

The same type of weighted average may be needed if unit variable costs differ by payer or product.

Alternatively, a weighted average contribution margin may be used instead of the revenue approach described above. An example of this approach is shown in Exhibit 5-6. It provides an example of determining the number of outputs needed to achieve a financial goal where four products are produced and prices and unit variable costs differ for each product. More complex situations where there are both multiple payers and multiple products can also be analyzed. A multi-payer, multi-price and multi-service environment only makes the math more complicated. The basic intuition and concepts are the same as in the simple models presented in this chapter.

Cost-Volume-Profit Analysis Under Capitation Payment

A provider paid a capitation rate is paid a flat amount per member per month (PMPM) to provide services for the member. Thus, capitated revenues are based on the number of enrollees who choose a provider not on the number of patients treated and services provided. The simplest possible assumption is that all revenues are derived from a single contract with a fixed number of enrollees. If so, revenues are fixed with respect to the number of services provided and they can be represented by a horizontal line (Figure 5-3). Note in such cases, that the concepts of profit and loss are completely reversed (as compared to Figure 5-1). Now, under capitated revenues, the profit area is to the left of the break even point and the loss area is to the right. Many provider organizations under capitated revenues would thus have an incentive to provide fewer patient services in order to remain at or below break even.

When multiple sources of revenues exist, then the graphical relationships will become more complex. For example, if some small amount of FFS revenues are also available to the provider (Figure 5-3), how will the total revenue be adjusted? [Answer: total revenues will be

Exhibit 5-6   Application of Weighted Average Contribution Margin to Multiple Product Case.

National Urgent Care Centers, Inc. is planning for the next fiscal year. Its staff projects the following visit types, prices and product mix for Urgent Care Center #2450.

Visit	Percent of Total Visits	Avg. Payment per Visit	Variable Cost per Visit	Direct Fixed Costs
Short	60%	$40	$30	$100,000
Intermediate	25	60	40	60,000
Long	10	80	55	125,000
Seriously Long	5	125	80	90,000
	100%			$375,000

In addition, the staff projects $246,000 fixed costs that are indirect with respect to the visits. Assume that the marginal tax rate is 34 percent and that Urgent Care Center #2450 must realize $75,000 in after tax profits.

A. The number of visits that must be produced for Center #2450 to achieve its goal is determined as follows:

Weighted CMU:				
Short	.60(40-30)	= 6	Direct Fixed Costs =	$375,000
Intermediate	.25(60-40)	= 5	Indirect Fixed Costs =	246,000
Long	.10(80-55)	= 2.5	Total Fixed Costs =	$621,000
Seriously Long	.05(125-80)	= 2.25		
Total CMU		15.75		

Before Tax Profit = $75,000/(1− .34) = $113,636 $$Q = \frac{621,000 + \$113,636}{\$15.75 \text{ per visit}} = 46,644 \text{ visits}$$

B. The number of each type of visit that must be produced.

Short	46,644 x .60 =	27,987
Intermediate	46,644 x .25 =	11,661
Long	46,644 x .10 =	4,664
Seriously Long	46,644 x .05 =	2,332
		46,644

C. Now consider what management might also consider to reduce the number of break even visits. For Example: Reduce total fixed costs, increase CMU or decrease VCU or change mix.

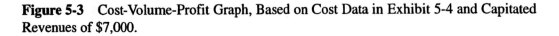

Figure 5-3   Cost-Volume-Profit Graph, Based on Cost Data in Exhibit 5-4 and Capitated Revenues of $7,000.

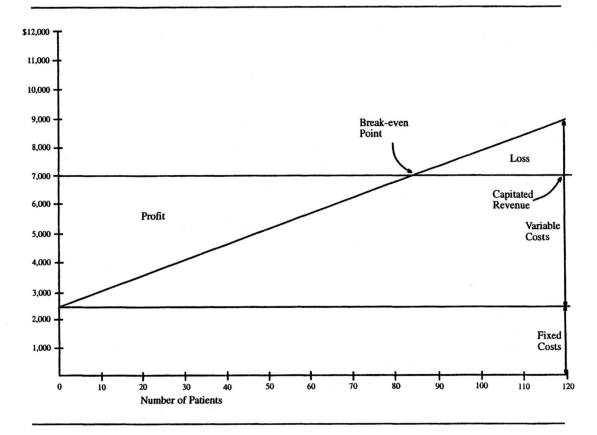

a sloping line, upwards to the left, perhaps intersecting the total cost line at a higher break even point.] What will happen to the total revenue line if the provider also receives significant FFS revenues? [Answer: total revenues will be a steeply sloping line, upwards to the right, perhaps never intersecting the total cost line, at least within our relevant range.]

Application of Cost-Volume-Profit Concepts

Exhibit 5-7 illustrates many of the equations developed earlier as well as demonstrating some of the basic arithmetic "checks" or "proofs" that can be used to verify the accuracy of your calculations. The example provides information that the manager of the radiology department might find useful in preparing her budget or in evaluating alternative price or volume levels. This comprehensive example integrates many of the concepts and equations discussed in this chapter. While somewhat redundant, it does provide a summary that many students will find helpful.

Exhibit 5-7 Application of Cost-Volume-Profit Concepts to Radiology Department.

Monthly budgeted fixed costs (FC)	$110,000
Variable costs per X-ray (VCU)	$85
Budgeted revenues per X-ray (RU)	$165
Expected monthly X-ray volume (Q)	4,000

1. Develop the Total Cost equation at the expected monthly volume:

   Total Cost = Fixed Costs + Variable Costs
   Total Cost = TFC + (VCU x Q)
   Total Cost = $110,000 + ($85 x 4,000)
   Total Cost = $110,000 + $340,000 = $450,000

2. Develop the break even equation:

   Total Revenue = Total Cost
   Total Revenue = Total Fixed Costs + Variable Costs
       RU x Q = FC + VCU x Q
       165 x Q = 110,000 + 85 x Q

3. Determine the break even number of X-rays by solving the break even equation:

   165 x Q = 110,000 + 85 x Q
     80 Q = 110,000
       Q = 1,375 X-rays

4. Using per unit data, calculate the contribution margin ratio and the variable cost ratio. Show that they are complementary.

$$\text{Contribution Margin Ratio} = \frac{\text{Contribution Margin per Unit}}{\text{Revenue per Unit}}$$

$$\text{CMR} = \frac{\text{CMU}}{\text{RU}} = \frac{80}{165} = 48.5\%$$

$$\text{Variable Cost Ratio} = \frac{\text{Variable Cost per Unit}}{\text{Revenue per Unit}}$$

$$\text{VCR} = \frac{\text{VCU}}{\text{RU}} = \frac{85}{165} = 51.5\%$$

Contribution Margin Ratio + Variable Cost Ratio = 100%

$$48.5\% + 51.5\% = 100\%$$

Exhibit 5-7   continued

5. Using dollars of revenues, at the expected monthly X-ray volume, calculate the contribution margin ratio and variable cost ratio. Show that they are complementary. Use the cost-volume-profit equation to develop the revenue and cost estimates:

$$\text{Total Revenue} = \text{Total Cost} + \text{Profit}$$

$$\text{Revenue per Unit x Quantity} = \text{Total Fixed Cost} + (\text{Variable Cost per Unit x Quantity}) + \text{Profit}$$

$$RU \times Q = TFC + (VCU \times Q) + \text{Profit}$$

$$165 \times 4{,}000 = 110{,}000 + 85 \times 4{,}000 + \text{Profit}$$

$$\$660{,}000 = 110{,}000 + 340{,}000 + \text{Profit}$$

Therefore, contribution margin, at the expected monthly X-ray volume, is:
Contribution Margin = Total Revenue – Variable Costs
Contribution Margin = $660,000 – $340,000 = $320,000

$$\text{Contribution Margin Ratio} = \frac{\text{Contribution Margin}}{\text{Total Revenue}} = \frac{\$320{,}000}{\$660{,}000} = 48.5\%$$

$$\text{Variable Cost Ratio} = \frac{\text{Variable Costs}}{\text{Total Revenue}} = \frac{\$340{,}000}{\$660{,}000} = 51.5\%$$

$$\text{Contribution Margin Ratio} + \text{Variable Cost Ratio} = 100\%$$
$$48.5\% + 51.5\% = 100\%$$

6. Determine the target profit at the expected monthly X-ray volume. Use the cost-volume-profit equation to develop the revenue and cost estimates:

$$\text{Total Revenue} = \text{Total Cost} + \text{Profit}$$

$$\text{Revenue per Unit x Quantity} = \text{Total Fixed Cost} + (\text{Variable Cost per Unit x Quantity}) + \text{Profit}$$

$$RU \times Q = TFC + (VCU \times Q) + \text{Profit}$$

$$165 \times 4{,}000 = 110{,}000 + 85 \times 4{,}000 + \text{Profit}$$

$$\$660{,}000 = 110{,}000 + 340{,}000 + \text{Profit}$$

$$\$210{,}000 = \text{Profit}$$

Exhibit 5-7   continued

7. Using the information in the preceding step, prepare a simple income statement, using contribution margins.

Total Revenue	$660,000
Less, Variable Costs	340,000
Contribution Margin	$320,000
Less, Fixed Costs	110,000
Profit (before taxes)	$210,000

8. Calculate the break even point (in X-ray units), using a different method than in Step #3 above. Do the two answers agree?

$$\text{Break - even level of Activity} = \frac{\text{Total Fixed Costs} + \text{Desired Profit}}{\text{Contribution Margin per Unit}}$$

$$\text{BEQ} = \frac{\text{Total Fixed Costs} + \text{Desired Profit}}{\text{Contribution Margin per Unit}}$$

$$\text{BEQ} = \frac{\text{TFC} + \text{P}}{\text{CMU}}$$

$$\text{BEQ} = \frac{\$110,000 + 0}{80} = 1,375 \text{ X - rays}$$

The two answers (in #3 vs. #8) must agree because the short-hand version of the break even equation is derived from the basic equation that was used earlier.

9. Calculate the point of equality, in dollars, including a desired profit objective. Verify your answer by multiplying the BEQ by the price per unit (RU).

$$\text{Point of equality (in dollars)} = \frac{\text{Total Fixed Costs} + \text{Desired Profit}}{\text{Contribution Margin Ratio}}$$

$$\text{Point of equality} = \frac{\text{TFC} + \text{P}}{\text{CMR}} = \frac{\$110,000 + 0}{48.5\%} = \$226,804$$

Alternatively, this point of equality (in dollars) = BEQ x RU = 1,375 x $165 = $226,875

Note that these two answers are not exactly the same. However, the slight differences are due to rounding. The careful reader will observe that the contribution margin ratio (CMR) requires rounding, which results in the slight differences between these two results. The astute analyst would probably report that the point of equality, in dollars, was "about" $227,000, or "just under" $227,000, so as not to convey an aura of precision that is not usually justified in these types of cost calculations.

Cost-Volume Profit Analysis and Other Managerial Objectives

While break even is often not a goal to which managers aspire, it is useful to know whether the department or the organizational unit is operating above or below break even. It is also useful to know how close one is to the break even point. A department that operates far above break even presents less risk than a department that is operating only slightly above or at break even. Similarly, a department that continually operates slightly above break even might be viewed as more stable and more consistent than a department that fluctuates wildly above and below break even.

A department operating near break even might be meeting the overall goals of a not-for-profit organization, as compared to a department that operates either way above or way below break even. In other words, it is the department's position relative to break even that is important. Trends in actual revenues, costs and profits are also important. Trends in the break even point for particular departments might also be monitored across different periods or under different strategies.

We have also seen in this chapter how prices can be set and financial goals other than break even can be achieved. Managers may also use the cost-volume-profit formula to check the effects of different strategies under different environmental conditions. This is the third use of cost-volume-profit analysis cited at the beginning of the chapter. For example, managers can assess the effect of decreasing total fixed costs on required volumes or prices. They can determine what would happen to break even quantities if payers discounted prices further. Managers may also evaluate the effect of payer or product mix changes on relevant variables. These are but a few examples of how cost-volume-profit analysis may be used in analyzing managerial actions and the effects of environmental changes.

Differential or Incremental Analysis for Non-Routine Decision-Making

In this section, we examine short-term **non-routine decisions**, which are also often called **alternative choice decisions**. We consider only decisions that are short-term and do not require the purchase of any long-lived equipment. They are non-routine because they are not a part of the everyday operations of the organization.

There are three general types of short-term non-routine decisions. The first type involves deciding whether to produce some product or service within the organization or sub-contract it to another vendor. These are also called **make-or-buy decisions**. The second type of decision involves **adding new services or products or dropping an existing service**. Similar alternative choices might reflect situations where the health care organization must decide whether to expand or contract a particular service or product line. Finally, accepting a price that is less than a list price or even less than the full cost of producing an output (**minimum pricing**) is also considered a short-term non-routine decision.

To make these decisions, the manager must compare **incremental (differential) revenues**, and **incremental (differential) costs**, or incremental (differential) profits. As discussed in Chapter 4, differential or incremental costs are those that differ with respect to a decision. Recall that differential costs may be variable or fixed. For example, if the decision is to double the size of a clinic, additional fixed as well as variable costs are likely to be incurred.

Sunk costs are irrelevant to the decision. They do not change if a particular decision is made. As a result, in any analyses, sunk costs must be identified and eliminated from consideration. Opportunity costs, the lost benefit of the next best alternative, are relevant. They are typically considered by explicitly comparing the two best alternatives.

The goal of the analyst in making these types of decisions is to maximize income or minimize costs for the organization as a whole. Therefore, the analyst must be careful to use the entire organization, not a subunit, to identify differential revenues and costs. Actions that lower (or increase) costs for one part of an organization may also affect another part of the organization. The organization is not well served if the benefit to one section of a decision is outweighed by the costs to another section. It is also important for the analyst to avoid using average, or costs per unit of output, since they vary with the volume of output.

In the remainder of this section, we present examples of the three types of short-term non-routine decisions.

Make-or-Buy Decisions

Consider the following cost comparisons between in-house laboratory testing versus an external vendor that will perform the same lab tests.

Total Costs of 5,000 Tests	In-House	Outsourcing	Difference
Lab Technicians @ $10 per test	$50,000	$0	$50,000
Chemicals @ $20 per test	100,000	0	100,000
Utilities	1,000	1,000	0
CEO Salary	2,000	2,000	0
External Vendor Contract	0	145,000	(145,000)
Total	$153,000	$148,000	$5,000

The two alternatives are compared side by side so that the opportunity cost of the next best alternative can be incorporated implicitly into the analysis. This presentation also shows clearly which costs differ with each alternative and which are sunk costs. If the lab tests are performed in-house, the organization must pay lab technicians on a piece rate and pay for chemicals. If the tests are outsourced, the organization will not incur these costs. However, the costs of the utilities and portion of the CEO's salary are incurred regardless of which alternative is chosen. Analysts must be careful to identify costs that are differential costs and sunk costs. The last column shows the costs that are differential with respect to the two alternatives. On the basis of the differential, or incremental, costs, the organization should choose to outsource the tests.

This analysis only shows financial considerations. There may be valid reasons not to outsource including better quality control, control of timing and scheduling, and potential economies of scale and synergy with other testing processes. The relevant question is whether these potential benefits are worth the $5,000 in incremental costs associated with the in-house lab tests. If they are not worth $5,000, then the provider should outsource the tests.

Exhibits 5-8 and 5-9 provide data for analyzing another make or buy decision. The health care organization can continue making its own medical records or accept a bid from an information processing specialist (Poirett Systems) that will shift all of a clinic's medical records processing to an external vendor. Exhibit 5-8 presents the current costs of processing medical records by the organization.

The bid from Poirett Systems is for $13.00 per record. While the proposed price seems attractive ($13.00 vs. $15.50), the saving is illusory. Average costs are rarely, if ever, the most relevant factors for making alternative choice decisions. Managers must look at costs that will change, incremental costs, and/or incremental revenues that will change under the proposed decision. The clinic must determine which costs continue regardless of who does the medical records processing. Alternatively, the clinic can examine the costs that will be saved (avoided) as another way of examining incremental benefits of outsourcing.

Compounding the difficulty of this decision is the realization that the volume of medical records will increase next year. The external vendor (Poirett Systems) has already incorporated the expected volume of 12,000 records in its bid price.

Exhibit 5-9 is based on the cost behavior patterns originally shown in Figure 5-8, assuming that labor and supplies are the only variable costs. The first column of Figure 5-9 is based on the new volume estimate. Extending the projected costs to 12,000 records results in total projected costs of $167,000 and an average cost of $13.92, which is certainly higher and less attractive than the $13.00 bid price. However, neither the $167,000 or the $13.92 can be used as the basis for evaluating the vendor's bid.

Exhibit 5-8   Current Costs in Medical Records Department.

	Current Costs (10,000 records)
Labor ($5.00 per record)	$50,000
Supplies ($1.00 per record)	10,000
Office Space	20,000
Other Administrative Costs	30,000
Supervisors	45,000
Total Costs	$155,000
Divide by Number of Records	10,000
Average Cost per Record	$15.50 per record

Exhibit 5-9   Incremental Analysis of Proposed Medical Records Processing.

	Projected Costs (12,000 records)	Incremental Costs or Costs Avoided (12,000 records)
Labor (5.00 per record)	$ 60,000	$ 60,000
Supplies ($1.00 per record)	12,000	12,000
Office Space	20,000	2,000
Other Administrative Costs	30,000	—
Supervisors	45,000	30,000
Total Costs	$167,000	$104,000
Divide by Number of Records	12,000	12,000
Average Cost per Record	$13.92	$8.67

Poirett Systems proposed to provide these services at a cost of $13.00 per record. Should the proposal be accepted?

The second numerical column in Exhibit 5-9 is designed to show which costs will be avoided if the medical records processing is transferred to the external vendor. It assumes that the $30,000 of administrative costs are allocated to medical records, and cannot be avoided. Assume that several supervisors will actually be declared "redundant" and those costs will decrease by $30,000 (column 2). All of the variable costs can be avoided if the service is not performed internally. The final question concerns the office space which can be used for some other productive purpose. If the vacant space can be rented to an optician at a net revenue of $2,000 per month, then the $2,000 becomes a cost of not outsourcing.

In this case, the costs avoided are most relevant. How much will the clinic save if the medical records processing is taken "off-site"? They will only save the "costs avoided" as shown in Column 2, which average $8.67 per record. So, the $13.00 bid is much higher than the incremental costs of medical records processing in the clinic. On an incremental basis, one could compare incremental costs of $156,000 (12,000 records multiplied by $13.00 per record) from the vendor versus the costs avoided of $104,000. In other words, why spend $156,000 to save $104,000? The incremental costs are, therefore, $156,000 versus the incremental costs of $104,000 which comprise $102,000 of costs avoided plus $2,000 of incremental rent revenue. Both items, together, are less than the cost of the external bid; therefore, the external bid should be rejected. Note that the improper comparison here would be the total projected costs of $167,000 versus the bid costs of $156,000. Even though that comparison seems to favor the vendor, it is an incorrect comparison. The $167,000 includes sunk costs but the $156,000 does not. The analysis below illustrates how such a comparison should be made.

Total Costs of 12,000 Records	Process Records	Contract with Poirett	Difference
Labor	$60,000	0	$60,000
Supplies	12,000	0	12,000
Office Space	20,000	20,000	0
Other Administrative Costs	30,000	30,000	0
Supervisors	45,000	15,000	30,000
Poirett Contract	0	156,000	(156,000)
Lost Rental Revenue	2,000	0	2,000
Total	$169,000	$221,000	($52,000)

The last column shows that it is more costly to contract for the medical records processing. The firm would spend $52,000 more than to process the records itself.

This section has shown that average costs can be very misleading when used for deciding whether to accept an external bid for a service that is now being conducted internally. The proper comparison for such decisions is to compare the incremental costs under the bid with the incremental costs of producing the service in-house. The astute manager would not want to pay $13.00 per record in order to save only $8.67 per record.

Adding or Dropping Products or Services

Differential or incremental analysis is also useful in deciding whether to add or drop products or services. The following data are for a pain clinic.

Income Statement (9,000 visits)	
Revenues ($100 per visit)	$900,000
Expenses:	
Therapists (3 @ 60,000 per year)	180,000
Supervisors	160,000
Other Administration	600,000
Supplies ($2.00 per visit)	18,000
Net Loss	($58,000)

This income statement shows that the Pain Clinic is operating at a net loss of $58,000. On this basis, management wants to eliminate the clinic's services. However, the majority of costs are shown as administrative costs. The manager who has studied this chapter and the preceding chapter will ask the pertinent question: How many of these costs will continue, even if the clinic is closed? It is clear that not all of the administrative costs can be saved if the clinic is closed. Eliminating services often means that the administrative costs are just re-allocated (transferred) to another part of the organization.

Exhibit 5-10 provides the relevant details concerning whether a provider should discontinue a pain management clinic. The analysis assumes that none of the administrative costs can be saved. It shows that the firm is $542,000 better off if it keeps the clinic. Thus, the Pain Clinic should not be eliminated. Alternatively, the analyst could determine that some of the administrative costs could be saved. However, it would take a savings of greater than $58,000 in administrative costs to change the decision.

Accepting Discounted Prices (Minimum Pricing)

The last type of decision for which differential (incremental) analysis is useful is for deciding whether to accept (or offer) a price that is below the regular price or even the full cost of producing the service or product. The rule for making such decisions is that the price should cover the differential costs of producing the product.

An example of minimum pricing may occur when an obstetrics physician practice must decide whether to accept Medicaid patients in a managed care program. Assume that the Medicaid payment per visit is $30 but the practice's usual charge is $60. A manager has compiled the following data concerning the costs of accepting 500 Medicaid patients who will generate 2500 visits.

Exhibit 5-10   Analysis of Whether to Discontinue a Pain Clinic.

	Continue (9,000 visits)	Discontinue	Difference
Revenues ($100 per visit)	$900,000	$0	$900,000
Expenses:			
Therapists			
(3 @ 60,000 per year)	180,000	0	180,000
Supervisors	160,000	0	160,000
Other Administration	600,000	600,000	0
Supplies			
($20.00 per visit)	18,000	0	18,000
Net Loss	($58,000)	(600,000)	$542,000

<u>Revenues</u>	
(2500 @ 30 per Visit)	$ 75,000
Expenses:	
Physicians	$ 80,000
Nurses	12,500
Supplies	25,000
Utilities	500
Administration	4,000
Total Expenses	<u>122,000</u>
Net Loss	($47,000)

Based upon the revenues and full costs of the visits, the practice would not want to take the new clients. It would want to charge at least $48.80 ($122,000/2500 visits) per visit. However, further analysis is necessary. We must ask if new staff must be hired to serve the new patients, whether any of the administrative costs could be avoided and if the utilities costs would still be incurred without the clients. In Exhibit 5-11, the analysis assumes current physicians can handle the additional volume and that they are paid 50 % of the net revenue per visit, no new nursing personnel would be hired, a part-time administrative employee would have to be added, earning $2,000 and utilities costs cannot be avoided. The last column shows the differential costs and revenues for accepting the lower Medicaid price. The practice would be $10,500 better off by taking the lower price, given the assumptions noted. It should be willing to take a minimum price of $25.80, which exactly covers the differential costs of the patients.

Exhibit 5-11   Minimum Pricing Example.

	Accept Clients (and Medicaid Price)	Do Not Accept Medicaid Clients	Difference
Revenues			
(2500 @ $30 per Visit)	$75,000	$0	$75,000
Expenses:			
Physicians	$80,000	$42,500	$37,500[1]
Nurses	12,500	12,500	0
Supplies	25,000	0	25,000
Utilities	500	500	0
Administration	4,000	2,000[2]	2,000
Total Expenses	122,000	57,500	64,500
Net Loss	($47,000)	($57,500)	$10,500

[1] Physicians are paid 50% of net revenue per visit ($15 per Medicaid visit).
[2] New part-time administrative personel.

Minimum Price per Visit = $64,500/2500 = $25.80.

There is also a materiality factor that must be considered in making alternative choice decisions. Very few responsible managers would eliminate a health care service just to save $10,000; maybe not even to save $100,000. The notion of materiality, in terms of the significance of the results to the entire organization, and to the health of its clients, must also be considered along with the more objective measures of costs and revenues. These, more subjective considerations, must be included in the manager's final analysis. The equations and methods illustrated in this chapter are most useful for obtaining a preliminary determination of the relative costs and benefits associated with particular choices. These methods will never provide all the inputs; they will not provide all the answers. Most decisions involve both qualitative and quantitative considerations; our approach is most useful for analyzing the quantitative factors.

Summary

An understanding of fixed and variable costs (cost behavior), contribution margins, break even and cost-volume-profit relationships is fundamental to good financial management. The applicability of cost behavior in cost-volume-profit analysis was discussed and illustrated. Cost-volume-profit analysis can help managers determine the quantity of output required to achieve financial goals, set prices and determine the effects of various managerial actions and environmental conditions. The chapter discussed alternative cost-volume-profit relationships using equations or graphical approaches.

The second part of the chapter showed how differential (incremental) costs and revenues are used in making short-term non-routine decisions and why sunk costs are not. These decisions, often called alternative choice decisions, may involve make or buy decisions, decisions about services and products to offer, and minimum prices to accept.

Notes

1. See Long, H. W., and Silvers, J. B. "Medicare Reimbursement is Federal Taxation of Tax-Exempt Providers" *Health Care Management Review* 1(1): 9-23, 1976.

Bibliography

Kolb, D.S. and J.L. Horowitz. "Managing the Transition to Capitation" *Healthcare Financial Management* (February): 64-69, 1995.

Krueger, D. and T. Davidson. "Alternative Approaches to Cost Accounting" *Topics in Health Care Financing* 13(4): 1-9, 1987.

Terms and Concepts

add or drop product or service
alternative choice decisions
break even
break even analysis
break even equation
break even quantity
contribution margin
contribution margin per unit
contribution margin ratio

cost-volume-profit equation
differential analysis
differential costs and revenues
incremental analysis
incremental costs and revenues
make-or-buy decisions
minimum pricing
non-routine decisions
variable cost per unit
variable cost ratio

Questions and Problems

5-1   In general, how does decreased occupancy and number of visits for a health care institution affect both costs and revenues (assuming 75% of the costs are fixed)?

5-2   If the volume of clients seen at Dr. Franklin's eye center increases from 100 in February
to 120 in March, how will total fixed costs be affected? What about fixed costs per unit?

5-3   If Dr. Franklin's client volume changes from 120 in March to 93 in April, how will total
variable costs be affected? What about total variable costs per unit?

5-4   How can the break even formulas described in this chapter be used to improve manager's
decisions? Which decisions?

5-5   The contribution margin depicts how much each unit of charges (or sales price) contrib-
utes toward covering fixed cost and profit. How does one determine the contribution
margin and the contribution margin ratio?

5-6   Discuss the difference between break even quantity (BEQ)and the point of equality (in
dollars).

5-7   The West End Mental Health Center received a one-year grant of $53,000 to hire a social
worker to conduct marriage counseling sessions. It is estimated that the new therapist will
add about $400 per month in overhead expenses and that each therapy session will add an
additional $20 to the center's expenses. The center would like to retain about $5,000 of
the grant to be able to continue to provide therapy to some of the couples in the following year. What is the maximum amount they can pay the social worker per month and
not exceed $53,000/year? The program is expected to see 53 couples per month. Begin
by separating and calculating revenue, fixed costs, variable costs, and profit.

5-8   Laurel Valley Hospital is considering providing one of three new services next year. Below is an analysis of three possible programs.

   A.   Using incremental cost analysis, which program should it choose? Would your answer change if total costs, instead of incremental costs, were analyzed? Limit your analysis to year 1.

	Well-Baby Clinic	Sports Medicine Clinic	Prenatal Clinic
Start-up costs	$25,000	$5,000	$42,000
Monthly expenses	13,000	22,000	12,000
Monthly revenues	24,000	31,000	17,000

   B.   Taking opportunity cost into account, how much does the well-baby clinic contribute to the hospital? What is the link between opportunity cost and incremental costing analysis?

5-9   The income statement for Dr. Pepper's private medical practice is summarized as follows:

Net revenue	
(8,000 patient visits)	$225,000
Expenses	
(including $40,000 fixed expenses)	$105,000
Profit	$120,000

Dr. Pepper believes that adding a nurse practitioner to his medical team would increase patient volume and patient revenues. The nurse practitioner would increase expenses by $45,000 ($25,000 in salary and fringe benefits and $20,000 in additional equipment and overhead).

   A.   How many patients (on average) must be seen to add the nurse practitioner and realize the same profit as before?

   B.   Dr. Pepper wants to increase his profit by $20,000 if he adds a nurse practitioner. How many patients would have to be seen to achieve this increase?

   C.   Graphically represent the situations in A and B.

5-10 The Community Medical Center offers a weekly hypertension clinic. Clients receive information on diet and exercise and a personal hypertension evaluation. The clinic is currently being funded through a federal grant, which is going to be cut in the next fiscal year. The directors are examining cost-volume data before trying to locate another source of funding.

Fixed Monthly Expenses	
Equipment depreciation expense	$ 240/month
Space rental, 2 locations ($5,160 center city, 1,500 shopping mall)	$6,660/year
Wages (3 RN's, 2 days per week)	$ 540/month
Travel expense	$ 35/month
Variable cost per client	$3

A. If the clinic is currently being reimbursed at $25 per client, what is the break even point in number of clients? In dollars?

B. What is the break even point in clients if the clinic only receives $20 per client?

C. The administrators are considering a plan to close the center at the shopping mall. Volume is expected to drop to 35 clients a month; $125 a month in rental expenses will be eliminated, the nurses will work only 1 day a week, and travel expenses will be cut to $20 a month. If they receive the $20 per client as assumed in B, will they break even?

5-11 Dr. Cary, a dentist for the County Health Department, submitted the following costs for the first year of operations of a dental clinic:

Dentist's salary	$ 5,000 + 20% of gross receipts
Hygienists' and clerical salaries	$29,000
Other fixed costs	$10,000
Depreciation	$ 2,000
Utilities and supplies	$5/patient
Charges	$35/patient
Patients	2,300

Dr. Cary proposes to expand the dental clinic by adding another examining station (purchase of equipment would be $30,000; expected life: 8 years) and hiring a full-time x-ray technician ($19,000). Additional variable costs per patient would be $2. This would allow the clinic to see 1,000 more patients per year. Charges would remain the same.

A. Determine the break even point in new patient visits for the clinic as it is set up now.

B. How much did the patients' visits contribute as "profit" to the dental clinic during the first year? (This might also be called a contribution to overhead expenses for the entire health department.)

C. Determine the break even point in patient visits if Dr. Cary is able to implement the changes he wants to make.

D. Assuming the dental clinic implements the plan and sees an additional 1,000 patients over current volume, how much will the clinic contribute to the health department's overhead?

5-12 Washington Memorial Hospital is a small community hospital with 3 departments: Medical-Surgical, Pediatrics, and Obstetrics. Each department is billed for some services based on patient volume and for other services on a flat rate based on number of beds. Below are the expenses charged to the Medical- Surgical Department in 19X7.

	Expenses Based on Patient-Days	Expenses Based on Number of Beds	Total
Meals	$63,420		
Laundry	31,000		
Pharmacy	84,220		
Laboratory	106,420		
Nursing	243,800	$83,280	
Maintenance/			
Janitorial	14,800	17,210	
Rent		186,420	
Other	8,042	22,640	
	$551,702	$309,550	$861,252

The Medical-Surgical Department has a bed capacity of 50 and did not expect to change this number for the coming year. During 19X7 each patient was charged, on average, $186 per day. The Department charged $2,715,600 in gross patient revenues.

A. How many patient-days were required in 19X7 to break even? Washington Memorial is planning to contract with a management firm to supply all administrative services for the hospital in 19X8. The hospital will charge the departments for administrative expense on a patient-day basis or on the number of beds. The budgeting office is trying to determine whether to charge $430 per bed in each department (administrative) or $41.20 per patient-day.

Assuming all expenses in the Medical-Surgical Department increase by 20% in 19X8 and charges increase to $225:

B. What is the break even point in patient-days for 19X8 if the department is charged administrative services on a per-bed basis?

C. What is the break even point if the department is charged per patient-day?

5-13 The Shadetree Outpatient Clinic has the following patient mix:

Percent	Patient Type	Reimbursement
30%	Private-Pay	Charges
35%	Medicaid	Cost
35%	Other	90% of charges

Total fixed costs are $55,000
VCU = $15/visit
Charge = $50/visit

A. The clinic would like to make a $50,000 profit this year. What break even volume is necessary for this to occur?
B. What is the break even point in total revenue?
C. Which patient type is the most profitable (per visit)?

5-14 The Guardian Home Health Agency offers four different services to the homebound ailing elderly. Price and cost information relevant to these services is presented below:

	A	B	C	D
Price	$30	$35	$48	$55
Contribution Margin%	65	70	55	45
% of Total Revenue	20	15	35	30

Total revenue (for all services) = $95,000
Total costs (for all services)   = $65,000

A. Find contribution margin per unit, variable cost per unit, revenue per service, and total fixed costs.
B. What total amount of revenue dollars is required for the Guardian Home Health Agency to earn $35,000 a year?
C. How many units of each service are sold?
D. If you had to eliminate all services but one, which would you choose to retain?

5-15 The Williams Company produces three different types of sutures. The sales mix and cost structure are given below:

	A	B	C
Price	$25	$35	$40
VCU	15	23	26
Sales Mix	35%	45%	20%

A. If fixed costs are $550,000, and 50,000 units are sold, what is the net income?
B. Which suture is more profitable per dollar sold?
C. Which suture is more profitable per unit sold?
D. During 19X6, the Williams Company had sales of $2,500,000 in the following break-down: 50% A, 30% B, and 20% C. Given this scenario, what is the break even point in sales dollars for each suture type?

5-16 The Island Health Center offers two distinct services: a dental clinic and a sports medi-cine clinic. Each clinic operates 40 hours a week, 50 weeks a year. The following costs reflect last year's operations:

	Dental Clinic	Sports Medicine Clinic
Charge	$35/visit	$45/visit
Utilities and Supplies	$5/patient	$7/patient
Salaries	$70,000	$95,000

A. If the sports medicine clinic averages 40 patients a week, what volume of dental clinic patients is necessary for the Island Health Center to break even?
B. The Island Health Center would like to realize a $50,000 profit without increasing charges or cutting costs. How can this be done?
C. Suppose the Island Health Center were divided into two separate entities (i.e., treat the dental clinic and the sports medicine clinic as individual units). Calculate the break even point in dollars for each clinic, using the contribution margin approach.

5-17 The Pineridge Urgent Care Center charges $55 per visit, has fixed costs of $300,000, and variable costs of $30 per visit. In addition, the center has the following cost struc-ture and patient mix:

Type of Patient		Reimbursement Basis Per Visit	
Self-pay	35%	Revenue rate	$55.00
Private insurance	20%	Revenue rate	$55.00
Medicaid	25%	Specified costs or	
		Revenue rate	$45.00
HMO	20%	90% of revenue rate	$49.50

A. What total patient volume is required for the center to break even?
B. The center would like to realize a $75,000 profit. How many patients of each type must be seen for this to occur?

C. If the percentage of private insurance patients drops to 10% and the percentage of HMO patients increases to 30%, what happens to the center's profitability? Use the total patient volume figure you obtained in Part B.

5-18 The Laurel Valley Hospital provides three services in approximately equal proportions every month. Total sales revenue for 1996 was $600,000. Cost data by service type are as follows:

	Well-Baby Clinic	Sports Medicine Clinic	Prenatal Clinic
Charge Per Visit	$55	$50	$40
Contribution Margin %	45	50	25
% of Sales	33	33	34
Fixed Costs	$10,000	$15,000	$25,000

A. For each clinic, calculate the variable cost per unit and the patient volume.
B. What profit or loss did the center realize in 1996?

5-19 Apply Cost-Volume-Profit concepts to a radiology department using the same format as in Exhibit 5-7 to answer the following questions, using the data as shown:

Monthly budgeted fixed costs (FC)	$225,000
Variable costs per X-ray (VCU)	$78
Budgeted revenues per X-ray (RU)	$195
Expected monthly X-ray volume (Q)	5,000

1. Develop the Total Cost equation at the expected monthly volume:

   Total Cost = Total Fixed Cost + Total Variable Cost

   Total Cost = TFC + (VCU x Q)

2. Develop the Break even Equation:

   Total Revenue = Total Cost

   Total Revenue = Total Fixed Cost + Total Variable Cost

   RU x Q = TFC + VCU x Q

3.   Determine the break even number of X-rays by solving the break even equation.

4.   Using per unit data, calculate the Contribution Margin Ratio and the Variable Cost Ratio. Show that they are complementary.

$$\text{Contribution Margin Ratio} = \frac{\text{Contribution Margin per Unit}}{\text{Revenue per Unit}}$$

$$CMR = \frac{CMU}{RU}$$

$$\text{Variable Cost Ratio} = \frac{\text{Variable Cost per Unit}}{\text{Revenue per Unit}}$$

$$VCR = \frac{VCU}{RU}$$

Contribution Margin Ratio + Variable Cost Ratio = 100%

5.   Using dollars, at the expected monthly X-ray volume, calculate the Contribution Margin Ratio and Variable Cost Ratio. Show that they are complementary. Use the cost-volume-profit equation to develop the revenue and cost estimates:

Total Revenue = Total Cost + Profit

Revenue per Unit x Quantity = Total Fixed Cost + (Variable Cost per Unit x Quantity) + Profit

$$RU \times Q = TFC + (VCU \times Q) + Profit$$

Contribution margin, at the expected monthly X-ray volume, is:

Contribution Margin = Total Revenue – Variable Costs

$$\text{Contribution Margin Ratio} = \frac{\text{Contribution Margin}}{\text{Total Revenue}}$$

$$\text{Variable Cost Ratio} = \frac{\text{Variable Costs}}{\text{Total Revenue}}$$

Contribution Margin Ratio + Variable Cost Ratio = 100%

6. Determine the target profit at the expected monthly X-ray volume. Use the cost-volume-profit equation to develop the revenue and cost estimates:

$$\text{Total Revenue} = \text{Total Cost} + \text{Profit}$$

$$\text{Revenue per Unit x Quantity} = \text{Total Fixed Cost} + (\text{Variable Cost per Unit x Quantity}) + \text{Profit}$$

$$\text{RU x Q} = \text{TFC} + (\text{VCU x Q}) + \text{Profit}$$

7. Using the information in the preceding step, prepare a simple income statement, using contribution margins.

8. Calculate break even stated in X-ray units, using a different method than in Step #3 above. Do the two answers agree?

$$\text{Break even level of Activity} = \frac{\text{Fixed Cost} + \text{Desired Profit}}{\text{Contribution Margin per Unit}}$$

$$\text{BEQ} = \frac{\text{Fixed Cost} + \text{Desired Profit}}{\text{Contribution Margin per Unit}}$$

$$\text{BEQ} = \frac{\text{FC} + \text{P}}{\text{CMU}}$$

9. Calculate the point of equality, in dollars. Verify your answer by multiplying the BEQ by the price per unit (RU).

$$\text{Point of equality (in dollars)} = \frac{\text{Fixed Cost} + \text{Desired Profit}}{\text{Contribution Margin Ratio}}$$

$$\text{Point of equality} = \frac{\text{FC} + \text{P}}{\text{CMR}}$$

5-20 As an application of Cost-Volume-Profit Concepts to a laboratory department, use the same format as in Exhibit 5-7 to answer the following questions, using the data as shown:

Monthly budgeted fixed costs (FC)	$435,000
Variable costs per test (VCU)	$34
Budgeted revenues per test (RU)	$170
Expected monthly volume of tests (Q)	35,500

1. Develop the Total Cost equation at the expected monthly volume:

   Total Cost = Total Fixed Cost + Total Variable Cost

   Total Cost = TFC + (VCU x Q)

2. Develop the Break even Equation:

   Total Revenue = Total Cost

   Total Revenue = Total Fixed Cost + Total Variable Cost

   RU x Q = TFC + VCU x Q

3. Determine the break even number of X-rays by solving the Break even Equation.

4. Using per unit data, calculate the Contribution Margin Ratio and the Variable Cost Ratio. Show that they are complementary.

$$\text{Contribution Margin Ratio} = \frac{\text{Contribution Margin per Unit}}{\text{Revenue per Unit}}$$

$$CMR = \frac{CMU}{RU}$$

$$\text{Variable Cost Ratio} = \frac{\text{Variable Cost per Unit}}{\text{Revenue per Unit}}$$

$$VCR = \frac{VCU}{RU}$$

Contribution Margin Ratio + Variable Cost Ratio = 100%

5. Using dollars, at the expected monthly X-ray volume, calculate the Contribution Margin Ratio and Variable Cost Ratio. Show that they are complementary. Use the cost-volume-profit equation to develop the revenue and cost estimates:

$$\text{Total Revenue} = \text{Total Cost} + \text{Profit}$$

$$\text{Revenue per Unit x Quantity} = \text{Total Fixed Cost} + (\text{Variable Cost per Unit} \\ \text{x Quantity}) + \text{Profit}$$

$$RU \times Q = TFC + (VCU \times Q) + \text{Profit}$$

Contribution margin, at the expected monthly X-ray volume, is:

$$\text{Contribution Margin} = \text{Total Revenue} - \text{Variable Costs}$$

$$\text{Contribution Margin Ratio} = \frac{\text{Contribution Margin}}{\text{Total Revenue}}$$

$$\text{Variable Cost Ratio} = \frac{\text{Variable Costs}}{\text{Total Revenue}}$$

$$\text{Contribution Margin Ratio} + \text{Variable Cost Ratio} = 100\%$$

6. Determine the target profit at the expected monthly X-ray volume. Use the cost-volume-profit equation to develop the revenue and cost estimates:

$$\text{Total Revenue} = \text{Total Cost} + \text{Profit}$$

$$\text{Revenue per Unit x Quantity} = \text{Total Fixed Cost} + (\text{Variable Cost per Unit} \\ \text{x Quantity}) + \text{Profit}$$

$$RU \times Q = TFC + (VCU \times Q) + \text{Profit}$$

7. Using the information in the preceding step, prepare a simple income statement, using contribution margins.

8. Calculate break even stated in X-ray units, using a different method than in Step #3 above. Do the two answers agree?

$$\text{Break even level of Activity} = \frac{\text{Fixed Cost} + \text{Desired Profit}}{\text{Contribution Margin per Unit}}$$

$$BEQ = \frac{\text{Fixed Cost} + \text{Desired Profit}}{\text{Contribution Margin per Unit}}$$

$$BEQ = \frac{FC + P}{CMU}$$

9. Calculate the point of equality, in dollars. Verify your answer by multiplying the BEQ by the price per unit (RU).

$$\text{Point of equality (in dollars)} = \frac{\text{Fixed Cost} + \text{Desired Profit}}{\text{Contribution Margin Ratio}}$$

$$\text{Point of equality} = \frac{FC + P}{CMR}$$

5-21 Apply Cost-Volume-Profit concepts to a laboratory department using the same format as in Exhibit 5-7 to answer the following questions, using the data as shown:

Monthly budgeted fixed costs (FC)	$298,000
Variable costs per test (VCU)	$58
Budgeted revenues per test (RU)	$145
Expected monthly volume of tests (Q)	17,875

1. Develop the Total Cost equation at the expected monthly volume:

$$\text{Total Cost} = \text{Fixed Cost} + \text{Variable Cost}$$

$$\text{Total Cost} = FC + (VCU \times Q)$$

2. Develop the Break even Equation:

$$\text{Total Revenue} = \text{Total Cost}$$

$$\text{Total Revenue} = \text{Fixed Cost} + \text{Variable Cost}$$

$$RU \times Q = FC + VCU \times Q$$

3. Determine the break even number of X-rays by solving the Break even Equation.

4. Using per unit data, calculate the Contribution Margin Ratio and the Variable Cost Ratio. Show that they are complementary.

$$\text{Contribution Margin Ratio} = \frac{\text{Contribution Margin per Unit}}{\text{Revenue per Unit}}$$

$$CMR = \frac{CMU}{RU}$$

$$\text{Variable Cost Ratio} = \frac{\text{Variable Cost per Unit}}{\text{Revenue per Unit}}$$

$$VCR = \frac{VCU}{RU}$$

Contribution Margin Ratio + Variable Cost Ratio = 100%

5. Using dollars, at the expected monthly X-ray volume, calculate the Contribution Margin Ratio and Variable Cost Ratio. Show that they are complementary. Use the cost-volume-profit equation to develop the revenue and cost estimates:

$$\text{Total Revenue} = \text{Total Cost} + \text{Profit}$$

$$\text{Revenue per Unit x Quantity} = \text{Fixed Cost} + (\text{Variable Cost per Unit} \\ \text{x Quantity}) + \text{Profit}$$

$$RU \text{ x } Q = FC + (VCU \text{ x } Q) + \text{Profit}$$

Contribution margin, at the expected monthly X-ray volume, is:

$$\text{Contribution Margin} = \text{Total Revenue} - \text{Variable Costs}$$

$$\text{Contribution Margin Ratio} = \frac{\text{Contribution Margin}}{\text{Total Revenue}}$$

$$\text{Variable Cost Ratio} = \frac{\text{Variable Costs}}{\text{Total Revenue}}$$

Contribution Margin Ratio + Variable Cost Ratio = 100%

6. Determine the target profit at the expected monthly X-ray volume. Use the cost-volume-profit equation to develop the revenue and cost estimates:

$$\text{Total Revenue} = \text{Total Cost} + \text{Profit}$$

$$\text{Revenue per Unit x Quantity} = \text{Fixed Cost} + (\text{Variable Cost per Unit} \\ \text{x Quantity}) + \text{Profit}$$

$$RU \times Q = FC + (VCU \times Q) + \text{Profit}$$

7. Using the information in the preceding step, prepare a simple income statement, using contribution margins.

8. Calculate break even stated in X-ray units, using a different method than in Step #3 above. Do the two answers agree?

$$\text{Break even level of Activity} = \frac{\text{Fixed Cost} + \text{Desired Profit}}{\text{Contribution Margin per Unit}}$$

$$BEQ = \frac{\text{Fixed Cost} + \text{Desired Profit}}{\text{Contribution Margin per Unit}}$$

$$BEQ = \frac{FC + P}{CMU}$$

9. Calculate the point of equality, in dollars. Verify your answer by multiplying the BEQ by the price per unit (RU).

$$\text{Point of equality (in dollars)} = \frac{\text{Fixed Cost} + \text{Desired Profit}}{\text{Contribution Margin Ratio}}$$

$$\text{Point of equality} = \frac{FC + P}{CMR}$$

5-22 Apply Cost-Volume-Profit concepts to a laboratory department using the following data:

Monthly budgeted fixed costs (FC)	$354,000
Variable costs per test (VCU)	$117
Budgeted revenues per test (RU)	$260
Expected monthly volume of tests (Q)	9,450

1. Develop the Total Costs equation at the expected monthly volume.

2. Use this data in the Break even Equation.

3. Determine the break even number of tests by solving the Break even Equation.

4. Using per unit data, calculate the Contribution Margin Ratio and the Variable Cost Ratio. Show that they are complementary.

5. Using dollars of revenue, at the expected monthly level of activity, calculate the Contribution Margin Ratio and Variable Cost Ratio. Show that they are complementary. Use the cost-volume-profit equation to develop the revenue and cost estimates.

6. Determine the target profit at the expected monthly volume. Use the cost-volume-profit equation to develop the revenue and cost estimates.

7. Using the information in the preceding step, prepare a simple income statement, using contribution margins.

8. Calculate break even stated in units, using a different method than in Step #3 above. Do the two answers agree?

9. Calculate the point of equality (in dollars). Verify your answer by multiplying the BEQ by the price per unit (RU).

5-23 Apply Cost-Volume-Profit concepts to a laboratory department using the same format as in Exhibit 5-7 to answer the following questions, using the data as shown:

Monthly budgeted fixed costs (FC)	$635,000
Variable costs per test (VCU)	$117
Budgeted revenues per test (RU)	$180
Expected monthly volume of tests (Q)	23,500

1. Develop the Total Costs equation at the expected monthly volume.

2. Use this data in the Break even Equation.

3. Determine the break even number of tests by solving the Break even Equation.

4. Using per unit data, calculate the Contribution Margin Ratio and the Variable Cost Ratio. Show that they are complementary.

5. Using dollars of revenue, at the expected monthly level of activity, calculate the Contribution Margin Ratio and Variable Cost Ratio. Show that they are complementary. Use the cost-volume-profit equation to develop the revenue and cost estimates.

6. Determine the target profit at the expected monthly volume. Use the cost-volume-profit equation to develop the revenue and cost estimates.

7. Using the information in the preceding step, prepare a simple income statement, using contribution margins.

8. Calculate break even stated in units, using a different method than in Step #3 above. Do the two answers agree?

9. Calculate the point of equality (in dollars). Verify your answer by multiplying the BEQ by the price per unit (RU).

5-24 Apply Cost-Volume-Profit concepts to a laboratory department using the following data to answer these questions:

Monthly budgeted fixed costs (FC)	$145,000
Variable costs per test (VCU)	$42.50
Budgeted revenues per test (RU)	$100
Expected monthly volume of tests (Q)	8,750

1. Develop the Total Costs equation at the expected monthly volume.

2. Use this data in the Break even Equation.

3. Determine the break even number of tests by solving the Break even Equation.

4. Using per unit data, calculate the Contribution Margin Ratio and the Variable Cost Ratio. Show that they are complementary.

5. Using dollars of revenue, at the expected monthly level of activity, calculate the Contribution Margin Ratio and Variable Cost Ratio. Show that they are complementary. Use the cost-volume-profit equation to develop the revenue and cost estimates.

6. Determine the target profit at the expected monthly volume. Use the cost-volume-profit equation to develop the revenue and cost estimates.

7. Using the information in the preceding step, prepare a simple income statement, using contribution margins.

8. Calculate break even stated in units, using a different method than in Step #3 above. Do the two answers agree?

9. Calculate the point of equality (in dollars). Verify your answer by multiplying the BEQ by the price per unit (RU).

5-25 Using the format in Exhibit 5-8 and 5-9, conduct a cost analysis of a proposed re-organization of the Medical Records Department.

	Current Costs (11,000 records)	Incremental Analysis (15,000 records)
Labor (5.00 per record)	$55,000	$75,000
Supplies ($1.00 per record)	11,000	15,000
Office space	30,000	(9,000)
Other Administrative Costs	45,000	———
Supervisors	65,000	35,000
Total Costs	$206,000	$116,000
Divide by number of records	11,000	15,000
Average Cost per record	18.727	7.733

Perott Systems proposed to provide these services at a cost of $14.00 per record. Should the proposal be accepted? Why? At what price might this proposal be desirable? Why?

5-26 Conduct a cost analysis of a proposed re-organization of the Medical Records Department.

	Current Costs (18,000 records)	Incremental Analysis 22,000 records)
Labor (5.00 per record)	$90,000	$110,000
Supplies ($1.00 per record)	18,000	22,000
Office space	65,000	(29,000)
Other Administrative Costs	66,000	—
Supervisors	87,000	43,500
Total Costs	$326,000	$146,500
Divide by number of records	18,000	22,000
Average Cost per record	18.111	6.659

Ross Systems proposed to provide these services at a cost of $11.00 per record. Should the proposal be accepted? Why? At what price might this proposal be desirable? Why?

5-27 Using the format developed in Exhibit 5-10, conduct an incremental analysis of whether to discontinue a Pain Clinic.

	Income Statement (8,000 visits)	Incremental Analysis (8,000 visits)
Revenues ($100 per visit)	$800,000	$800,000
Therapists (3 @ 50,000 per yr.)	150,000	150,000
Supervisors	140,000	140,000
Other Administration	500,000	?
Supplies ($2.00 per visit)	16,000	16,000
Net Loss	($ 6,000)	?

Should the Pain Clinic be discontinued? Why? Under what considerations might you recommend that the Pain Clinic be discontinued? If you later find that clients from the Pain Clinic have also utilized other health services at a contribution margin averaging $300,000 per year, how would that affect your recommendations?

5-28 Using the format developed in Exhibit 5-10, conduct an incremental analysis of whether to discontinue a Pain Clinic.

	Income Statement (7,000 visits)	Incremental Analysis (7,000 visits)
Revenues ($100 per visit)	$700,000	$700,000
Therapists (3 @ 55,000 per yr.)	165,000	165,000
Supervisors	135,000	135,000
Other Administration	500,000	?
Supplies ($2.00 per visit)	14,000	14,000
Net Loss	($114,000)	?

Should the Pain Clinic be discontinued? Why? Under what considerations might you recommend that the Pain Clinic be discontinued? If you later find that clients from the Pain Clinic have also utilized other health services at a contribution margin averaging $100,000 per year, how would that affect your recommendations?

5-29 Using the format developed in Exhibit 5-10, conduct an incremental analysis of whether to discontinue a Pain Clinic.

	Income Statement (8,500 visits)	Incremental Analysis (8,500 visits)
Revenues ($120 per visit)	$1,020,000	$1,020,000
Therapists (3 @ 75,000 per yr.)	225,000	225,000
Supervisors	245,000	245,000
Other Administration	700,000	?
Supplies ($2.00 per visit)	17,000	17,000
Net Loss	($167,000)	?

Should the Pain Clinic be discontinued? Why? Under what considerations might you recommend that the Pain Clinic be discontinued? If you later find that clients from the Pain Clinic have also utilized other health services at a contribution margin averaging $200,000 per year, how would that affect your recommendations?

5-30 National Urgent Care Centers, Inc. is planning for the next fiscal year. Its staff projects the following visit types, prices and product mix for Urgent Care Center #2450.

Visit	Percent of Total Visits	Avg. Payment per Visit	Variable Cost/Visit	Total Fixed Costs
Short	60%	$40	$30	$100,000
Intermediate	25	60	40	60,000
Long	10	80	55	125,000
Seriously Long	5	125	80	90,000
	100%			$375,000

In addition, the staff projects $246,000 fixed costs that are indirect with respect to the visits. Assume that the marginal tax rate is 34 percent and that Urgent Care Center #2450 must realize $75,000 in profit.

a. How many visits must be produced for Center #2450 to achieve its goals?

b. How many of each type of visit must be produced?

c. Before presenting your results to top management, describe and test an alternative scenario to decrease the number of visits needed.

5-31 You have been asked to assist a physician group practice in negotiating with an HMO. If the group accepts the contract, it will supply all of its revenues. The following annual information has been supplied for 5,000 visits.

Revenue per Member per Month	$ 35
Physician Salaries	400,000
Nursing Salaries	225,000
Office Staff Salaries	65,000
Office Supplies	20,000
Building and Equipment Leases	20,000
Utilities	5,500
Miscellaneous	16,600
Profit	50,000
Medical Supplies	$25 per visit

(All salaries include benefits)

Assume that 50% of the nursing and miscellaneous expenses are variable. Also assume that each member is expected to make .5 visits to the group each year. (Therefore, to convert the visit data to cost per member month, multiply the cost per visit by .5 and divide by 12.)

   a. Determine the number of member months required to break even. EXCLUDE TAXES.

   b. Convert the member months to covered lives.

5-32 You have been asked to assist a physician group practice in negotiating with an HMO. If the group accepts the contract, it will supply all of its revenues. The following annual information has been supplied for 5,000 visits.

Revenue per Member per Month	$ 40
Physician Salaries	410,000
Nursing Salaries	180,000
Office Staff Salaries	80,000
Office Supplies	15,000
Building and Equipment Leases	35,000
Utilities	5,500
Miscellaneous	18,600
Profit	70,000
Medical Supplies	$27 per visit

(All salaries include benefits)

Assume that 50% of the nursing and miscellaneous expenses are variable. Also assume that each member is expected to make .5 visits to the group each year. (Therefore, to convert the visit data to cost per member month, multiply the cost per visit by .5 and divide by 12.)

   a. Determine the number of member months required to break even. EXCLUDE TAXES.

   b. Convert the member months to covered lives.

5-33 Insurance firm ABC contracts with medical providers for services. It provides the following data:

	Quantity	Variable Fixed or Variable Cost
Revenue pmpm	$125	NA
Member Months	50,000	NA
Administrative Costs pmpm	$17	FC
Medical Expenses pmpm	$69	VC
Other Professional Expenses pmpm	$14	VC
Outside Referral Expenses pmpm	$17	VC
Emergency and Out of Area Expenses pmpm	$2	VC

   a. What is the BEQ in member months?

5-34 Use the following projections to estimate the BEQ for the newly formed Integrated Delivery System (you must decide which items are fixed and which are variable costs:

Revenue pmpm	$125
Member months	50,000
Administrative Costs pmpm	$17
Medical Expenses pmpm	$69
Other Professional Expenses pmpm	$14
Outside Referral Expenses pmpm	$17
Emergency and Out of Area Expenses pmpm	$2

a. What is the BEQ in member months?

5-35 Your ambulatory surgery center has just received its reimbursement rates from its payors for the upcoming year. Medicare, Medicaid, and Blue Cross all group outpatient surgical procedures into categories. Assume that each payor uses the following three categories for reimbursement purposes.

a. Determine the overall breakeven quantity of cases required to break even.
b. Determine the quantity of cases in each category required to break even.
c. If a study reveals that the number of cases required to break even is unlikely, list the actions that you, as manager, could take.

	Percent of Cases	Payor	Net Rate	Variable Cost	Fixed Cost*
I.	10	Medicare	1000	500	
	10	Medicaid	750	500	$140,000
	5	Blue Cross	900	500	
	9	Other	1200	500	
II.	4	Medicare	750	450	
	16	Medicaid	600	450	$40,000
	7	Blue Cross	800	450	
	12	Other	700	450	
III.	2	Medicare	1000	750	
	10	Medicaid	800	750	$150,000
	9	Blue Cross	1250	750	
	6	Other	1350	750	

Joint Fixed Costs: $200,000**

  * Total direct fixed costs of each category.
**Additional fixed costs of the center.

5-36 The Outpatient Surgical Hospital (OSH) performs three levels of procedures. The expected mix, unit variable cost and reimbursement rate for each level of procedure is presented below. All payers reimburse at the same rate based upon the level of complexity of the procedure. Total fixed costs for OSH for the year are expected to be $470,000.

Proc. Level	Expected Mix	Unit Variable Cost	Reimbursement Rate
I	0.50	$1,500	$2,400
II	0.40	$2,250	$3,000
III	0.10	$3,000	$4,000

a. How many procedures must be performed for OSH to break even?

b. How many of each procedure level must be performed for OSH to break even?

c. If the managers of OSH wanted to earn $100,000 in after tax profits, how many total procedures would have to be performed? Assume a tax rate of 34 percent.

d. Suppose that market competition makes achieving the total number of procedures to reach the goal in part c unlikely. Briefly, list and explain the actions you could take.

e. Using the information from part c, if the planning department estimated that only 600 procedures would be demanded by patients in the market area, how would that estimate affect earnings after taxes?

5-37 Health Care Providers, Inc. (HCP, Inc.) has accepted a global capitation contract to provide a full range of health care services to a defined population group. One of the service types it does not currently provide is men's health services. Use the following information to determine if HCP, Inc. should make the services or should subcontract with Men's Health, Inc. to provide these services. Men's Health, Inc. has submitted a bid of $45,000. To produce the services in-house, HCP would have to hire new clinicians on a part-time basis to provide the services. No new equipment would be needed. The following costs are projected for providing the services in-house.

Cost Item	Amount
Clinicians	$40,000
Supplies	$ 750
Depreciation	$ 2,000
Administration	$ 2,500
Pharmacy	$ 600
Telephone, Office Supplies	
Computer Services	$ 1,500

Pharmacy includes the costs of pharmaceuticals plus a 20 percent markup for indirect costs.

Should HCP, Inc. make or buy the services? Why?

5-38 A hospital is evaluating potential contracts with two emergency physician groups. Both groups would bill and collect for all physician services. The hospital will pay them nothing and will incur no additional billing costs. The full costs associated with the Emergency Room follow.

Expense	Amount
ER Administration	$65,000
Other Hospital Admin.	40,000
Depreciation	100,000
Supplies	58,000
Labor	300,000

Group 1 would also like the hospital to purchase $50,000 in new equipment. Group 2 has promised to increase non-ER hospital net revenues by $75,000 but would require $25,000 in supplies expenses above those required by Group 1.

With which group should the hospital contract? Why?

5-39 Should a provider necessarily drop out of the Medicaid program if its payment only covers 75 percent of the average cost of a Medicaid patient day? Use differential and fixed and variable cost concepts in responding.

5-40 The managers of Viceroy, Chateleine and Chancellor, Inc. are considering self-insuring for employee medical expenses. For administrative services (to process the claims), they could either contract with ROBDA, Inc. or handle the processing in-house. Alex Soothsayer, head of the Management Information Systems Dept., projects the following costs for processing the claims in-house.

Labor	$100,000
Computer time	25,000
Postage and supplies	77,000
Travel	12,500
Training	35,000

The MIS Dept. owns all of its computer equipment and pays no fees for computer usage. Alex estimates that only two new employees would have to be hired at a cost of $75,000. In addition, several existing personnel would assume some new responsibilities. He plans to spend ten percent of his time on the project. However, he feels that he will have to attend two more conferences this year and send several of his staff to others. To train his staff for the project, he will require $25,000 in additional funds to upgrade their skills.

ROBDA has submitted a bid of $180,000 for the project.

Should the firm contract with ROBDA to handle administrative services? Show how you made your decision.

5-41 Rehab Hospital must evaluate whether to contract with Physical Therapists Unlimited, Inc. (PTUI) for $200,000 to cover staffing shortfalls. An estimated 3,900 physical therapy outpatient visits generating an average of $50 per visit would be produced by the group if the contract is signed. Current staffing produces 6,000 visits. Rehab Hospital expects an additional $75,000 in inpatient revenue.

The extra visits will require an additional $50,000 in inpatient and outpatient supplies. Senior management staff will spend approximately 5 percent of their time, costing $25,000 on the project. Billing costs are expected to increase by $5,000 and depreciation expenses for the Physical Therapy Dept. are expected to be $36,000. The hospital's corporate headquarters will charge $25,000 more in management (overhead) fees to the hospital.

Should Rehab Hospital contract with PTUI? Why?

5-42 The Surgery Center must decide whether to continue offering training programs for its staff or to hire WeTeachUm (WTU) to provide the services. Currently, the center employs an educator whose annual salary and benefits total $40,000. The Director of Nursing also typically spends ten percent of his time, amounting to $7,000 on educational programs. Other current staff time totals $15,000. In addition, materials costs $5,000, depreciation on the classroom space is $7,500 and utilities are estimated to cost $1,000 per year. WTU has offered a contract price of $55,000.

Should the Surgery Center contract with WTU? Why?

6 Cost Allocation

In previous chapters, we introduced several different cost concepts and we showed how different kinds of costs are used for different purposes at hand. Costs must be relevant for the particular decision or question. In this chapter, we show how to determine the full cost of an organizational unit. The organizational unit may be a division, a department, or an individual staff member, such as an individual physician in a group practice.

The most relevant costs for determining the full cost of a cost object, in this case, an organizational unit, are direct and indirect costs. **Direct costs** can be traced directly to a cost object. **Indirect costs** are those that cannot be easily traced to a cost object. The **full cost** is the sum of direct costs plus a share of indirect costs. **Cost allocation** determines the share of the indirect costs that are added to the direct costs of the cost object. Cost allocation is necessary because it is not economically feasible for an accounting system to turn all indirect costs to direct costs.

In this chapter, we discuss the objectives and purposes of cost allocation, describe the process of cost allocation, focusing on three methods, and discuss the relationship of cost allocation to reimbursement and payment issues. Although we illustrate cost allocation with a simple example for a provider organization, it is important to remember that the cost allocation process and methods are relevant to a range of payer, provider and integrated organizations of all size.

Objectives and Purposes of Cost Allocation

The basic objectives of cost allocation were eloquently stated in the American Hospital Association's (AHA) monograph, *Cost Finding and Rate Setting*[1]:

1. To provide full cost information as a basis for establishing rates for services and for assessing the adequacy of existing rates,
2. To provide information in negotiating reimbursement contracts with contracting agencies, and in determining the amount of reimbursable costs,
3. To provide information for hospital associations, government agencies, and other external groups, and
4. To provide information for use in managerial decision-making in areas other than rate setting.

These objectives have been broadened considerably since the AHA monograph appeared. A contemporary cost accounting text[2] expresses them as:

1. To justify costs or compute reimbursement.
2. To provide information for economic decisions.
3. To measure income and assets for reporting to external parties.
4. To motivate managers and employees.

These objectives are much broader than the AHA's earlier approach to cost allocation because they include a behavioral dimension, a broader focus on cost measurement, and a tie-in to financial reporting (through both income determination and asset valuation).

Thus, the full cost information generated by cost allocation may be useful for many purposes. The firm may use it for reimbursement purposes as with cost-based reimbursement. Here, cost allocation procedures must satisfy the requirements of health care purchasers and reimbursing agencies who often have detailed rules about how indirect costs should be calculated. A health care firm may also use this full cost information as "building blocks" for the output costing that we describe in the next chapter. A markup may then be added to the output cost to set a price. A multidivisional health care firm may want to know the full cost of a division such as a nursing home subsidiary. An insurance firm may want to know the full cost of a contract with an employer. Another use of full cost information is for determining practice costs for individual physicians to enable the net income of each member of a group practice to be determined and distributed. The reader is challenged to think of other purposes.

Before getting into the technical details surrounding cost allocation issues, we want to frame this discussion in a slightly larger context. Specifically, many of the issues pertaining to cost allocation are a special case of a larger issue called **transfer pricing**. Transfer pricing is simply the dollar amount assigned to any transfer of services or goods between two organizational units. Transfer prices are "internal" prices that are used to record goods or services exchanged within an organization. Because transfer prices are often a source of much discussion, if not conflict and negotiation, we want to look at the broad objectives that must be satisfied under any transfer pricing scheme. They are:

1. Transfer prices should induce or increase **goal congruence**, so as to motivate or induce decisions that are in the best interests of individual organizational subunits as well as the organization as a whole.
2. Transfer prices should contribute to reliable and accurate evaluation of the organizational unit and its managers.
3. Transfer prices should facilitate the communication of organizational goals throughout the organization.

In other words, transfer prices should enhance performance evaluation, should decrease conflicts between individual and organizational goals, and should facilitate the communication of organizational goals. There are several methods for determining transfer prices. The cost allocation methods described in this chapter are transfer prices based on full costs. As such, they should assist in achieving the behavioral objectives of transfer pricing.

We now move to a discussion of the technical aspects of cost allocation. First, we define cost centers, the basic accounting unit for cost allocation. Then, we discuss statistics for allocating indirect costs. Finally, we describe and illustrate three methods of cost allocation.

Cost Centers

The first step in cost allocation is to divide the organization into cost centers. **Cost centers** are subunits of the organization for which costs are accumulated. They may be departments, parts of departments, divisions, or individual practitioners in health care organizations. The identification of cost centers is at the discretion of management unless they are used for reimbursement purposes. In this case, the third party payers specify how costs must be accumulated. Once cost centers are identified, the next step is to trace direct costs to each cost center.

Next, the cost centers must be further classified as either service or revenue centers. A **service center** is a cost center that does not generate revenue. An example is the administrative unit of an outpatient surgical center. A **revenue center** is a cost center that does generate revenue. The operating room of the outpatient surgical center is generally a revenue center. The focus of this chapter is how to allocate costs from supporting or service centers to revenue centers. Therefore, revenue centers are the cost objects of interest in this chapter. The costs of the service centers, which are indirect to the revenue centers, must be allocated to each revenue center. Thus, each revenue center will receive a share of the indirect costs.

Although cost allocation in health care organizations has traditionally only allocated costs from service to revenue centers, with integration of providers and payers, this may change. In integrated organizations, patient care departments may no longer generate revenue directly. Instead, it may be the insurance contract that generates revenues for the firm. The firm may still want to know the full cost of each of its patient care units. Thus, it may choose certain cost centers rather than revenue centers as the cost objects. This modification is recognized in Chapter 7 where cost allocation is used as a "building block" for determining the full cost of individual services or products.

A modest example of direct and indirect costs is shown below. Building and equipment service centers are common to most organizations, as are administrative services. Hospitals would also generally treat their laundry and linen services, as well as dietary and cafeteria services, as service centers. Other health care organizations, such as an insurance company or an HMO, might treat their client billing and claims centers as service centers. A physician would generally treat the receptionist and janitorial services as service centers. The general rule is if a cost center generates revenue from patients or clients, then it is a revenue center. If there is no revenue, then by definition it can be called a **non-revenue center** or service center. To illustrate these concepts, we will use an example of a small clinic that has two service centers and two revenue centers. These cost centers and their costs are shown below:

Service Centers	
Rent	$ 200,000
Administration	100,000
Subtotal	$ 300,000
Revenue Centers	
Medical Care	$ 400,000
Pediatrics	600,000
Subtotal	$1,000,000
Total Costs	$1,300,000

In this example, the direct costs of the medical care and pediatric centers total $1 million. The $300,000 of costs in the two service centers are all considered to be indirect costs relative to the two revenue centers and will be allocated on some basis to the revenue centers. The fundamental question is how to allocate the $300,000 costs to the revenue centers. When the allocation process is complete, the entire $1,300,000 will be in the revenue centers. While some obvious choices might be not to allocate any costs to the revenue centers, or to allocate the costs equally, managers generally use more sophisticated allocation criteria.

Allocation Criteria

Several criteria can be used to determine the amount of indirect costs to allocate to a revenue center. Managers must first decide how the costs will be used and which objectives to satisfy, and then choose cost allocation techniques that are based on the appropriate criteria. Three decidedly different criteria might be applied:

1. **Cause-and-effect**. A causal criterion would be based on activities or services that cause the costs to be incurred. The resources consumed, such as hours of labor or square feet of floor space, are often causally related to the costs incurred. Managers often find that causal criteria are more credible and better understood.

2. **Benefits received**. This criterion requires managers to identify who benefits by receiving particular services. By identifying such beneficiaries, costs are expected to be incurred in proportion to such benefits.

3. **Fairness, equity, and ability to pay**. Fairness and equity are based on some underlying notion of reasonableness or acceptability. Ability to pay is similar in that if the cost center has sufficient resources, or is sufficiently profitable, then it has a greater ability to pay for such services.

These possible criteria have been listed in order of preference with the cause-and-effect criterion being the most preferred. In many instances, benefits received will be highly correlated with the cause-and-effect variables. While different measures might be used under each of these criteria, the most common measures of both benefits and causal relationships are some measure of the services conducted in each cost center. The last category, based on fairness, might be judgmentally determined based on perceptions and negotiation. Since the cause-and-effect criterion is preferred, it is discussed in more detail.

Using Allocation Statistics Based on Services Provided

The services provided by service centers to the revenue centers form the **allocation basis** of indirect costs to the revenue centers. Note that a service center may provide services to other service centers as well as to revenue centers.

In any particular case, there are a variety of measures of services that might be used. The basis of allocation may range from square feet of space to number of employees. In a laundry, services might be measured by the pounds of "wet" laundry or by the pounds of "dry" laundry. In a cafeteria, the service might be counted as the number of persons served or the number of meals prepared or the dollar value of items sold. Managers must choose which statistical indicators of service are most relevant for the organization. The choice must be one for which accurate data regarding the services provided are available.

In some areas, the basis for allocation is pre-specified by payers. For example, under cost-based reimbursement, Medicare requires that administrative and general costs must be segregated into six components, each of which must be allocated on a designated basis:

Administrative and General Costs	Allocation Basis
Nonpatient telephones	Number of (nonpatient) lines or instruments
Data processing	CPU time (hours)
Inventory management	Supplies expense ($)
Admissions	Gross inpatient billing ($)
Accounts receivable management	Gross billings ($)
Other administrative and general costs	Accumulated cost center costs ($)

This example illustrates some of the limitations of choosing any particular allocation basis. These administrative categories and allocation bases ignore some essential elements of working capital management. They do not separate malpractice insurance or other insurance costs; they lump utility costs into the "other" category. They ignore the costs of telecommunications systems. Printing costs are lumped with data processing costs. Using accumulated cost center costs as the basis for allocating other administrative and general costs has some significant weaknesses. One may question the accuracy of allocating any category of indirect costs simply on the basis of direct costs. Medicare does allow a simpler approach: the institution can treat all administrative costs as one single cost center provided that the institution has not previously elected the component approach.

When not limited by third party payers, allocation bases are open to managerial discretion with appropriate justification. Figure 6-1 illustrates several alternative allocation bases using AHA recommendations for providers. Whenever a cost allocation basis that reflects costs more realistically or results in a more accurate cost allocation is identified, that new allocation base may be aggressively pursued by the health care manager. However, the manager must first determine whether the benefit exceeds the cost of using a different allocation base.

It is not our purpose here to discuss all of the alternative allocation bases for all types of providers and payers. However, it is important to suggest that managers look carefully at the cost-benefit trade-off associated with alternative measures. While it may be nice to have more accurate measures, is it worth the expense? Will more accurate service and product cost measures result? More relevant costs? All of these questions must be considered when the service statistics are first chosen. Is it more beneficial for managers to spend more time gathering more accurate statistics or on solving some other more critical issue concerning quality of patient care and outcomes?

The allocation bases are used to form ratios or proportions of each service center's costs that will be allocated to a particular cost center. To illustrate forming ratios, consider the small clinic described earlier. For the moment, assume that the landlord bills the clinic in two equal parts for the space used by the medical care center and by the pediatrics center. Also assume that the administrators estimate that the majority of their time is spent on matters concerning the pediatric center. After some further reflection, they agree that one-third of their time is spent on the medical care unit and the rest is devoted to pediatrics. These estimates would result in the following allocation statistics:

	Rent	Administration
Medical Care	50%	33.3%
Pediatrics	50%	66.7%
Total	100%	100.0%

These percentages must sum exactly to 100%. If not, then the service center costs will not be fully allocated and the costs in some revenue centers will ultimately be understated or overstated.

Allocation Methods

There are three common allocation methods that we consider. Unless a particular payer or reimbursing agency requires one method, then managers may choose any appropriate cost allocation method according to their perceived relevance for different decisions. Since the choice is often a matter of managerial preference, we show how the methods differ and illustrate each method of cost allocation.

Figure 6-1 Alternative Allocation Bases.

Cost Center	Bases of allocation	Recommended by AHA
Depreciation: building and fixtures	1. Square feet (net or gross)	Yes
	2. Square feet by building component	Yes
Depreciation: movable equipment	1. Square feet (net or gross)	Yes
	2. Square feet by building component	Yes
	3. Dollar value of equipment department	Yes
	4. Actual depreciation by department	Yes
Interest expense (mortgage)	1. Square feet (net or gross)	Yes
	2. Square feet by building component if interest is specifically identifiable	No
Central service and supplies	1. Amount of costed requisitions	Yes
	2. Analysis of labor and supply usage	Yes
Pharmacy	1. Amount of costed requisitions	Yes
	2. Special studies requisitions	Yes
Medical records	1. Estimated time spent	Yes
	2. Number of patient days	Yes
	3. Number of admissions	Yes
Social services	1. Estimated time spent	Yes
Nursing school	1. Hours in curriculum	No
	2. Percentage of time spent	Yes
	3. Number of patient days	Yes
Housekeeping	1. Square feet (net or gross)	Yes
	2. Percentage of time spent in each department	Yes
	3. Actual costed work orders	No
Dietary and cafeteria	1. Number of meals served	Yes
	2. Number of trays distributed	No
	3. Accumulated costs	Yes
	4. Number of employees	No
Nursing service administration	1. Percentage of supervision time	Yes
	2. Number of nurses	No
	3. Number of nursing hours worked	Yes
Admitting	1. Number of admissions	Yes
	2. Gross impatient revenue	No
Operation of maintenance of plant	1. Square feet (net or gross)	Yes
	2. Percentage of time spent in each department	Yes
Purchasing	1. Supplies purchased in each department	Yes

Figure 6-1   continued

Cost cetner	Bases of allocation	Recommended by AHA
Laundry and linen service	1. Number of pounds of laundry (soiled, wet, clean)	Yes
	2. Number of pieces of laundry	Yes
	3. Specific dollar allocation (where served by outside service)	Yes
Maintenance personnel	1. Gross salaries	Yes
	2. Number of full-time equivalent employees	Yes
	3. Specific identification from department payroll records	Yes
Administrative and general*	1. Accumulated cost	Yes
	2. Number of full-time equivalent employees (hours worked)	No

* Usually should be broken down into several cost centers and allocated on different bases. *Source*: Adapted with permission from Frank, C.W. *Maximizing Hospital Cash Resources* (Germantown, MD: Aspen Systems Corporation), 1978.

Figure 6-2   Direct Cost Allocation Method.

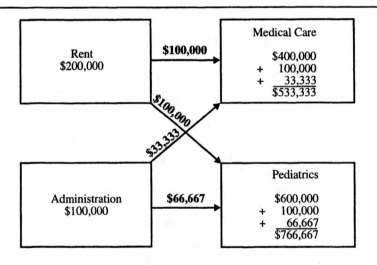

Total costs,

Medical Care = $533,333 = $400,000 + 100,000 + 33,333 = $ 533,333

Pediatrics = $766,667 = 600,000 + 100,000 + 66,667 = $ 766,667

Total costs, all departments = $ 1,300,000

Direct Allocation Method

The **direct allocation method** is simple and straightforward. Costs are allocated directly from service centers to each revenue center. No costs are ever allocated from one service center to another service center with the direct method. Therefore, the direct method is characterized by direct allocations from service centers only to revenue centers.

Figure 6-2 shows how the allocation statistics, or service percentages, discussed earlier are applied to the indirect costs in the administrative and rent cost centers. The $300,000 of service center costs are distributed or allocated directly to the two revenue centers. Half the rent costs are allocated to medical care and half to pediatrics ($100,000 in each case). One-third of the administrative costs are allocated to the medical care revenue center, while the remainder [(2/3)($100,000)=$66,667] is allocated to pediatrics. The costs of the medical care center now include its original direct costs of $400,000 plus the newly allocated (share of indirect) costs of $133,333, yielding total costs of $533,333. Similarly, the pediatrics revenue center now has its original direct costs of $600,000 plus allocated costs of $166,667, yielding total costs of $766,667. The direct costs of the revenue centers have been joined with the indirect costs allocated from non-revenue or service centers. The total cost of the two revenue centers is now $1,300,000.

Any further cost calculations with these data will now be based on both direct and indirect costs for the two revenue centers. For example, if cost per unit in each revenue center is now calculated, the results will now include both direct and indirect costs. This is a fundamental accomplishment of cost allocation: to join direct and indirect costs in a revenue center so that the full costs of each unit providing patient or client services can be determined.

The direct method, although conceptually and computationally simple, may not reflect how indirect costs affect larger and more complex health care organizations. Specifically, it does not consider the services provided by one non-revenue center to another. Services provided to other service centers are ignored! Consequently, either the step-down or the reciprocal method is used to capture the effects of services provided by service centers to other service centers. Where these relationships are numerous and complex, the reciprocal method best reflects these relationships.

Step-Down Allocation Method

The **step-down method** derives its name from the stairstep pattern of the step-down worksheet. The step-down method, also called the sequential method, is distinguished by three features:

1. A starting point, which refers to the first service center's costs to be allocated, and order of allocation are selected,
2. Service center costs are allocated to some other service centers as well as to revenue centers, and
3. There is no reallocation of costs to a service center after that center's costs have been allocated to other centers. This procedure is called **closing a cost center.**

The starting point and order of allocation are crucial variables in the step-down method. Changing either changes the resultant allocated costs, perhaps significantly. The starting point is usually the service center that provides services to the largest number of other cost centers. Alternatively, a second best choice for the starting point is the service center with the largest total costs. Depreciation expenses, including interest, are often the starting point in the step-down method because they are both large in amount and serve all other cost centers that occupy space in the organization's building. The last service center to be closed in the step-down method is normally the one that receives services from the largest number of other cost centers and, in turn, provides services to the fewest number of other cost centers.

Figure 6-3 illustrates a simple step-down allocation that is applied to the allocation of costs from two service centers to two revenue centers. Start first with the allocation statistics (as shown at the bottom of the figure) which reflect more accurate data than were used previously for direct cost allocation. Recall that under the direct method, we used some intuitive and subjective estimates as the basis for the allocation statistics.

Management has decided to use the number of square feet as the basis on which to allocate the costs in the rent center. The number of square feet outside of the rent center is used to determine the allocation statistics shown at the bottom of Figure 6-3. The service relationships are determined with ratios or proportions. These percentages, 30%, 45%, and 25%, serve as the basis for allocating costs from the rent center to the other three cost centers, one of which, administration, is also a service center. These allocation statistics are intended to represent the flow of services out of the service centers into the other cost centers. In this example, 30% of the rent is allocated to administration, 45% is allocated to medical care, and 25% to pediatrics.

The allocation is done in the step-down worksheet. The first step is to allocate $60,000 (or 30%) of the $200,000 total rent to administration. Correspondingly, 45% and 25% of total rent costs are allocated to two revenue centers (medical care and pediatrics). At this stage, administration has total costs of $160,000 ($100,000 of its original costs plus $60,000 in allocated costs).

The second step is to allocate costs from administration to the remaining cost centers. The entire $160,000 which is the sum of the administration direct and allocated costs is allocated to the two revenue centers served by administration. Rent has now been "closed," and no costs can be allocated into that service center, even if managers now might want to recognize that the administration service center also manages rental services. The reader can now recognize the importance of the starting point and order of allocation. The administration costs are now allocated at $96,000 (60% of $160,000) to medical care, and $64,000 (40% of $160,000) to pediatrics. These allocations can be traced through Figure 6-3.

All of the costs allocated to the revenue centers can now be added to the (original) direct costs in the revenue centers. For medical care, its direct costs of $400,000 are added to the costs allocated from the rent center ($90,000) and the costs allocated from the administration center ($96,000). This results in total costs in the medical care center of $586,000. The reader should verify the flow of costs resulting in pediatric costs of $714,000. The total costs of the two revenue centers are summarized in Table 6-1.

Figure 6-3   Step-down Cost Allocation Diagram, Worksheet, and Allocation Statistics.

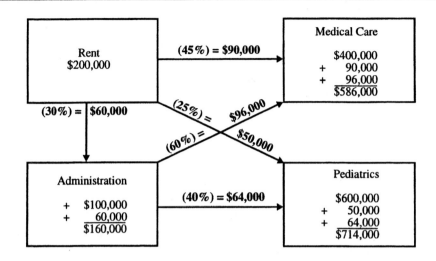

STEP-DOWN WORKSHEET

	Costs to be Allocated	Rent	Administration	Total Costs
Rent	$200,000	−200,000	—	0
Administration	100,000	+ 60,000	−160,000	0
Medical Care	400,000	+ 90,000	+ 96,000	$586,000
Pediatrics	600,000	+ 50,000	+ 64,000	714,000
Total	$1,300,000	0	0	$1,300,000

ALLOCATION STATISTICS

To Other Cost Centers	From Service Centers			
	Square Feet	Rent	FTE	Administration
Administration	30,000	30%	N.A.	N.A.
Medical Care	45,000	45%	42	60%
Pediatrics	25,000	25%	28	40%
Total	100,000	100%	70	100%

It should now be evident that the resultant costs of the revenue centers include all the indirect costs plus those costs that can be directly attributed to patient care and charged to those revenue centers. The total costs of $1,300,000 that were previously recorded in four different cost centers are now in the two revenue centers. Comparing the total costs after the allocation with the total costs before the allocation provides an important mathematical check on the arithmetic accuracy of the allocation procedures.

The step-down method is the predominant method used when provider reimbursement is cost-based. After allocation, the revenue center costs would then be apportioned to various cost-based reimbursing agencies in proportion to the number of beneficiaries served. The apportionment to third parties is fairly straightforward under any of the cost allocation methods, and it is not discussed further. However, for our purposes, we will use the results of these cost allocations as inputs to determining the full cost of health care outputs (see Chapter 7).

The step-down cost allocation method obviously becomes complex whenever many cost centers are involved. The examination and evaluation of different starting points and different allocation orders would be tedious and time consuming. Most reimbursing agencies specify a particular starting point and a particular order of allocation. However, alternatives are accepted as long as approval is received in advance and the information is submitted in an approved format.

Fortunately, this process is not as tedious as it might appear because service bureaus, accounting firms, and software vendors for microcomputers have all adapted the step-down cost allocation method to a simple computerized process. Such programs can be re-run with a variety of different data, assumptions, starting points, and allocation orders. The results can then be compared to determine how the cost allocation process might be altered to improve the accuracy and relevance of the costs allocated to revenue centers.

Reciprocal (Simultaneous Equation) Allocation Method

The **reciprocal method** relies on the simultaneous solution of a series of equations representing the patterns of services among cost centers. It is called the reciprocal method because it recognizes all services that cost centers provide to, and receive from, other cost centers. The step-down method closes out a service center at each step and does not recognize patterns of reciprocal services. Even though the closed cost center receives services from other cost centers, the step-down method does not recognize them.

The reciprocal method is considered to be more accurate and objective than the step-down method because it recognizes service interdependencies. It does not rely on an arbitrary starting point. No order of allocation is necessary because this method is a simultaneous solution using matrix algebra of *all* the cost flows between cost centers. Since it captures all of the service relationships, no information is ignored and no bias is introduced by the choice of a cost allocation method.

The reciprocal method is illustrated in Table 6-2 using most of the same data as under the step-down method (Figure 6-3). The only difference is that the allocation statistics for the administration center now include services received from the rent center. In other words, the allocation statistics have been recomputed to reflect the interdependencies between the two

Table 6-1   Total Patient Costs in Two Revenue Centers Using the Step-Down Method.

Costs	Medical care	Pediatrics
Departmental costs	$400,000	$600,000
Costs allocated from:		
Rent*	90,000	50,000
Administration*	96,000	64,000
Total costs	$586,000	$714,000

* See Figure 6-3.

cost centers. The careful reader will have noticed that the allocation statistics used in one method cannot be used under other methods. Therefore, one of the important differences between the allocation methods is the different definitions of service interactions that are captured in the allocation statistics.

Reciprocal computations involving two service centers are simply a matter of setting up two equations with two unknowns and solving them by algebraic substitution. The equation for rent includes $200,000 of original costs plus 25% of administration's costs. The solutions to the simultaneous equations are then posted to a cost allocation worksheet and allocated to all the cost centers that receive services from that particular service center.

Notice in Table 6-2 that the costs of rent now include costs of services provided to it by administration. The total cost to be allocated has "exploded" to a larger figure of $243,243, which is then distributed to administration (30%, or $72,973), medical care (45%), and pediatrics (25%). The **exploded costs** for rent and administration are then "canceled" in the process of completing the worksheet such that the only remaining costs are in the revenue centers. In this simple example, the results do not differ significantly from the results obtained under the step-down method (Table 6-3) but there are substantial differences between the full cost figures for the direct and step-down methods. Since these data are so simplistic, little generalizability can be inferred.

A more complex set of relationships (more cost centers, asymmetric patterns of service relationships) will usually lead to quite different results for the step-down and reciprocal methods. When more than two or three service centers exist, then the reciprocal method requires matrix algebra. Description of these matrix algebra computations used in the reciprocal method is beyond the scope of this text. The manual calculations needed to accomplish a complex reciprocal allocation are on the order of several months of work with a calculator. Fortunately, computers allow the analyst to avoid such a behemoth effort.

The differences may be immaterial, and not worth the extra effort or costs of using a different method. The astute analyst will usually evaluate both the step-down and the reciprocal methods over two or three periods before finally determining which to use. The inquisitive reader is referred to Chapter 9 of Suver, Neumann and Boles' more detailed book, *Management Accounting for Health Care Organizations* (see Bibliography). In each case, the

Table 6-2 Reciprocal Cost Allocations Using Two service Centers.

	Costs to be allocated	Rent	Administration
Rent (a)	$200,000	—	25%
Administration (b)	100,000	30%	—
Medical care (c)	400,000	45%	45%
Pediatrics (d)	600,000	25%	30%
	$1,300,000	100%	100%

Cost equations:
(a) = costs of rent after recognizing services provided by administration.
(b) = costs of administration after recognizing services provided by rent.
(a) = 200,000 + .25(b)
(b) = 100,000 + .30(a)

To solve, substitute (a) into second equation:

(b)   = 100,000 + .30(200,000 + .25(b))
(b)   = 100,000 + 60,000 + .075(b)
.925(b) = 160,000
(b)   = 172,973

(a) = 200,000 + .25(172,973)
(a) = 200,000 + 43,243
(a) = 243,243

Cost equations must also be prepared for each of the revenue centers. The numerical solutions to (a) and (b) will be substituted into the revenue center equations: e.g.,
(c) = 400,000 + .45(a) + .45(b)
(d) = 600,000 + .25(a) + .30(b).
(c) = 400,000 + .45(243,243) + .45(172,973)
(c) = 400,000 + 109,459 + 77,838 = 587,297
(d) = 600,000 + .25(243,243) + .30(172,973) = 600,000 + 60,811 + 51,892 = 712,703

---

analyst must look at both the numerical differences in costs under each method, as well as the cost-benefit trade-offs associated with gathering the necessary data and computing the allocated costs under each method. In other words, while the results are important, the effort needed to get those results is also important.

Generally, the step-down method is used for cost-based reimbursement puposes. The reciprocal method falls under Medicare's category of a "more sophisticated" method for which advance approval is required. There has been some reluctance to grant such approval because of past difficulties in trying to audit a reciprocal cost allocation. The mathematical computations are too voluminous to reproduce on paper and would be difficult to follow even if they were printed. The only audit mechanism available is to input the original data into an independently obtained computer program and compare the audit results with the institution's original cost allocation. Material differences would then be subject to explanation and examination. Because much Medicare auditing, has moved to an electronically-linked system, fewer barriers to use of the reciprocal method exist. If an institution is using a program prepared by an accounting firm, a service bureau, or any other independent organization that has already secured approval for the use of its software, then no major objection to use of the reciprocal method as a component of that software should be made. The provider must still justify the results as more accurate and more realistically reflective of the actual costs incurred on behalf of the third party's beneficiaries. Since the reciprocal method recognizes interdependencies and is not as arbitrary as other methods, such justification is not hard to substantiate.

From the description of cost allocation, it is easy to see that managers must make many decisions that affect the resulting full cost of revenue centers. Many of the choices involve arbitrary decisions by managers. The choice of allocation statistics and method are examples of such choices. Because there are so many choices to be made, we can conclude that cost allocations are inherently somewhat arbitrary. This is a fundamental attribute of cost allocation that must be considered when using the results. However, the full cost information is not useless. Reasonable choices lead to reasonable cost estimates.

Cost Allocation for Reimbursement and Pricing _____

One of the purposes of cost allocation is to compute reimbursement. In this section, the historical use of cost allocation in cost-based reimbursement for hospital providers is discussed. Since cost-based reimbursement is still used by some payers for some types of services, a current example, that of subacute care, is also discussed. Finally, the relevance of cost allocation for other payment methods and pricing for payers and providers is discussed. The latter are examples of other purposes—namely, other economic decisions—mentioned earlier.

Cost Allocation Under Cost-Based Reimbursement

As discussed in Chapter 1, most recipients of health care services in the United States typically do not pay the charges of health care providers directly. Instead, the provider is

Table 6-3   Comparison of Revenue Center Costs Using Three Alternative Allocation Methods.

Revenue Centers	Costs Under Each Allocation Method		
	Direct	Step-down	Reciprocal
Medical care	$ 533,333	$ 586,000	$ 587,297
Pediatrics	766,667	714,000	712,703
Total	$1,300,000	$1,300,000	$1,300,000

Source: Figures 6-2 and 6-3 and Table 6-2.

usually paid by a third party that has taken on a legal obligation (through social policy, insurance contract, etc.) to pay for some or all of the health care rendered to the third party payer's beneficiaries. Third parties include Medicare, Medicaid, Blue Cross, and commercial insurance companies.

One method of paying providers for services is **retrospective cost-based reimbursement (CBR).** With this method, costs related to patient care, called **allowable costs,** are defined by the payer. They generally include administrative, building, and interest costs in addition to nursing, diagnostic and other therapy costs. They usually do not include basic research and beauty shop costs, for example. Using the cost centers and allocation bases permitted by the payer, the provider applies the step-down cost allocation method to actual allowable costs incurred to determine the full costs of its revenue centers. The proportion of the revenue center's costs attributable to the payer's clients or beneficiaries is then determined. For acute care hospitals this may be done with the proportion of the revenue center's total patient days or revenues attributable to the payer's clients. Note that the costs of individual patients are not tracked as care is delivered. Instead, the cost of delivering care to all of the payer's clients using a provider is estimated.

Until the mid-1980s, Medicare, Medicaid and most other payers reimbursed hospital providers with cost-based reimbursement. They used CBR partially to ensure that their beneficiaries and clients received equal access to care. Since that time, the popularity of cost-based reimbursement among payers has declined.

There are several reasons why the popularity of cost-based reimbursement has declined. Payers became disenchanted with cost-based reimbursement because it created perverse incentives for providers. Since costs could be passed along to payers, there were no incentives for efficiency. Cost-based reimbursement also motivated providers to maximize revenues from government patients. **Revenue maximization** led to management policies that were designed to ensure that the full cost of providing a service to government patients was recognized in accordance with Medicare and Medicaid and other cost-based payer regulations.

Payers became disenchanted with CBR because of rapidly increasing costs. Originally, Medicare's objectives stated that the government was to pay the full cost of covered services on behalf of its beneficiaries. One means Medicare and other cost-based payers used to limit cost increases was to redefine allowable costs. Providers often reacted with **cost shifting** in which they allocated more costs to payers with looser regulations or that paid on the basis of charges. Conventional wisdom suggests that the private insurance companies and the private-pay patients have borne the brunt of cost shifting.

To alleviate the perverse incentives of cost-based reimbursement for providers, many payers designed payment systems that were not based on CBR. However, CBR is still used in payment programs for certain health care services. Therefore, many of the cost allocation techniques that were once widely used under CBR are still relevant. One example concerns skilled nursing facilities and sub-acute care units which are reimbursed by Medicare on the basis of routine, ancillary and capital costs.

Reimbursement for Sub-Acute Care Units

To take advantage of CBR, hospitals may consider converting acute care units into sub-acute care units (a type of Medicare-certified skilled nursing unit). Such a conversion helps control costs by providing care in a less expensive setting for patients who require less intensive services. It can also maximize the provider's payments for Medicare patients. Wilkes Kothmann[4] suggests the following:

> A subacute unit can greatly enhance Medicare reimbursement. The unit may obtain a "new provider" exemption from Medicare's routine cost limit for more than three, but less than four, years. As a result, the program is "cost-reimbursed" for this period....
>
> In addition to understanding Medicare cost-based reimbursement, individuals must understand the types of costs associated with cost-based programs. The components of costs include direct, overhead, capital and ancillary costs. Direct costs are those directly incurred by the subacute care unit and include such items as salaries, non-billable supplies and other expenses. *Overhead costs are costs allocated from non-revenue producing areas such as dietary services, laundry services, administration and medical records services* [emphasis added]. Medicare reimburses for the overhead costs of a subacute care unit (overhead costs are not reimbursed for acute care units). Benefits derived from reimbursed overhead allocations generally exceed any incremental overhead cost incurred by the addition of the subacute care unit....
>
> For many organizations and systems, a subacute care unit is a means to diversify services, control costs and enhance revenue at a time when these actions are critical for financial survival.

This long quotation indicates the continuing importance of cost allocation for certain sectors of the health care industry. Similar conclusions relevant to the home care sector are drawn by Church[5]:

> While Medicare still reimburses home care agencies for overhead costs, agencies should ensure that their accounting procedures permit them to produce comprehensive cost reports. Home care agencies need highly detailed financial reporting mechanisms to allocate costs precisely. For example, agencies should know the exact costs of office supplies charged to home health nurses or nurse's aides, be able to determine the amount spent for recruiting staff in each discipline, and document staff continuing education expenditures.... To support cost reporting and assist home care agencies in becoming low-cost providers, hospital financial managers must be willing to allocate sufficient resources for the collection and analysis of requisite data. The common denominator in home care is the home visit, which has three major cost components-labor, supplies, and overhead. Home care providers should be able to allocate the cost of each visit among these three components by capturing data on salaries, fringe benefits, travel allocations, and other information.

Allocation Strategies for Cost-Based Reimbursement

When providers are reimbursed with cost-based reimbursement, managers must consider several strategies that significantly affect the results of any cost allocation. Of course, they must assess whether these decisions are permitted by the payer and whether the benefits exceed the costs of managerial action.

The first part of any allocation strategy is to prepare a budget or pro forma cost allocation report two to three months in advance. Cost allocations must be tied to the operating budgets of the institution. The operations budgeting process should be used not only to predict direct costs of cost centers but also to forecast allowable indirect costs for pricing purposes. Cost implications of operating decisions are often not considered until well after the budget implementation date, or, in the worst case, at the end of the year. Budget cost allocations must involve both cost and utilization statistics. Utilization of services must first be forecast for all payment groups, and then the costs of those services can be predicted. Both cost and utilization statistics are essential inputs into the cost allocation process.

A second allocation strategy is to allocate costs to areas that reflect a higher proportional utilization by cost-based payers. An example would be to move costs from an outpatient surgical center, where most patients pay charges, to the operating room of the hospital, which has a higher incidence of use by cost-based patients. This type of managerial cost shifting must be justifiable by the achievement of a more accurate cost allocation. Payer auditors cannot strongly argue against cost allocation results that are more accurate or that "more realistically" reflect the costs of serving their beneficiaries or clients. However, a disadvantage of switching to a more sophisticated or more accurate cost allocation method is that the institution may not later revert to the previous method. This irreversible election must have prior approval from the payer and must be made in view of long-range strategies and plans. This type of permanent change in reimbursement methods cannot be made solely to achieve larger cash flows in the current period.

One method of managerial cost shifting involves reclassification journal entries. Journal entries are made to transfer costs from one cost center to another. For example, a laboratory connected to a blood bank can be reclassified out of the blood bank and into the general laboratory, or interest on long-term debt can be allocated on the same basis as depreciation instead of being included in the administrative and general account. Three general justifications for reclassification entries can be made:

1. Common personnel or linkages of other costs between several cost centers,
2. Achievement of a more realistic relationship between (statistical) allocation bases and cost center costs, and
3. More accurate identification and/or documentation of cost center costs.

Many health care institutions can maximize reimbursement by reviewing the organizational chart relative to the chart of accounts. To the extent that costs are being commingled in one account when they relate to several different cost centers or job responsibilities, such costs should be separated and recorded in separate accounts. The same general guidelines apply to patient revenues. A computerized spreadsheet or analytical model may assist in the pro forma calculations to determine whether the separations are advantageous. An example involving a blood bank and a general laboratory follows:

	Blood Lab	General Lab	Combined
Operating Expenses	$20,000	$250,000	$270,000
% Inpatient Utilization	100%	75%	78%
Costs Allocated to			
Inpatients	$20,000	$187,500	$210,600

In this example, it would be better to keep the cost centers combined because the costs that could be assigned to inpatient services would be greater on a combined basis ($210,600) versus when not combined ($20,000 + $187,500 = $207,500). This conclusion assumes that inpatients have a greater representation of cost-based patients than do outpatients.

A third major allocation strategy concerns the choice of an **allocation sequence**. The allocation sequence determines which cost center costs are allocated first. Most standardized reporting forms suggest an order of allocation beginning with depreciation. This sequence is only a recommended one, based on the rule-of-thumb that the cost center that serves the most other cost centers should be allocated first. Other sequences may be more advantageous. For example, it may be more accurate to begin with cost centers with low utilization by CBR patients. In any event, choice of an allocation sequence requires experimentation.

A final allocation strategy is the choice of allocation method. A manager must forecast the impact of various alternatives on total financial requirements, and this requires simulating the effects of the various methods to determine which one accomplishes the desired objectives. With the availabilty of computers, this simulation has become less costly and more feasible.

Cost Allocation and Other Payment Methods

Cost allocation is also relevant for payers and providers in setting prices of individual outputs, whether they are patient care services or insurance contracts. As noted previously, cost allocation is a "building block" for determining the costs of individual outputs. Chapter 7 discusses costing of a variety of types of health care outputs using the results of cost allocations. A markup can be added to the full cost of an output to set its price.

Cost allocation is also useful for providers that must accept payer or market prices. That is, they cannot set the prices they are paid. For example, since 1983, the Medicare program has reimbursed acute care hospitals for operating costs on the basis of a prospective price determined by the patient's diagnosis. Some state governments have adopted similar prospective payment systems for Medicaid patients as have other payers for their clients. Outpatient services may also be purchased under similar approaches, using Ambulatory Visit Groups (AVGs) or Ambulatory Patient Groups (APGs). Some Blue Cross plans, which in the past may have paid on the basis of full charges, now pay only a share of full charges or a prospectively negotiated rate. Under managed care, many payers are implementing capitation payment in which the provider is paid a flat amount per enrolled member per month. Such payment shifts the risk of losses to providers if their costs exceed revenues.

Determining whether the payment exceeds the provider's costs requires more sophisticated cost analyses than we have described in this chapter. Some of these analyses, those that involve full costing of outputs, are explained in Chapter 7.

However, allocated costs also have a significant potential to affect adversely financial and managerial decisions in health care organizations. Recall that cost allocation is at least somewhat arbitrary. Cost allocations may produce the illusion that some services are being provided at a loss. Or, they may lead to setting contract bid prices too high and thereby losing a managed care contract with an employer or insurer. Differential analysis, described in Chapter 5, is usually a more relevant tool for making contracting decisions than full cost analyses.

Even more important is the broad emphasis on cost control and cost management. Rather than just concentrating on cost allocations to achieve the organization's financial goals and cash flow requirements, managers must look broadly at how costs influence the organization's strategy and competitive position. Cost data may identify the need to reduce costs to be competitive in the market. This topic is discussed further in Chapter 7.

Cost Allocation and Other Managerial Decisions

Managerial decisions other than payment and pricing may also involve cost allocation. It can be used to determine allocation of expenses to individual physician members of a group practice. The physician's costs can then be subtracted from revenues to determine his or her income. Cost allocation may also be useful in motivating managers to align their goals with those of the organization when it is used to determine performance incentives. Cost allocation uses full costs as transfer prices within the organization. Managers must evaluate whether other transfer pricing methods are more useful in accomplishing goal congruence. A complete discussion of the latter is beyond the scope of this text.

Managers must also exercise care in using fully allocated costs. As noted throughout the book, costs must be relevant to the decision at hand. Full cost information is not useful in making some types of decisions. One such type of decision is the alternative choice (and minimum pricing) decision. As discussed in Chapter 5, the analyst should use differential costs and revenues and ignore sunk costs in making these decisions. Full costs typically include both differential and sunk costs. Therefore, they are not useful in making alternative choice or minimum pricing decisions.

Similarly, cost allocations may also lead to improper performance evaluations of managers. It should be obvious that allocated costs are not controllable by the recipient cost center; they are only controllable at the cost center where they originate. Therefore, cost allocations and performance measures derived from allocated costs should not be used to evaluate managerial performance. Only controllable costs and controllable revenues should form the foundation of managerial performance evaluations.

In addition, allocated costs may appear to be variable when they are not. For example, when computer system costs are allocated with a rate per hour of use, the rate typically includes both variable and fixed costs for the computer services department. Managers of cost centers using computer services may attempt to minimize the cost to their departments by finding a cheaper source outside of the organization. Although the cost allocated to the department may decline, the cost to the organization as a whole declines by far less because of the fixed costs that remain. Thus, cost allocation may contribute to lack of goal congruence if managers are not fully educated with respect to cost allocation and if their performance evaluations depend upon full costs.

Summary

Cost allocation is a means of determining the full cost of an organizational unit. The full cost includes both direct costs for the unit and a share of indirect costs. Any measure of "full" or total costs must include some portion of allocated costs, because it is too expensive to trace each separate cost through the organization to every possible service or procedure. The allocation method may be as complex as the reciprocal method, or it may be a simple average, equally apportioned across all services and products.

The cost allocation process is extremely important to most health care providers because of the continuing need to determine accurate cost data for decision-making and reimbursement. Some cost-based reimbursement mechanisms are still used by many third-party payers or purchasers. The sizable indirect costs incurred by most health care providers require that sophisticated allocation techniques be used whenever possible to determine the full cost of each unit of service.

However, managers must be knowledgeable about the relative strengths and weaknesses of cost allocation and the different allocation techniques. They must recognize how their decisions during the cost allocation affect the full cost results. They must also recognize that such full cost information is not relevant for many types of decisions.

Notes

1. American Hospital Association (AHA). *Cost Finding and Rate Setting*. Chicago: AHA, 1968.
2. Horngren, C.T., G. Foster and S.M. Datar. *Cost Accounting: A Managerial Emphasis*. Englewood Cliffs, New Jersey: Prentice-Hall, 1994, p. 499.
3. *Ibid.*, p. 501
4. Kothmann, W.L. "Is Subacute Care Feasible?" *Healthcare Financial Management* (October): 62-63, 1996.
5. Church, L. "Positioning Hospital-Based Home Care Agencies for Managed Care" *Healthcare Financial Management* (February): 31-32, 1996.

Bibliography

Canby IV, J.B. "Applying Activity-Based Costing to Healthcare Settings" *Healthcare Financial Management*, (February): 50-56,1995.

Carpenter, C.E. et al. "Cost Accounting Supports Clinical Evaluations" *Healthcare Financial Management* (April): 40-44, 1994.

Church, L. "Positioning Hospital-Based Home Care Agencies for Managed Care" *Healthcare Financial Management* (February): 29-32, 1996.

Duncan, D. G. and C. S. Servais. "Preparing for the New Outpatient Reimbursement System" *Healthcare Financial Management* (February): 42-49, 1996.

Feuerstein, T. and C.A. Anderson. *Budgeting and Cost Management for Medical Groups*. Englewood, CO: Center for Research in Ambulatory Health Care Administration, 1990.

Fogel, L.A. and K. Gossman-Klim. "Getting Started with Subacute Care" *Healthcare Financial Management* (October): 64-74, 1995.

Granof, M.H., P.W. Bell, and B.R. Neumann. *Accounting for Managers and Investors*. Englewood Cliffs, NJ: Prentice Hall, 1993.

Kothmann, W.L. "Is Subacute Care Feasible?" *Healthcare Financial Management* (October): 60-63, 1995.

Murray, M.J. and D.J. Anderson. "How Should Hospitals Relate to Medicare HMOs?" *Healthcare Financial Management* (January): 40-46, 1996.

Suver, J.D., B.R. Neumann, and K. Boles. *Management Accounting for Healthcare Organizations*. Oak Brook, IL: Pluribus Press, 1993.

Terms and Concepts

allocation basis
allocation sequence
allowable costs
"closing" a cost center
cost allocation
cost center
cost shifting
direct cost
direct method
"exploded" costs
full costs

goal congruence
indirect cost
non-revenue center
reciprocal method
retrospective cost-based reimbursement
revenue center
revenue maximization
service center
step-down method
transfer pricing

Questions and Problems

6-1   Distinguish between cost-based and charge-based payments for health care services.

6-2   From current news sources such as the *Wall Street Journal, Healthcare Financial Management,* or other business or management journal, identify ways in which reimbursement by diagnostic-related grouping (DRG) will affect cash flows to health care providers.

6-3   Discuss, in your own words, the distinction between "direct" costs and "full" costs.

6-4   What is meant by the term "cost allocation"?

6-5   Identify three different cost allocation methods and discuss the relative advantages and disadvantages of each.

6-6   Under any of the cost allocation methods discussed in this chapter, there is no association of costs with specific patients. Why not?

6-7   Why are the choice of starting point (cost center) and order of allocation important under the step-down method? Why are they irrelevant under the reciprocal method?

6-8 Discuss how financial modeling might aid in the choice between different cost allocation methods.

6-9 What is meant by "closing out" a cost center in the step-down method?

6-10 What is meant by an "exploded" cost in the reciprocal method?

6-11 Under what circumstances would health care financial managers try to move costs out of outpatient units and into inpatient units? Construct an example in which this would not be advisable.

6-12 What does cost shifting mean? What research or proof is necessary to prove the existence and scope of cost shifting?

6-13 Discuss the pre-planning that is necessary prior to preparing a cost report.

6-14 What is meant by an allocation sequence? An allocation basis?

6-15 Discuss each of the allocation strategies discussed in this chapter and indicate why they are important.

6-16 Discuss the behavioral aspects associated with cost allocations. For this purpose, start with the objectives of transfer pricing discussed in the early part of this chapter. Indicate how you think any of the cost allocation methods discussed in this chapter will contribute to, or diminish, any of these objectives.

6-17 A. Using the following data, complete a step-down cost allocation using the maintenance cost center as a starting point.

	Costs	Square Feet	Meals	Full-time Employees
Maintenance	$ 300,000	1,000	--	10
Dietary	400,000	10,000	100	20
Administrative	600,000	30,000	1,000	30
Nursing	1,200,000	100,000	20,000	80
Ancillary	800,000	60,000	1,000	40
	$3,300,000	201,000	22,100	180

B. What order of allocation did you use in part (a)? Why? Recompute the step-down using a different allocation order, still starting with maintenance. What differences are observed? Why?

6-18 Construct simultaneous equations for the following simple cost system and allocate service center costs using the reciprocal method.

	Costs	Number of Requisitions	Supply Full-Time Employees
Supply costs	$ 30,000	—	2
Administration	100,000	3,000	3
Patient screening	300,000	4,000	6
Laboratory	200,000	3,000	4
	$630,000	10,000	15

6-19 Allocate service center costs using the step-down method and starting with the administration cost center.

Service Centers	Costs	Square Feet	Employees
Administration	$200,000	2,000	6
Housekeeping	50,000	—	6
Revenue Centers			
Nursing	600,000	20,000	18
Home Care	300,000	8,000	6
	$1,150,000	30,000	36

6-20 A. Why wouldn't housekeeping be a good starting point in problem 6-19?
 B. What is the effect of housekeeping on the home care program?
 C. Use the reciprocal method (equations) for the data in problem 6-19 and allocate the service center costs.

6-21 A. Using the step-down method, what would happen to the cost allocations in Problem 6-19 if no service center costs were allocated to the home care program?
 B. Using the reciprocal method, what would happen to the allocations in Part A if the administrative cost center was not allocated any costs of housekeeping?

6-22 Allocate service center costs to each of the three revenue centers using the step-down method.

	Costs	Square Feet	Meals	Full-time Employees
Service Centers				
Maintenance	$ 150,000	—	2,500	10
Dietary	400,000	10,000	—	15
Administrative	600,000	20,000	2,500	10
Revenue Centers				
Laboratory	600,000	30,000	2,500	20
Radiology	800,000	40,000	2,500	30
Nursing	2,000,000	100,000	30,000	50
	$4,550,000	200,000	40,000	135

6-23 Contact health care providers in your community who are using DRG-based payment systems and AVG-based payment systems. Compare and contrast these two systems. Based on interviews with managers in these organizations, discuss the advantages and disadvantages of each payment system.

6-24 Based on the prior problem, ascertain what cost allocation methods were used in each organization. Compare and contrast these methods relative to those described in this chapter. Note particularly any improvements that these managers have identified, relative to the methods described in the chapter.

6-25 Contact a local health care provider which has evaluated the costs and benefits of offering a sub-acute care unit. Interview them about the types of calculations necessary for such an evaluation. If possible, review these calculations, concentrating on the different types of cost allocations that were used. Compare and contrast their methods with those described in this chapter.

6-26 Determine the full cost of the life insurance and health insurance divisions of Large Insurer, Inc. Use the number of policies to allocate marketing costs, FTEs to allocate administration and square feet to allocate depreciation.

Cost Center	Direct Costs	Square Feet	Number of Policies	Number of FTEs
Marketing	14,000,000	7,500	—	100
Administration	15,000,000	12,000	—	250
Depreciation	1,000,000	—	—	—
Life Insurance	30,000,000	20,000	50,000	50
Health Insurance	48,000,000	15,000	75,000	50
Total	$108,000,000	54,500	125,000	450

7

Costing of Outputs

Care providers and payers are interested in knowing the cost of the products and services they provide for several reasons. The first reason involves pricing. When market conditions permit, firms set prices or negotiate reimbursement rates that exceed the full cost of each output. Even if firms are unable to control prices in this way, they still need to determine if the market price exceeds the full cost of an output. Second, providers and payers need to budget for costs and to plan for cost control in advance of a fiscal year. Finally, firms can use cost information to evaluate performance and to control costs during the fiscal year by comparing the actual cost of outputs with the planned, or standard, cost.

As was discussed in Chapter 4, costs can be classified in several ways. The classification that is relevant varies with the cost object or objective. Thus, not surprisingly, the cost information needed for each of the three purposes listed above is different. In Table 7-1, the most relevant classifications of cost data for each of the purposes are shown. The table is divided into two sections. The first section shows uses of projected, planned or standard costs for a time period. The second section highlights uses of actual costs generated during a time period. As can be seen from the table, direct and indirect costs are the most relevant types of costs for determining prices or negotiating reimbursement rates. To budget or plan for costs and their control, the manager needs to have information concerning fixed and variable costs and controllable and uncontrollable costs. When trying to control costs or when evaluating

Figure 7-1 Classifications and Uses of Cost Information.

	Most Relevant Cost Classification		
Purpose	Direct / Indirect	Fixed/ Variable	Controllable / Noncontrollable
Planned/Standard Costs			
Pricing and negotiating reimbursement	X		
Cost planning and budgeting		X	X
Actual Costs			
Controlling costs and performance evaluation			X

management performance during the year, it is important to understand which costs are controllable and who controls them.

Many organizational costing systems, however, are limited in the types of cost information they provide to managers. Often, these systems report only direct and indirect cost information. Thus, they serve the first purpose in our discussion.

In this chapter, we, too, begin with direct and indirect costs. We show how direct and indirect costs are used to develop full cost information for pricing or negotiating reimbursement rates for various outputs of health care firms. The outputs include individual services, groups of services or, in the case of capitation costing, the availability of health care services during a time period. Since this information is frequently used for pricing and negotiating reimbursement rates for an upcoming year, we use planned or projected costs throughout the discussion.

We begin by reviewing the definitions of direct and indirect costs. Next, methods of determining direct costs and of assigning indirect costs for individual and groups of health care services are discussed. An introduction to costing for the availability of services during a time period, or capitation costing, is then presented. Finally, since cost control is required for organizations to be competitive in today's health care environment, we briefly discuss using cost information for cost control.

Direct and Indirect Costs

To determine the full cost of an output, its direct costs should be added to a *share* of the costs that are indirect to the output. **Direct costs** are defined as costs that are directly traceable to a cost object. In this chapter, the cost object is an output. **Indirect costs** are costs that are not directly traceable to a cost object. They provide resources for more than one cost object. Such expenses are often called **overhead**.

To determine direct and indirect costs for an output, the output must be defined precisely. An output may be an individual service such as a laboratory test or a group of services delivered to a patient during a specific time period such as an outpatient visit, all-inclusive per diem, or patient stay in a facility. Once the output is defined, its **full cost** can be determined by identifying its direct costs and adding a share of the costs that are indirect to the output.

The costs that are direct and indirect depend not only on the cost object but also on the sophistication of the organization's information system. Frequently, tracing direct costs to an individual output type in health care organizations may be difficult or very costly because of the number and variety of different outputs. For example, the direct costs for a specific laboratory test would include supplies but, since it may be difficult to trace depreciation and labor expenses to the specific test, these would be indirect costs. The extra investments necessary to improve information systems to identify other direct expenses may be deemed too costly for the benefit provided. Therefore, some direct cost information may not be readily available.

General Model for Full Costing of Outputs _____

In Figure 7-1, a general model for determining the full cost of outputs is presented. For purposes of this chapter, the outputs produced by an organization's cost or revenue centers are costed. A cost center is simply an organizational subunit for which costs are collected. It may be a hospital department or the entire hospital. A revenue center is a subunit of the organization for which both costs and revenues are collected. As with a cost center, a revenue center may be defined in alternative ways. Revenue centers include a department such as a laboratory in the physician group practice, a product line division of a hospital or a health maintenance organization.

In the cost or revenue center, as is shown in Figure 7-1, both direct costs and the share of indirect costs assigned to the output must be determined. Note that two categories of indirect costs are included. There are those that are indirect to the cost or revenue center as well as those that are direct to the center. Costs that are indirect to the revenue or cost center, such as general administrative costs, have been allocated to it from other cost centers of the organization. Although the second type of indirect costs can be traced to the cost or revenue center, they are difficult or impossible to trace to specific outputs. For example, salaries of supervisors in the laboratory are direct to the laboratory but difficult to trace directly to specific tests. Thus, these costs are indirect to the output itself. Some indirect costs can become direct costs if more resources are devoted to the information system or if estimates are made.

Figure 7-1 General Model for Determining the Full Cost of an Output.

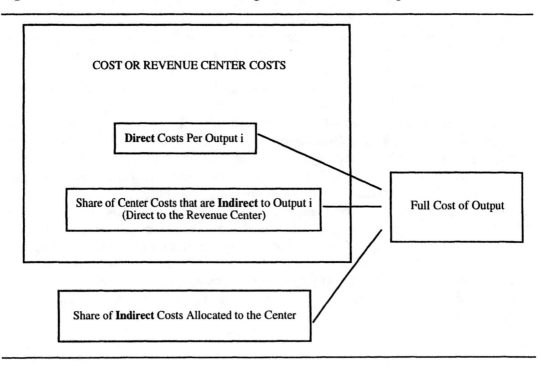

In the majority of cases, cost and revenue centers produce more than one output. The model shows that, first, direct costs for the output (Output i) are identified. Then a share of indirect (overhead) costs is added to the direct cost per output. Shares of indirect costs are also added to the center's other outputs.

Costing Individual or Groups of Health Care Services

In this section, we begin with the ratio of cost to charges method in which direct and indirect costs are not separated in determining the full cost of an output. Next, we show methods of identifying direct costs and move to assigning indirect costs to individual or groups of health care services. All of the methods discussed in this section are applicable to a variety of health care organizations. Two methods for determining direct costs are discussed below. The first method uses relative value units to determine the direct cost of an output. The second method measures the direct costs. Next, two methods for assigning indirect costs to outputs are summarized. They use: (1) quantity of output and (2) relative value units. The direct and indirect costing methods may be combined in any way to determine the full cost of an output.

No Direct Cost Determination—The Ratio of Cost to Charges Method

The ratio of cost to charges method of costing health care outputs does <u>not</u> require separating direct and indirect costs. Instead, it involves multiplying the charge, or list price, for the health care service by the **ratio of cost to charges (RCC)** for a revenue center of an organization. In this manner, the full cost (direct plus indirect) of the output is determined.

The ratio of cost to charges for a center is defined as:

$$RCC = \frac{\text{Total Revenue Center Expenses}}{\text{Total Revenue Center Charges}}$$

For the revenue center, the total expenses are summed as are the total list prices of the services produced or expected to be produced during a time period. The RCC is then multiplied by the list price of the service to determine its full cost as in:

Full Cost of Output = Charge for Output x RCC.

For example, assume that the laboratory of MD Practice, Inc. has an RCC of .60 and that the list price for a test is $80. The estimated full cost of the test is:

Full Cost of Test = $80 x .60 = $48.

In addition to generating cost estimates for individual services, the RCC method is used in estimating the full cost of a group of services for a patient stay or for a patient stay of a particular type in a hospital. Here, however, it is necessary to recognize that during a patient stay, services are provided to patients by a variety of revenue centers. The RCC is usually different for each of these revenue centers. Thus, for the patient stay, the charges generated in each revenue center must be summed and multiplied by that center's RCC. The simplified example in Table 7-2 demonstrates how a patient's total charges generated during a hospital stay can be converted to full costs. The full cost of this patient's stay is estimated to be $9410.

The same process can be used to determine the average cost of a type of patient stay, such as for a specific diagnosis, for a number of patients. Table 7-3 shows that the total charges generated in each revenue center by all patients with an XYZ type stay are multiplied by the RCC of the revenue center. The cost estimates from each revenue center are summed and divided by the number of patients to determine an average cost per patient.

The RCC method of costing is a simple and inexpensive way to estimate the full cost of a service or of a group of services. It uses information that is readily available in the majority of health care provider organizations. List prices or charges for each output, and total charges

Table 7-2   Costing a Patient Stay Using the Ratio of Cost to Charges (RCC).

Revenue Center	Total Charges Generated During Patient Stay	RCC of Revenue Center	Total Cost of Stay
ICU	$5,000	1.25	$6,250
Medical/Surgical	2,000	1.10	2,200
Laboratory	800	0.70	560
Radiology	500	0.80	400
		Total	$9,410

Table 7-3   Determining the Average Cost of a Patient Stay of Type XYZ Using the Ratio of Cost to Charges.

Revenue Center	Total Charges Generated During Stay of All XYZ	RCC of Revenue Center	Total Cost of All XYZ Stay
CCU	$600,000	1.20	$720,000
Medical/Surgical	300,000	1.10	330,000
Laboratory	100,000	0.70	70,000
Radiology	80,000	0.80	64,000
		Total	$1,184,000

$$\frac{\$1,184,000}{122 \text{ Patient Stays}} = \$9,704.92 \text{ Full Cost per each XYZ Patient Stay}$$

and expenses for a revenue center are typically recorded. In addition, with this method, no additional expenses are incurred to identify direct and indirect costs for an individual output.

There are some disadvantages associated with the RCC method as well. An important disadvantage is that the accuracy of the cost estimate produced by the RCC method is questionable. Since costs that are directly traceable to the output are not identified, some irrelevant costs may be included in the cost estimate. In addition, when using this method, the analyst assumes that the RCC for each output of the revenue center is the same. Finally, it is necessary to have list price, or charge, data for all individual service outputs. Although most health care organizations currently collect this information, list prices may no longer be kept for individual services as integrated delivery systems evolve and as fee-for-service payment becomes less common.

It is also important to remember that the cost estimate produced is an average full cost for the output. It includes variable and fixed costs. Total variable costs increase when more outputs are produced but total fixed costs do not increase within the relevant operating range of the firm. Although the average variable cost for an output is constant, the average fixed cost per output declines with increasing volume. Therefore, the average cost of the output is not particularly useful for budgeting at different volumes of output. As is noted in Table 7-1, fixed and variable cost categories, instead of direct and indirect costs, are needed for planning and budgeting.

Determining Direct Costs

Relative Value Units. As noted previously, it may be difficult for some health care firms to trace costs directly to outputs. The difficulty may arise from the number and variety of outputs they produce or from limitations in information systems. Therefore, it may be necessary to estimate direct costs.

One common method of estimating the direct cost of outputs is to assign relative value units to them. **Relative value units (RVUs)** reflect resource intensity differences required to produce an output relative to those required for other outputs. A base value of one is assigned to an output and all other outputs are assigned a relative value. The differences are identified through a study or series of studies. Studies may be done internally or RVUs from studies done by others may be used.

In Figure 7-2, some examples of health care RVUs developed by the federal Medicare program for reimbursement purposes are shown. The case weights for the Medicare Diagnosis Related Groups may be considered relative value units. In addition, examples of RVUs developed for the Resource Based Relative Value Scale (RB-RVS) for physician reimbursement for Medicare patients are shown.

The example in Figure 7-3 illustrates how relative value units may be used to determine direct costs. In this case, total direct nursing care costs for this patient care unit are not routinely traced to the two different types of patient days. Therefore, the hours of nursing care per patient day on the patient care unit are used to determine the relative resource intensity, thus, the relative value units, for each of the two outputs. As can be seen from Figure 7-3, a Level I patient day has a relative value of 1.0 and a Level II patient day has a relative value of 1.51.

Figure 7-2   Examples of Relative Value Units (RVUs).

A. Case Weights for Selected Medicare Diagnosis Related Groups (DRGs)

DRG Number	Title	Case Weight for FY 1995
36	Retinal Procedures	0.5989
64	Ear, Nose, Mouth & Throat Malignancy	1.1419
78	Pulmonary Embolism	1.4211
103	Heart Transplant	13.5495
148	Major Small & Large Bowel Procedures with Complications	3.2220
243	Medical Back Problems	0.7122
317	Admit for Renal Dialysis	0.5149
373	Vaginal Delivery Without Complicating Diagnoses	0.3387
462	Rehabilitation	1.6623

B. RVUs for Selected Medicare Resource Based Relative Value Scale (RB-RVS)

Current Procedure Terminology (CPT) Code	Description	Total RVUs for 1994
11100	Biopsy of Skin Lesion	1.38
33860	Ascending Aorta Graft	72.93
33510	CABG, Single	58.69
50590	Fragmenting of Kidney Stone	20.93
67141	Treatment of Retina	13.72
71260	Contrast CAT Scan of Chest	7.24
99295	Neonatal Critical Care	21.67
99354	Prolonged Service, Office	1.74

Figure 7-3   Using RVUs to Determine the Direct Nursing Cost by Patient Acuity Level.

I. Data

Acuity Level	Patient Days	Hours of Nursing Care	Number of RVUs	Total Direct Nursing Care Costs
1	6,675	5.10	1.0	---
2	1,994	7.70	1.51	---
				$829,212

II. Develop RVUs—Acuity Level 2 Relative to Acuity Level 1

$$\frac{7.70 \text{ hours}}{5.10 \text{ hours}} = 1.51 \text{ RVUs}$$

III. Determine the Total Number of RVUs

Acuity Level	Patient Days	Number of RVUs	Acuity Weighted Patient Days (RVUs)
1	6,675	1.0	6,675
2	1,994	1.51	3,011
		Total	9,686

IV. Determine Cost per RVU or Weighted Day

$$\frac{\$829,212}{9,686 \text{ RVUs}} = \$85.61 \text{ per RVU}$$

V. Determine Cost per Type of Patient Day

Level 1   1.00 RVU x ($85.61 per RVU) = $85.61 per day

Level 2   1.51 RVU x ($85.61 per RVU) = $129.27 per day

Next, the total number of relative value units is determined by multiplying the number of each output (days) by its number of RVUs. Then, total direct nursing care costs are divided by the sum of the RVUs (acuity weighted days) to determine the cost per RVU. Finally, the cost per RVU is multiplied by the RVUs for each output to determine the direct cost for each type of patient day.

Use of relative value units (RVUs) improves the ability to identify direct costs. For the RVUs to be useful, however, the original study to determine the RVUs must be accurate. Moreover, the RVU scales should be updated periodically. Costing based upon RVUs is more expensive than with the RCC method. More of the analyst's time is required for this costing method. In addition, conducting or updating a relative value study can require considerable resources.

As with the RCC method, the direct cost produced using the RVU method may not be particularly useful for planning and budgeting purposes. Because fixed costs are likely to be averaged into the full cost estimate, the full cost of the output may not be useful for projecting total costs for different volumes of output.

Measurement of Direct Costs. To improve the accuracy of direct cost data for service outputs, direct costs can be measured instead of being estimated with relative value units. The direct variable costs of outputs can be determined by record-keeping while an output is produced or by conducting special studies. Both will show the actual labor time, supplies and the like used to produce an output. For example, the production of a service may require one unit of Input A, which costs $1.00 each, plus two hours of Labor Type B at $20 per hour. Therefore, the direct cost of this service is $41 ($1.00 + $20.00 + $20.00).

In Figure 7-4, an example from an outpatient diagnostic imaging center is summarized. As can be seen from the figure, the average time required by radiological technicians and office services personnel for each procedure is measured in minutes. The number of minutes is multiplied by the average hourly wage to determine the direct personnel costs. (Benefits are excluded in this example.) Then, the film and other medical supplies required for each procedure are costed. The labor and supplies costs are added to determine the direct cost of each procedure.

Measurement improves the accuracy of the direct cost estimate, but it is the most costly of the methods we discuss. Resources must be devoted to the record-keeping required. Thus, it may be necessary to limit its use to outputs that are the most costly or highest in volume. As with the RVU method, the underlying record-keeping and the cost analysis must be accurate for the method to produce accurate results. Costs must reflect the work process realistically. For example, the normal costs of spoiled, wasted and broken supplies or materials must be included. Studies must be updated periodically as technology, patient type, or personnel change.

Measuring direct costs has the potential to improve the usefulness of the cost estimate for planning purposes by documenting variable and fixed costs. However, managers must act to make costs variable or fixed in practice. For example, although this method may identify the time required by personnel to produce an output, direct labor costs are not variable unless managers use only the amount needed to produce the outputs. If, for example, staff are not told to go home when there is no work to do, the total labor cost is really fixed, not variable.

Figure 7-4 Using Measured Direct Variable Costs for Determining the Direct Cost of Diagnostic Imaging Procedures.

Procedure	Technician Time Per Procedure (in minutes)	Office Services Time Per Procedure (in minutes)	Technician Cost at $15.47/Hour	Office Services Cost at $8.16/Hour	Medical Supplies	Direct Cost Per Procedure*
1	70	20	$18.05	$2.72	$80.17	$100.94
2	40	20	10.31	2.72	18.03	31.06
3	50	20	12.89	2.72	10.87	26.48
4	90	20	23.21	2.72	74.80	100.73
5	70	20	18.05	2.72	10.87	31.64
6	80	20	20.63	2.72	83.89	107.24
7	90	20	23.21	2.72	83.89	109.82

* Direct Cost = Technician Cost + Office Cost + Medical Supplies

Now, we turn to determining how to assign a share of the indirect costs to service outputs. We combine the information with the direct costs to produce an estimate of the full cost of a service or a group of services.

Assigning Indirect Costs

Quantity of Output. Perhaps the simplest means of assigning indirect costs to outputs is to divide the total indirect costs by the quantity of outputs to be produced in the revenue center. In this way, each service to be produced is assigned an equal amount of indirect costs or overhead.

Figure 7-5 illustrates an equal assignment of indirect costs to each of two laboratory tests. In this example, the direct variable cost has already been measured for each laboratory test. The costs direct to the laboratory revenue center but indirect to each test are divided by the total volume of tests to be produced. Additional costs allocated to the laboratory are also divided by the volume of output. Then, equal amounts of indirect costs are added to the direct costs of each test to determine the full cost of each.

Assigning equal amounts of indirect costs to each output is inaccurate if the outputs are not homogeneous in their resource requirements. For example, some service outputs require more supervisory time than other outputs. In this case, the equal assignment of indirect costs may underestimate the cost of some outputs and overestimate the cost of others.

As is true with direct costs, it is important not to confuse the fixed costs assigned to each output with variable costs. The total of the fixed costs does not increase when additional outputs are produced. Nor, does the total decrease when fewer outputs are produced.

Figure 7-5   Assigning Equal Amounts of Indirect Costs to Laboratory Tests.

I. Data

	Volume	Direct Variable Cost Per Test	Other Laboratory Costs (Indirect to Each Test)	Costs Allocated to the Laboratory (Also Indirect to Each Test)
Test 1	8000	$4	---	---
Test 2	2000	$10	---	---
Total	10,000	---	$100,000	$200,000

Cost Per Test = Direct Cost Per Test + Other Costs Per Test + Allocated Costs Per Test

II. Per Unit Cost of Test 1

$$\$4 \text{ per test} + \frac{\$100,000}{10,000 \text{ tests}} + \frac{\$200,000}{10,000 \text{ tests}} = \$34 \text{ per test}$$

III. Per Unit Cost of Test 2

$$\$10 \text{ per test} + \frac{\$100,000}{10,000 \text{ tests}} + \frac{\$200,000}{10,000 \text{ tests}} = \$40 \text{ per test}$$

Relative Value Units. The assignment of indirect costs to outputs can be improved by recognizing differences in the resource requirements of outputs. One way to recognize such differences in costing is to use relative value units (RVUs) to determine the share of indirect costs to add to the output's direct costs.

Figure 7-6 returns to the laboratory example in Figure 7-5 and assigns RVUs, based upon a prior study, to each test. As before, when using RVUs for direct cost estimation, it is necessary to determine the total number of RVUs expected to be produced during the time period. The volume of each test is, thus, multiplied by its number of RVUs. The total number of RVUs is summed and divided into the indirect costs to determine the indirect cost per RVU. Then, for each test, the indirect cost per RVU is multiplied by the number of RVUs used to conduct each test. This indirect cost amount is added to the test's direct cost to determine its full cost.

Using RVUs improves the accuracy of assigning indirect costs. The extra study and effort, however, does add to the cost of producing the full cost of outputs.

As before, it is important not to confuse the fixed cost assigned to each output with variable costs. Total fixed costs are constant for any level of output in the relevant range.

Figure7-6 Assigning Indirect Costs to Laboratory Tests Using Relative Value Units.

I. Data

	Volume	Direct Variable Cost Per Test	Relative Value Units per Test	RVUs Generated
Test 1	8,000	$4	1	8,000
Test 2	2,000	$10	2	4,000
			Total RVUs	12,000

Other Laboratory Costs = $100,000
Allocated Indirect Costs = $200,000

Cost Per Test = Direct Variable Costs Per Test + Indirect Costs Per RVU

II. Determine the Indirect Cost Per RVU

$$\frac{\$100,000}{12,000\ RVUs} + \frac{\$200,000}{12,000\ RVUs} = \$25.00\ per\ RVU$$

III. Determine Cost of Test 1

$4 per test + ($25 per RVU x 1 RVU) = $29.00 per test

IV. Determine Cost of Test 2

$10 per test + ($25 per RVU x 2 RVUs) = $60.000 per test

Costing the Availability of Services During a Time Period ———

The definition of the service or output is not always an individual service or even groups of services delivered to patients for payers, for fully integrated delivery systems, and, increasingly, for care providers. Instead, the output may be the availability of a specified group of services for enrollees for a period of time, usually a month. The cost of the availability of services is relevant for payers, such as health maintenance organizations (HMOs), that enroll subscribers in health plans. It is also relevant for providers who accept fixed payments from payers or employers for agreeing to make available specified services for a group of enrollees in a health plan.

The cost of making these services available is determined on an average per member per month basis. A **member month** occurs when one member is enrolled in a health plan for one month. The cost per member per month (pmpm) is also called a capitation rate.

In this section, we demonstrate how to determine the average (full) cost per member per month. As before, a share of the indirect costs is added to the direct costs of the output. We use two methods to identify direct costs. The first is the cost or budgetary method. It is useful for providers or payers who deliver, or "make," health care services for patients. The second method is the fee-for-service, or "buy," method. It is useful for organizations that do not deliver the services. Instead, these organizations contract with providers to deliver services. They pay at least some providers for each service delivered on a fee-for-service basis. An example would be a health maintenance organization (HMO) that contracts with physicians, hospitals, home health agencies, and other health care providers to deliver services to its enrollees. Alternatively, a physician group practice could use this method when subcontracting with other providers to deliver services that the group does not produce.

For both costing methods, the cost of the availability of services during the time period is determined by the cost of services expected to be used. To determine the average cost, however, the analyst must precisely define the package of covered services and the expected utilization of each. Expected utilization depends upon many factors including the demographic characteristics of the enrollees, services covered in the benefit package, incentives for providers, and medical management ability of providers. Past utilization data may be trended to the future and adjusted for changes in coverage to derive expected utilization rates. Given the complexity and importance of this task, however, the assistance of an actuary may be necessary to help with projecting utilization.

Cost or Budgetary Method

With the cost or budgetary model, expected utilization is translated into the components required to make the services that are expected to be used. The numbers of full-time equivalent physicians, nurses, laboratory technicians, medical records staff, and other personnel are determined. Then, the direct costs of each of the components are identified and summed. This direct cost total is divided by the total number of member months expected for the time period to determine the cost per member per month.

An example for ophthalmology physician office services for an enrolled population of 100,000 is shown in Table 7-4. Direct costs include the costs of physician salaries and benefits, staff salaries and benefits, and supplies. As can be seen from the table, based upon expected utilization data and health plan requirements, one physician is required for every 25,000 covered lives (enrollees). Other staff for the office are listed as well. For all personnel, the total annual cost is determined and then is divided by the total number of expected member months. In this case, 100,000 enrollees for 12 months amounts to 1,200,000 member months. Supply costs are averaged for a visit and multiplied by the number of visits expected per year. Each member is expected to average 0.25 visits to the offices every year.

In addition to the direct costs, indirect costs for building and equipment depreciation, interest expenses, utilities and other costs are summed. They are divided by the quantity of output, the number of expected member months. Finally, the average cost per member per month for each component is summed to determine the average cost per member per month, or the **capitation rate**.

Table 7-4   The Cost or Budgetary Method for Determining the Average Cost Per Member Per Month for Ophthalmology Office Services for 100,000 Covered LIves.*

Physicians	Covered Lives Per Physician	Number of Physicians	Annual Cost per Physician	Total Cost Per Year	Average Cost Per Member Per Month**
Ophthalmologists	25,000	4	$150,000	$600,000	$0.50
Other Staff	**Personnel per Physician**	**Total Number of Staff**	**Annual Cost per Staff Member**		
Registered Nurses	1	4	$35,000	$140,000	$0.12
Nursing Assistants	2	8	20,000	$160,000	$0.13
Receptionists	.5	2	22,000	$ 44,000	$0.04
Fiscal and Administrative	.75	3	34,000	$102,000	$0.09
Other	.25	1	18,000	$ 18,000	$0.02
				Staff Subtotal	$0.40
	Visits per Member per Year	**Average Cost Per Visit**			
Supplies	0.25	$25		$625,000	$0.52
Depreciation, Interest, Utilities, Etc.				$165,000	$0.14
Total Capitation Rate					$1.56

* The number of member months per year is 1,200,000 (100,000 members x 12 months).
** Average cost per member per month equals total annual cost/number of member months.

   This method of costing requires careful planning and relies heavily upon reliable and complete data. Accurate data are needed to project the expected utilization and the resources required to produce the services expected to be used during a time period.

   As before, it is important not to assume that the average cost per member per month is a variable cost. Fixed costs are typically included in both the direct and indirect costs. For example, physician and other staff salaries may be fixed if they are paid for a set number of hours per week even if there are no patients seen. In addition, many facility (indirect) costs, such as the depreciation expense, are fixed. Therefore, the average cost per member per month should not be used to project total costs when the number of member months is different from the original quantity used to determine the average cost.

Fee-For-Service Method

The cost per member per month of the availability of services may also be determined by multiplying the expected utilization for each service by the average cost per service. Again, the total is summed and divided by the number of member months to determine the expected direct cost per member per month. The indirect cost is divided by the number of member months and added to the direct cost.

This method is useful for payers, such as HMOs, that purchase services for their enrollees from providers rather than producing the services themselves. They may use this method either to determine the expected cost when payment to providers is on a fee-for service basis or to help set a flat per member per month payment rate for a provider group. Similarly, providers who contract with payers to provide a package of services, some of which they produce and some of which they do not produce may use this method in contracting with other providers. As with payers, providers may use the fee-for-service method to determine the expected cost if they pay other providers on a fee-for-service basis or they may use flat rates to pay the other providers.

As discussed for the cost or budgetary method, first, expected utilization must be determined. With this method, however, the utilization for each type of service in the benefit package, usually per 1000 members, is multiplied by the average payment per service. The average payment is determined from market data or from rates negotiated with providers. These rates may be from discounted charges, all-inclusive per diem rates, or other payment methods. Sources of data for these rates include negotiations with the providers, state data bases, cost report data from the federal Health Care Financing Administration, and professional organizations.

The cost per member per month is the sum of the following across all services:

$$\frac{\text{Annual Utilization per 1000 x Unit Cost}}{12 \text{ x } 1000 \text{ Members}} = \text{Cost per Member per Month}$$

An example for determining the cost per member per month for physician services is shown in Table 7-5. In the table, annual utilization data per 1000 members are multiplied by the average cost per service. When that amount is divided by 12,000 (1000 members x 12 months), the expected, or average, direct cost per member per month is shown. Expected co-payment and co-insurance amounts are subtracted for the net cost per member per month. Then, the net cost per member per month for each service is summed to produced the average cost per member per month for physician services.

In contrast to the budgetary method, the fee-for-service method does produce an average direct variable cost per member per month. As the payer or provider covers an additional life, or enrolls a new member, the total expected medical care (direct) costs increase by the aver-

Table 7-5 The Fee-For-Service Method for Determining the Cost Per Member Per Month for Physician Services.

Type of Service	Annual Utilization Per 1000	Average Cost	Cost Per Member Per Month(1)	Co-Pay	Co-Pay PMPM(2)	Net Cost PMPM(3)
Inpatient Surgery	43 proced.	$1068.38	$3.83			$3.83
Outpatient Surgery	401 proced.	317.13	10.60			10.60
Anesthesia	85 proced.	788.46	5.58			5.58
Inpatient Visits	271 visits	73.05	1.65			1.65
Office Visits	3924 visits	37.89	12.39	5.00	1.64	10.75
Consults	95 consults	125.00	0.99	5.00	0.04	0.95
ER Visits	125 visits	52.30	0.54			0.54
Immunizations & Injections	555 proced.	17.98	0.83			0.83
Allergy Tests & Injections	302 proced.	22.54	0.57	5.00	0.13	0.44
Well Baby Visits	113 exams	39.14	0.37	5.00	0.05	0.32
Physical Therapy	336 exams	34.77	0.97			0.97
Obstetrics—Deliveries	15.5 cases	2242.74	2.90	5.00	0.01	2.89
Obstetrics—Other	19.3 cases	589.32	0.96	5.00	0.01	0.95
Radiology	992 proced.	100.28	8.29			8.29
Pathology	3500 proced.	24.04	7.01			7.01
Outpatient Mental Health	351 visits	73.39	2.15	10.00	0.29	1.86
Outpatient Substance Abuse	38 visits	67.41	0.21	10.00	0.03	0.18
Diagnostic Testing	416 proced.	51.69	1.79		____	1.79
Total			$61.63		2.20	$59.43

(1) (Utilization per 1000 x Average cost)/12,000.
(2) (Co-Pay x Utilization per 1000)/12,000.
(3) Cost PMPM – Co-Pay PMPM.

age cost per member per month. Thus, this cost estimate can be used to determine total direct costs of care as the number of outputs (member months) increases.

When indirect costs, many of which are fixed, are added, total costs no longer increase by the average cost per member per month. This is because many of the administrative costs are fixed. In Table 7-6, the example in Table 7-5 is expanded to show additional types of medical care (variable) costs as well as the indirect fixed costs. The indirect fixed costs include administrative costs, such as information system costs, and profits.

Prices and Full Costs

The full cost per output for individual services, groups of services, and the availability of services can be used in setting prices or in negotiating reimbursement rates. However, in today's health care environment, price is not always under the control of the health care firm. As Figure 7-7 shows, the pricing environment of the firm may allow it to be a price setter, price taker, or somewhere in between.

For example, health care firms are **price setters** when they are paid the full charges they set or when they are paid on a cost basis. When paid charges, firms use their full cost information for outputs and add a markup to generate a profit. In contrast, when markets set prices, care providers and payers are **price takers**. Markets, not the health care firms, set the prices. Although prices in most health care markets are not totally market driven, many observers feel the U.S. is moving in this direction.

When prices are negotiated, as some payers or employers do with care providers, firms fall in-between price setting and price taking. Providers are also in-between price setting and price taking if prices are regulated or set by a payer because the payer often uses data from care providers to set the prices it pays. Since the data typically come from many firms, the provider has less control over the price than when payment is based upon charges or costs.

In any of these cases, full cost information helps the provider or payer avoid the risk that the full cost of the health services output will exceed the price of the output. It helps managers set prices that exceed the full cost of the output and it helps managers identify when cost control is necessary to keep costs under a market price. Unfortunately, the direct and indirect cost information used in determining the full cost of an output is usually not very helpful in identifying means of controlling costs.

Using Full Cost Information for Cost Planning and Control

Knowing the average full cost of outputs is not enough to be competitive in today's health care environment. Payers and providers must also be able to control costs. As noted previously, the direct and indirect cost information used to determine the cost of an output is not enough to control its cost.

Throughout the chapter we have noted that fixed and variable cost information is needed for planning total costs. Although fixed and variable cost information is important in project-

Table 7-6 The Fee-For-Service Method for Determining the Average Cost Per Member Per Month for All Medical Services and All Indirect Costs.

Type of Service	Annual Utilization Per 1000	Average Cost	Cost Per Member Per Month (1)	Co-Pay	Co-Pay PMPM(2)	Net Cost PMPM(3)
Hospital Inpatient						
Medical	145 days	$1068.90	12.92			12.92
Surgical	127 days	1793.41	18.98			18.98
Psychiatric	36 days	596.97	1.79			1.79
Alcohol & Drug	22 days	437.03	0.80			0.80
Maternity	31 days	1509.30	3.90			3.90
Subtotal	361 days		38.39			38.39
Hospital Outpatient						
Emergency Room	150 visits	202.00	2.53	25.00	0.31	2.22
Surgery	92 cases	1504.18	11.53			11.53
Other	445 serv.	187.83	6.97			6.97
Subtotal			21.03		0.31	20.72
Other						
Home Health Care	28 visits	150.00	0.35			0.35
Ambulance	14 runs	350.00	0.41			0.41
Infertility	4.4 serv.	2134.00	0.78	5.00	0.00	0.78
Dental	133 visits	96.00	1.06	5.00	0.06	1.00
Subtotal			2.60		0.06	2.54
Physician Costs			59.43			59.43
Total Medical Costs			121.45		0.37	121.08
Profit (5%)			6.07			6.07
Less Coordination of Benefits (4%)			4.86			4.86
Administration (15%)			18.22			18.22
Total			$140.88		$0.37	$140.51

(1) (Utilization per 1000 x Average cost)/12,000.
(2) (Co-Pay x (Utilization per 1000))/12,000.
(3) Cost PMPM – Co-Pay PMPM.

Figure 7-7   The Range of the Pricing Environment for Health Care Providers and Payers.

Firm As:	Pricing based on:
Price Setter	Costs or Charges
	Negotiated Prices
	Regulated Prices
Price Taker	Market Prices

ing costs, it is not sufficient for controlling costs. To control costs, as well as to evaluate performance, costs must be identified as controllable and noncontrollable. (See Table 7-1.) Further, who does or can control the cost must be identified.

During the planning or budgeting process, controllable costs are used to plan operations for the upcoming year. During and at the end of the fiscal year, actual and planned controllable costs are compared to assess cost control performance. In the remainder of this section, we discuss how controllable and noncontrollable cost information can help to control the costs of outputs.

Individual and Groups of Services

As mentioned previously, to control the costs of individual or groups of services, managers must first identify which costs are controllable for managers. In addition, they must identify factors, or **cost drivers**, which act alone and in combination, to influence these controllable costs. In Table 7-7, six factors or cost drivers for hospital costs are identified[1]. Similar cost drivers influence costs for other types of health care services. In addition the figure shows examples of controllable costs and who controls them. Since space is limited, the costs are only illustrative of the types of cost items for each cost driver. The examples are limited to the length of stay and laboratory test components of care. As can be seen from the table, both clinicians and managers can exert influence over costs and some of the groups exerting control are external to the organization. Next, each cost driver is briefly discussed.

As the *case-mix* of patients increases, resources per case and input unit prices are likely to increase. In contrast, as the *volume* of patients increases, the fixed costs of the provider may be spread over more patients, thereby reducing the cost per case. In addition to management, physicians and insurers exert control over the case mix and patient volume. Physicians admit and discharge patients to the facility. Insurers direct patients to certain facilities with which they have contractual arrangements.

Table 7-7 Examples of Cost Drivers, Controllable Costs, and Groups Exerting Control for a Patient Stay in an Acute Care Hospital.

Cost Drivers and Cost Items	*Groups Exerting Control*				
	Physicians	Other Clinical Staff	Senior Management	Managers of Clinical Services	Insurer
I. Case Mix	X		X		X
II. Patient Volume	X		X		X
III. Resources Per Case					
Length of Stay	X	X	X	X	X
Number of Diagnostic Exams	X			X	
IV. Input Unit Prices					
Cost of Labor			X	X	
Cost of Laboratory Supplies	X		X	X	
V. Input Efficiency					
Hours of Labor per Stay		X	X	X	
Laboratory Supplies per Test		X		X	
VI. Fixed Facility and Administrative Costs					
Building and Equipment	X		X	X	
Administrative Overhead			X		

Using more *resources per case* clearly drives costs up as does low *input efficiency* in delivering services. Senior management exerts influence over length of stay by working with clinicians to develop treatment protocols and expected lengths of stay for particular types of cases. Managers of clinical services, including nursing and ancillary services, as well as the clinical staff working in these areas, can influence the length of stay through efficient management and performing procedures in a timely and efficient manner. Similarly, clinical staff and management of laboratory services can control the supplies used per test by purchasing high quality supplies, setting standards, and performing efficiently. Insurers monitor and control the patient's length of stay as well.

Finally, high *fixed facility and administrative* costs will increase costs because they are indirect costs added to each output. Both management and clinicians exert control over building and equipment costs. Physicians demand certain equipment to produce services, but management evaluates the financial feasibility of each piece of equipment.

Availability of Services

At least some of the cost drivers for the cost of the availability of services overlap with those for health care services, especially if payers also are producers of services. In Table 7-8, using the insurer's perspective, seven cost drivers for the availability of health care services for an enrolled population are listed. As for services, each cost driver may influence costs alone as well as costs in combination with other cost drivers. These cost drivers and related costs are summarized below.

Demographic and socioeconomic characteristics of the enrolled population are related to the health status and the type of services that are needed. For example, an elderly population will use different services than a younger population. Further, an insurer may experience adverse selection if its enrollees are sicker than expected. These characteristics and the *volume* of enrollees are influenced by the insurer's marketing and enrollment efforts as well as by the willingness of primary care physicians to participate in the health plan.

Increasing the volume of enrollees, or covered lives, is an important way to control the average cost per member per month. Some members have high costs and some members have low costs but many members' cost per month lies in-between the extremes. When the number of enrollees is low, any extreme case, high or low, will influence the average quite a bit. In contrast, when the number of enrollees is high, a few extreme cases are not likely to influence the average cost per member per month as much.

This logic is also supported by some basic statistical concepts. The payer or health plan does not typically enroll all of the population of a geographic area. Instead, it "samples" from the population as it accumulates its enrollees. The cost per member per month is likely to be normally distributed for the underlying population. That is, the probability of any enrollee having an extremely high or low cost per month is likely to be low. The probability of any enrollee having a cost per month in the middle of the extremes is much higher. The plot of the probabilities and the cost per member per month takes on the characteristic bell-shaped normal curve.

Each possible sample of enrollees drawn from the population has a different average, or mean. Basic statistical concepts indicate that the average, or mean, of the sample means equals the population mean. In addition, the distribution of the means of the samples narrows as the number in each sample increases. For health plans and providers, this means that the risk of the average cost per member per month of its enrollees being much higher or lower than the expected, or population, mean decreases as enrollment increases. Figure 7-8 illustrates this phenomenon with the average total medical costs per member per month determined in Table 7-6.

The third cost driver, *utilization of services*, is influenced by the primary care physician as well as by specialist physicians and the insurer, which must approve utilization of services. Control over *input unit prices* paid to hospitals and specialist physicians depends upon their ability to negotiate as well as the payer's market power. However, if the payer adjusts pay-

Table 7-8 Examples of Cost Drivers, Controllable Costs, and Groups Exerting Control for Payers Who Are Not Providers.

Cost Drivers and Cost Examples	Groups Exerting Control			
	Hospital	Primary Care MD	Specialist MD	Insurer
I. Demographic and Socioeconomic Characteristics of Enrolled Population		X		X
II. Volume of Member Months		X		X
III. Utilization of Services				
Number of Primary Care Office Visits		X		X
Number of Specialist's Office Visits		X	X	X
Number of Hospitalizations		X	X	
IV. Input Unit Prices				
Hospitalization Payment	X			X
Specialist Visit Payment			X	X
V. Efficiency Per Episode of Care				
Number of Ancillary Tests per Visit or Stay		X	X	
Length of Hospital Stay	X	X	X	
VI. System Efficiency				
Clinical Complications	X	X	X	
Cost of Late Intervention in Disease Process		X	X	
Cost of Preventable Diseases		X		X
VII. Fixed Administrative Costs				X

ment for the severity of the illness, the demographic and socioeconomic characteristics of the enrolled population influence input unit prices. *Efficiency per episode* of care is controlled by the provider organizations but is also influenced by the needs of the enrolled population.

System efficiency affects costs through appropriate treatment of existing conditions and avoiding preventable conditions. Finally, insurers who administer health plans exert control over *administrative costs*.

Figure 7-8   Example of Distribution of Average Medical Service Cost per Member per Month by Number of Members.

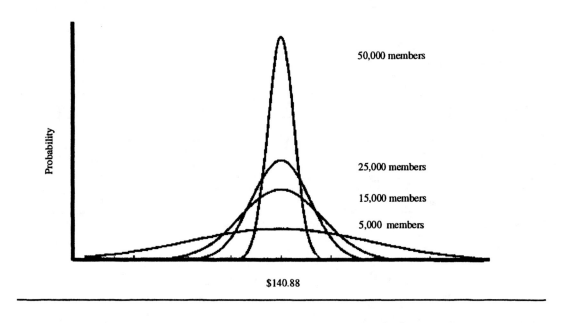

50,000 members

25,000 members

15,000 members

5,000 members

Probability

$140.88

Summary

Costing health care outputs involves estimating the direct cost per output and adding a *share* of the organization's costs that are indirect, or not readily traceable, to the output. The full cost information produced is useful in setting prices or in negotiating reimbursement rates. It also provides information on whether expected prices are likely to exceed the full costs of each output.

In this chapter, we have presented common methods of determining direct and indirect costs that can be used in a variety of health care organizations. Each method has strengths and weaknesses with regard to accuracy and costliness. For example, measurement of direct costs is the most accurate but also the most expensive method. The RCC method, in contrast, is not very costly, but it is also not very accurate. The more costly and accurate methods are most likely to be used with the organization's high volume and revenue outputs. Less costly, but usually less accurate, methods are likely to be used for low volume or low revenue outputs.

All of the full cost figures are *estimates* that reflect many accounting decisions. The estimates change if different accounting decisions are made. They also reflect the quality of the data used. Good accounting decisions and data of high quality enable the firm to improve the accuracy and, therefore, the usefulness of the cost estimates for pricing.

Managers should remember that these cost estimates are average costs. Since many health care costs are fixed, if the volume of output changes, the full cost of the output will also change. Similarly, the average full cost of an output can not simply be multiplied by a new volume to derive total costs. To do so would ignore the constancy of total fixed costs within a relevant operating range.

We have also discussed that direct and indirect cost information is not particularly useful for cost planning and control. Simply knowing the (average) full cost of outputs is not enough to be competitive in today's health care environment. Payers and providers must also be able to control costs. As noted previously, the direct and indirect cost information used to determine the cost of an output is not enough information on which to control any costs.

Fixed and variable cost information, which is important in projecting costs, is also not sufficient for controlling costs. To control costs, as well as to evaluate performance, organizations must identify controllable and noncontrollable costs. With this information, providers and payers can identify cost drivers and the activities to control costs.

Notes

1. Young, D.M. and L.K. Pearlman. "Managing the Stages of Hospital Cost Accounting" *Healthcare Financial Management* (April): 58-80,1993.

Bibliography

Aczel, A.D. *Complete Business Statistics*. Homewood, IL. : Irwin, 1989.

Awasthi, V.N. and L. Eldenburg. "Providing Cost Data to Physicians Helps Contain Costs" *Healthcare Financial Management* (April): 40-42, 1996.

Berlin, M.F. "Using Cost Accounting in a Medical Group Practice" *Medical Group Management Journal* (May-June) 42(3): 22-32, 1995.

Canby, J.B., IV. "Applying Activity-Based Costing to Healthcare Settings" *Healthcare Financial Management* (February): 50-56, 1995.

Cleverley, W.O. "Product Costing for Health Care Firms" *Health Care Management Review* 12(4): 39-48, 1987.

Federal Register, 42 CFR Parts 405 and 414, Thursday December 2, 1993.

Hill, N.T. "Adoption of Costing Systems by U.S. Hospitals" *Hospital and Health Services Administration* (Winter) 39(4): 521-537, 1994.

Karpiel, M.S. "Using Patient Classification Systems to Identify Ambulatory Care Costs" *Healthcare Financial Management* (November): 31-37, 1994.

Orloff, T.M., C.L. Littell, C. Clune, D. Klingman, and B. Preston. "Hospital Cost Accounting: Who's Doing What and Why" *Health Care Management Review* 15 (4): 73-78, 1990.

Prospective Payment Assessment Commission (ProPAC). 1995. *Report and Recommendations to the Congress*, March 1, 1995. Washington, D.C.: ProPAC.

Ramsey, R.H. "Activity-Based Costing for Hospitals" *Hospital & Health Services Administration* (Fall): 385-396, 1994.

Ryan, J. B. and S.B. Clay. "Understanding the Law of Large Numbers" *Healthcare Financial Management* (October): 22-24, 1995.

Schimmel, V.E., C. Alley and A.M. Heath. "Measuring Costs: Product Line Accounting Versus Ratio of Cost to Charges" *Topics in Health Care Finance* 13(4): 76-86, 1987.

Sutton, H.L., Jr. and A.J. Sorbo. *Actuarial Issues in the Fee-For-Service/Prepaid Medical Group*. Englewood, CO.: Center for Research in Ambulatory Health Care Administration, 1993.

Thorley Hill, N. and E. Loper Johns. "Adoption of Costing Systems by U.S. Hospitals" *Hospital & Health Services Administration* (Winter): 521-537, 1994.

Young, D.M. and L.K. Pearlman. "Managing the Stages of Hospital Cost Accounting" *Healthcare Financial Management* (April): 58-80, 1993.

Terms and Concepts

capitation rate	member month
cost driver	overhead
direct cost	price setter
full cost	price taker
indirect cost	ratio of cost to charges
	relative value units

Questions and Problems

7-1 How does the sophistication of an organization's information system affect its ability to identify direct costs?

7-2 Summarize the advantages and disadvantages of the following methods of identifying the direct costs of an output: a) RCC, b) RVU, and c) measurement.

7-3 Summarize the advantages and disadvantages of the following methods of identifying the indirect costs of an output: a) quantity of output and b) RVUs.

7-4 Explain why the full cost of an output derived using direct and indirect costs may not be particularly useful for planning or for cost control.

7-5 Which type of firms would be most likely to use the budgetary instead of the fee-for-service method of determining a capitation rate?

7-6 List some common examples of relative value units in health care.

7-7 False Cape Hospital wants to determine the cost of a patient day for the three levels of care it provides in its clinic. Direct nursing costs for the clinic for the fiscal year have been determined to be $187,000. Use the following data to determine the full cost each type of visit to the clinic.

Care Level	Patient Visits	Relative Weight
Subacute	2000	.75
Acute I	1500	1.0
Acute II	300	1.8
	3800	

7-8. An employer coalition in your state has cited the cost per patient day for cardiac care as being above the peer group standard. Your firm has argued that the patients are sicker so they spend more time in CCU than others and that it is the cost of the CCU part of the stay that drives up cost per day. To prove your point, you must cost days in the CCU, cardiac stepdown and medical/surgical units. Total costs for the cardiac care product line are $6,540,900.

Unit	Average Daily Supplies Cost	Average Daily Nursing Hours	Average Nursing Hourly Wage	Average Patient Intensity Level	Patient Days
CCU	$300	7.0	$20	4	1800
CCU Stepdown	200	5.0	19	2	2500
Med/Surg	100	3.0	18	1	3600

7-9. HMO, Inc. has offered a contract for hospital services for 6,000 covered lives to Hospital Health Network, Inc. (HHNI). HHNI plans to operate as a broker for hospital services in the region. The capitation rate HMO, Inc. has set is $50 per member per month. HHNI has gathered the following data regarding expected utilization and costs.

Service	Expected Utilization per 1000 members	Average Reimbursement ($)	Copay
Inpatient			
Med-Surg.	211 days	1259	
Maternity	57 days	1385	
ICU/CCU	31 days	2267	
Emergency Room	132 visits	275	50
Outpt. Surgery	50 surgeries	1649	
SNF	10 days	229	
Ambulance	40	258	25
Outpt. Hosp. Services	200	100	10

a. Evaluate the contract.
b. If HHNI found the capitation rate to be too low, what actions could the firm take to control costs?

7-10. The CFO of an HMO wants to use full cost information for pricing for the next fiscal year. Three types of contracts will be offered: (1) employee only, (2) family, and (3) employee and children. The COO has determined that the third type of contract is 2.3 times as resource intensive as the first and that the second type is 1.5 times as resource intensive as the first type. Projected full costs are $1,580,670. Determine the full cost of each type of contract using the following data.

Contract Type	Direct Variable Expected Volume	Cost per Contract
A	500	$ 60
B	1600	160
C	1400	140

7-11. Find the average cost per case for DRG 1200 using the following data from the hospitals in Hospital System, Inc. There were 500 cases during the last year.

Total Charges by Revenue Center

Dept.	Charges	Dept. RCC
Surgery	$1,250,000	0.90
ICU	900,000	0.75
Central Supply	25,000	1.20
Pharmacy	150,000	1.70
Laboratory	125,000	1.40
Radiology	300,000	1.30
Emergency	62,500	0.95

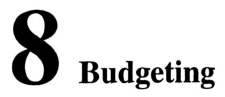

8 Budgeting

A budget is the basic financial document in most health care organizations. It is the fundamental tool for tying together the planning and control functions of management. Although novices to the budget process tend to approach budgeting with some trepidation, it can be understood relatively easily if it is thought of as a natural extension of the planning process.

In essence, the budget is the last product of the planning effort. A major outcome of planning is determining the organization's activities for the coming year. The budget converts activities into estimates of how many and what types of resources will be used, how these resources will be paid for, and how much revenue will be generated and received as a result of carrying out the planned activities.

This chapter begins with a discussion of the context within which budgeting takes place, considers the process by which a budget is formulated, and then presents a discussion of the four major types of budgets. Finally, an extensive budget preparation example for a not-for-profit community clinic is presented. The concepts and methods illustrated in this example are applicable to a wide range of health care provider and payer firms.

The Context of Budgeting

Planning

Planning can be viewed as a process by which a health care organization attempts to anticipate the future and determine the organization's role in shaping and reacting to a predicted set of events. Planning is comprised of three stages: (1) environmental assessment; (2) programming; and (3) budgeting.

Environmental Assessment. Because the future is uncertain, the success of planning rests upon how well providers and payers anticipate future events that will affect their ability to deliver services. In the past, with cost or charge based reimbursement for providers and with employers that were able to pay ever increasing premiums to payers, planning played a rather minor role in many health care organizations. However, in today's complex environment, many health care organizations are finding that systematic, formalized planning is not only a desirable activity, but a necessary prerequisite to both short- and long-term survival. In this vein, effective planning rests largely on the accuracy of an assessment of the environment.

The External Environment. It is useful to separate external from internal factors in the environmental assessment process. The **external environment** is comprised of those factors largely outside the jurisdiction or control of management that will have an effect upon the health care organization. These factors range from the international, national, and local economies to the physical environment and the rapidly changing world of health care technology. Examples of these factors for a provider organization are presented in Figure 8-1.

Theoretically, the results of an environmental assessment should be a set of assumptions concerning a series of narrowing levels of the environment: international, national, local, and organizational. For instance, because American firms face international competition in selling their goods and services, they are interested in controlling the cost of health care benefits they provide to their employees. Of course, international events affect day-to-day operations domestically as well. For instance, many health care organizations continue to be concerned with the effects of changes in the policies of oil-producing countries upon the prices paid domestically for energy. Assumptions about such conditions should be made in planning and developing budgets.

As with international events, changes in the national political and economic environments are important factors for health care firms to anticipate. The results of national elections can influence governmental policy toward health care providers and payers. Increasing competition among health care providers and changes in reimbursement methods and amounts are contributing to a change in the structures of provider organizations. The single physician practice is giving way to single and multispecialty group practices as well as a variety of physician-hospital organizations. Similarly, hospitals are no longer simply focusing on traditional in- and outpatient services, but are concerned with various forms of service delivery such as one-day surgicenters, health maintenance organizations (HMOs), and various non-health care endeavors. Some are forming joint ventures with insurance firms. These industry trends, although national in scope, become important marketing concerns at the local level and should be included in the assumptions made in planning the budget. Other national level concerns include certification procedures, the general economy, inflation, and employment.

The Marketing and Internal Environments. To determine how best to respond to the changing environment, health care organizations must also be concerned with their marketing and internal environments. As noted in Figure 8-1, the marketing environment includes both actual and potential patients, enrollees, payers, caregivers, and competing organizations.

The **internal environment** includes such factors as organizational structure, board composition, the traditional mission of the organization, and the personnel who manage and deliver health care services. All of these factors combine to become both resources and constraints with respect to which the organization plans its future (see Figure 8-1).

Programming. The actual process of planning for the future that follows environmental assessment is called **programming** (Figure 8-1). In programming, the organization translates its assumptions of what the future will be like into the steps it will implement to take advantage of the anticipated environment and accomplish its mission. At the most abstract level, this process begins with a mission statement that supplies an overall direction to the organiza-

Figure 8-1 Major Components in the Three Phases of Planning.

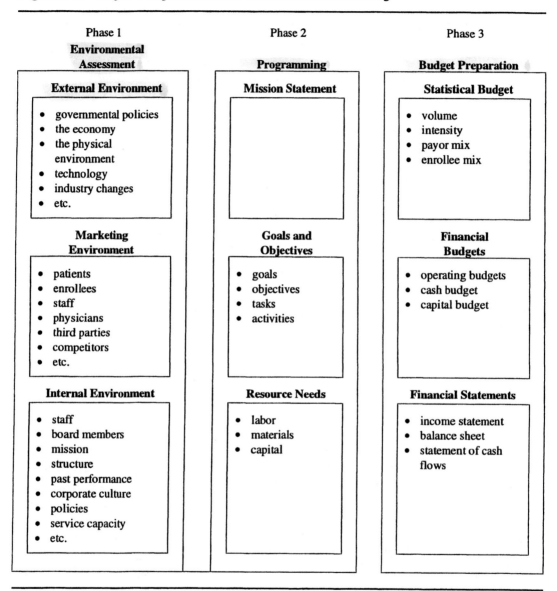

Phase 1 **Environmental Assessment**	Phase 2 **Programming**	Phase 3 **Budget Preparation**
External Environment • governmental policies • the economy • the physical environment • technology • industry changes • etc.	**Mission Statement**	**Statistical Budget** • volume • intensity • payor mix • enrollee mix
Marketing Environment • patients • enrollees • staff • physicians • third parties • competitors • etc.	**Goals and Objectives** • goals • objectives • tasks • activities	**Financial Budgets** • operating budgets • cash budget • capital budget
Internal Environment • staff • board members • mission • structure • past performance • corporate culture • policies • service capacity • etc.	**Resource Needs** • labor • materials • capital	**Financial Statements** • income statement • balance sheet • statement of cash flows

tion. The mission of governmental health care providers may be specified by law or regulation. Other health care providers and payers may have greater latitude in specifying their mission.

The mission statement, together with the environmental assessment, is translated into the goals and objectives of the organization or organizational unit. **Goals** are general statements concerning what the organization wants to accomplish (e.g., to develop a professional organization capable of meeting all health care needs of the service area at reasonable cost). **Objectives** are more specific statements of process or desired outcome (e.g., to decrease inpatient stays by 5% or decrease medical care expenses by 7.9%). Goals and objectives essentially answer questions related to what services are going to be offered, to whom, and how. In answering these questions, programming leads to budgeting. In determining how services are going to be offered, the firm must consider what resources will be needed and how they will be paid for. An example of a respiratory therapy department's objective and related resource requirements is presented in Exhibit 8-1.

Once goals, objectives, and resource requirements have been identified, the actual preparation of the budget may begin. **Budget preparation** is the process of translating goals, objectives, and activities into forecasts of anticipated volume, of the resources needed to provide services, and of the cost of those resources.

Postbudget Activities: Implementing and Controlling

Once the budget has been prepared, it serves as a guide to managers regarding the resources available to provide services. To the extent that the budget provides an accurate picture of how the organization intends to use its resources, any variances from the budget become important indicators of changes from anticipated levels of patient, service or resource mix. These variances can then be scrutinized to determine what courses of action are available for management to correct any problems that may exist. This concept is discussed in more detail in the next chapter.

The Budget Process _____

Who Budgets?

Many different approaches to budgeting exist. At one extreme, there are organizations in which a majority of the budgeting process takes place at the higher administrative levels of the organization. In this **authoritarian** or **top-down approach**, there is little involvement from the majority of the staff. This orientation toward budgeting has the advantages of being relatively expeditious and reflecting top management's perspective. On the other hand, it has the disadvantages of lacking the involvement, communication, and commitment that can result from a more participatory budget preparation endeavor. These disadvantages are usually not temporary. Morale problems and inefficiencies may result when staff are not aware of or feel they do not have control over the resources available to them. Similar problems may result when staff do not feel committed to management's goals as expressed in the budget. The authoritarian perspective toward budgeting seems to work best in small organizations where there is not a sharp division of labor, or where the organization has already developed a relatively authoritarian climate.

The **participatory approach** to budgeting, on the other hand, perceives the budgeting process from the point of view of **responsibility management**. This perspective assumes that authority and responsibility should be delegated to the lowest feasible level of manage-

Exhibit 8-1 An Example of a Respiratory Therapy Department Objective and Related Resource Specification.

Objective	Resource Requirements	Period Affected
Replace existing manual ventilation bags with continuous ventilators.	a. Receive supply budget funding (obj. Code 299) for purchase of new manual ventilation bags.	07/9X
Goals:	Cost: $7,000.00	
1. Increase patient safety	b. Authorize specifications for bid process.	07/9X
2. Decrease waste of liquid oxygen	c. Submit purchase request with specifications to purchasing.	08/9X
3. Inhibit unnecessary increase in liquid oxygen consumption	d. Complete bid process.	
	e. Receive and implement use of new manual ventilation equipment.	11/9X-12/9X 12/9X-01/9X

Objective Cost

299 expense	($7,000.00)
299 savings	9,821.00
Estimated net gain	$2,821.00

Explanation of Objective:

1. Cost of liquid oxygen has increased an average of 17% to 20% per year.

2. Cost of liquid oxygen is $.0041 per cubic foot.

3. 1 cubic foot of oxygen = 28.32 liters of oxygen

4. Adult manual ventilation bags placed with ventilators are used for patient care approximately 4 continuous hours per 24 hours.

5. Oxygen flow is left running to these manual ventilation bags by nurses at a rate of 10 liters per minute, 24 hours per day. Thus, 20 hours of gas flow is wasted per bag daily.

6. Consider the following:
   a. 10 liters per minute x 60 minutes = 600 liters per hour, 14,400 liters used per bag.
   b. 14,400 − 2,400 liters per day used in patient care = 12,000 liters wasted per day per bag.
   c. In fiscal year 1980-81, 5,590 patient days of manual ventilation bags used with ventilators.
   d. 12,000 liters divided by 28 liters per cubic foot = 428.5 cubic feet wasted per day per bag
   e. 5,590 patient days x 428.5 cubic feet wasted = 2,395,315 cubic feet wasted per year on all bags.
   f. 2,395,315 cubic feet x $.0041 = $9,820.8 cast of wasted gas per year.

ment in the organization. In this regard, responsibility center management attempts to include staff at numerous levels in the budgeting process. The belief is that, if people prepare their own budgets, a natural responsibility is built into the budget at each level at which the budget was prepared, and concurrently, there will be more commitment to the budget by those who prepared it. The main advantages of this approach are that it brings about a natural involvement, commitment, and communication among those involved. A major disadvantage is that the means (the budgeting process) can come to overshadow the ends (the budget); that is, time that could be spent on producing services and products may be spent in meetings and preparing forms related to the budget. A second disadvantage is that the final budget may not reflect top management's desires.

In fact, in many cases, balancing the authoritarian and participatory approaches is reasonable. Top administration should furnish the guidelines and parameters (such as the institutional goals and objectives for the year) and allow lower levels of management to work within them. Along with the administration and staff, representatives of the board of directors should be involved in the budget preparation process from its initial stages to its final approval. After all, the budget is ultimately the responsibility of the board.

Timing

Although some smaller organizations can complete the budgeting process in a relatively short time, larger health care organizations may be involved in some phase of the budgeting process during the entire year. A typical budgeting cycle begins with a distribution of a timetable and is followed shortly by top management's distribution of the institution's goals and objectives for the year. Next, the various departments are given time to prepare their volume projections and budgets and discuss them with various key personnel in the organization. Often several sessions are planned for top management to meet with each department so that the department can inform management of its thinking (no last-minute surprises!), and the department can be informed of and react to management's input and feedback. Finally, all department budgets are reviewed essentially simultaneously, modifications are made (usually after a highly political process), and the final budgets are prepared.

It should be noted that there is a trend toward supplementing annual budgeting with quarterly or monthly budgeting. Thus, the organization is continually looking a year ahead. These types of budgets which are continually updated are called **rolling budgets**. Since budgeting is an ongoing activity, it does not consume a large amount of resources all at once, but spreads the effort throughout the year.

Budgets

Although one often speaks of "the" budget, there are actually four major budgets in large organizations: the statistics budget, the operating budget, the cash budget, and the capital budget. In addition, a number of organizations also prepare income statements, balance sheets, and statements of cash flow on a pro forma basis (Figure 8-2). These budgets are illustrated later with an example for a not-for-profit clinic.

Figure 8-2 End Products of the Budgeting Process.

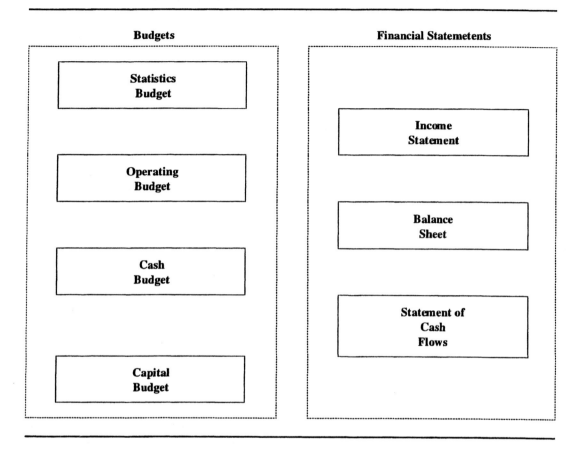

The Statistics Budget

The statistics budget is used to project the volume for the coming year. These volume estimates are then used to help forecast revenues and expenses on an accrual basis (the operating budget) and on a cash basis (the cash budget). The capital budget is used to project the costs associated with capital acquisitions. An example of a statistics budget can be seen in Table 8-1. This example forecasts volume using relative value units, (RVUs) which weight visits by the relative amount of time or resources they consume.

The Operating Budget

The operating budget is the second major type of budget (Table 8-2). It is comprised of two sub-budgets, the expense and revenue budgets, both of which are prepared on the accrual basis of accounting.

Table 8-1   Community Clinic Statistics Budget for 19X2 Relative Value Units of Service.

Payer Type	Jan	Feb	Mar	Apr	May	Jun	Jul	Aug	Sep	Oct	Nov	Dec	Total
Charge-Based													
Brief	34	45	61	56	53	46	38	39	50	55	46	40	563
Routine	522	698	938	858	814	712	590	610	772	842	710	610	8,676
Complex	752	1,008	1,356	1,240	1,176	1,028	852	880	1,116	1,216	1,028	880	12,532
Total	1,308	1,751	2,355	2,154	2,043	1,786	1,480	1,529	1,938	2,113	1,784	1,530	21,771
Cost-Based													
Brief	15	19	24	18	22	20	19	23	22	21	19	20	242
Routine	202	254	320	242	286	270	250	298	290	278	256	260	3,206
Complex	148	184	232	176	208	196	184	216	212	204	188	188	2,336
Total	365	457	576	436	516	486	453	537	524	503	463	468	5,784
Flat Fee													
Brief	6	6	6	6	6	6	6	16	15	6	6	6	91
Routine	80	80	80	80	80	80	80	190	174	80	80	80	1,164
Complex	36	36	36	36	36	36	36	84	76	36	36	36	520
Total	122	122	122	122	122	122	122	290	265	122	122	122	1,775
Capitation													
Brief	4	6	7	9	6	8	20	31	33	28	24	25	201
Routine	72	98	124	152	104	132	328	518	542	456	400	418	3,344
Complex	88	116	148	184	124	160	396	624	656	552	480	504	4,032
Total	164	220	279	345	234	300	744	1,173	1,231	1,036	904	947	7,577
Total RVUs	1,959	2,550	3,332	3,057	2,915	2,694	2,799	3,529	3,958	3,774	3,273	3,067	36,907

The Expense Budget. The expense budget is a dollar estimate of the amount of resources needed to provide products or services during the coming year. In large organizations, expenses are usually developed on a department-by-department basis and then consolidated into a single document. Currently, though, there is a trend to develop projections along product lines as well as by department. The expense budget comprises the bottom part of the operating budget (Table 8-2).

Each organization has its own unique types of expenses. A health maintenance organization typically lists expenses for hospital, physician, outpatient, Emergency Room, and out-of-area care as well as for administrative costs. For most provider organizations, the major item is the labor expense. In certain departments, such as pharmacy, or in smaller community health care organizations, labor expense may be relatively constant from month to month and from budget period to budget period. However, in larger organizations or those with large programmatic or seasonal fluctuations, personnel identification and scheduling may be a major undertaking. Nonlabor expenses for providers include materials and supplies, contractual ser-

Table 8-2 Community Clinic Operating Budget for 19X2.

	Jan	Feb	Mar	Apr	May	Jun	Jul	Aug	Sep	Oct	Nov	Dec	Total
Revenues													
Gross patient revenue	$45,786	$55,591	$68,739	$63,008	$62,788	$58,017	$56,251	$60,678	$68,674	$71,720	$66,400	$63,270	$740,922
Less deductions & allowances	2,781	3,582	4,646	3,847	4,103	3,742	3,324	3,740	4,045	4,107	3,638	3,435	44,990
Net patient revenue	43,005	52,009	64,093	59,161	58,685	54,275	52,927	56,938	64,629	67,613	62,762	59,835	695,932
Other revenue	2,486	2,272	2,532	2,471	2,654	2,681	2,661	2,690	2,647	2,886	2,763	2,911	31,654
Total revenue	$45,491	$54,281	$66,625	$61,632	$61,339	$56,956	$55,588	$59,628	$67,276	$70,499	$65,525	$62,746	$727,586
Expenses													
Labor	$25,538	$27,859	$31,163	$30,269	$30,489	$30,240	$31,412	$34,902	$36,788	$35,728	$35,412	$34,262	$384,062
Supplies	5,708	7,245	9,278	8,563	8,194	7,619	7,892	9,790	10,906	10,427	9,125	8,589	103,336
Interest	891	889	887	938	934	930	945	941	936	932	928	924	11,075
Penalties	110	7	0	0	0	0	0	0	0	12	0	0	129
Depreciation	792	792	792	792	913	913	713	744	744	744	744	744	9,427
Utilities	1,500	1,500	1,100	1,000	700	900	1,500	1,500	1,500	800	1,000	1,500	14,500
Rent	4,000	4,000	4,000	4,000	4,000	4,000	4,000	4,000	4,000	4,000	4,000	4,000	48,000
Cleaning	300	300	300	300	300	300	300	300	300	300	300	300	3,600
Telephone	350	350	350	350	350	350	350	350	350	350	350	350	4,200
Travel	67	67	67	67	67	67	67	67	67	67	67	67	804
Insurance	6,750	6,750	6,750	6,750	6,750	6,750	6,750	6,750	6,750	6,750	6,750	6,750	81,000
Maintenance	85	85	85	85	85	85	85	85	85	85	85	85	1,020
Provision for bad debts	1,195	1,574	2,088	1,846	1,824	1,620	1,380	1,484	1,764	1,864	1,603	1,425	19,667
Other	97	97	97	97	97	97	97	97	97	97	97	97	1,164
Total expenses	47,383	51,515	56,957	55,057	54,703	53,871	55,491	61,010	64,287	62,156	60,461	59,093	681,984
Excess of revenues over expenses	($1,892)	$2,766	$9,668	$6,575	$6,636	$3,085	$97	($1,382)	$2,989	$8,343	$5,064	$3,653	$45,602

vices, utilities, and depreciation. As with labor costs, the amounts needed in any of these items will be based on the forecasted volume of service to be delivered during the budget period.

The Revenue Budget. The second part of the operating budget is the revenue budget. The revenue budget comprises the top part of Table 8-2. Many health care organizations have many sources of revenue. A health maintenance organization reports revenues from premiums, coinsurance and interest income. Providers typically show patient and other revenues.

Traditionally, most health care providers have received the majority of their revenues from service-related activities, appropriations, or contributions. However, more and more providers are concerned with raising funds from non-health care activities such as investments, space rental, and various commercial enterprises. Because of the multiplicity of payers for health care services, the development of the revenue budget is somewhat more complex in many health care provider organizations than in traditional commercial enterprises. There are currently four major types of arrangements by which health care providers are paid: charges, costs, flat fee, and capitation.

Charges. Some patients or third party payers pay the charge the health care provider sets for the service. Usually the price is the cost of a service plus a markup. Some feel that this approach does not encourage efficiency, for it allows the health care provider to pass inefficiencies on to the consumer. On the other hand, to the extent that the provider is efficient, it can potentially recoup a larger margin at a given level of payment. It should be remembered that although a patient or a third party is billed for charges, it does not mean that they will pay the full amount. The difference between charges and the amount that will actually be paid is termed "deductions and allowances from revenue." This concept is further illustrated in the example of budget preparation that follows.

Cost-Based Reimbursement. A second means of payment is cost-based reimbursement. Under this arrangement, the patient or a third party agrees to pay for the "reasonable" costs of care. It was the predominant mode of payment by Medicare during the 1960s and 1970s and is still used by some third parties for some types of services. This method has the advantage of encouraging quality care, since the costs are paid for by the payer, but it tends to increase inefficiencies, in that inefficient and unnecessary costs may also be passed along to the payer.

Flat-Rate Reimbursement. A third means of payment is flat-rate reimbursement. Under this arrangement, the patient or third party determines in advance exactly what it will pay. This is the method now used by Medicare for inpatient operating costs under the prospective payment system (PPS), which is commonly referred to as the diagnosis-related groups (DRG) system of payment. Under PPS, the provider may keep the excess revenues beyond costs, but must absorb any loss. Thus, the provider is more at risk than under cost-based reimbursement. It is felt that this method tends to encourage efficiencies in the provision of care. Some feel it may have a detrimental effect on quality because the provider has incentives to provide fewer services to the patient to avoid a loss.

Capitated Payments. The fourth major means of payment is capitation. Under capitated payment arrangements, the provider receives a predetermined amount to take care of all or a portion of an enrollee's needs over a period of time, such as a month or a year. If the care that was provided costs less than the payments received, then the provider earns a profit. If the care costs more than the capitation, then the provider loses money. In general, capitated payment encourages efficiency and health promotion and disease prevention, but some feel it may have a detrimental effect on quality because providers have an incentive to provide too few services. Capitation is the payment method that is characteristic of HMOs and other managed care arrangements.

Together the revenue and expense budgets comprise the operating budget (Table 8-2). Note that since the operating budget is a forecast of revenues and expenses based on the accrual method of accounting, it is similar to the forecasted (pro forma) income statement for the next year. A forecasted income statement can be found later in this chapter.

The Cash Budget

Since the operating budget is prepared on the accrual basis of accounting, it does not tell an administrator the expected flow of cash in and out of the organization. That is the purpose of the cash budget (Table 8-3). The cash budget is derived by converting the operating budget from the accrual basis of accounting to cash flows.

As cash flows become more problematic in times of economic difficulties, the importance of an accurate projection of cash inflows and outflows increases. Although many health care organizations forecast cash flows on an annual or quarterly basis, it is becoming increasingly important to project cash flows on a daily or weekly basis at least a month in advance. The cash budget is discussed in Chapter 12 as well.

The Capital Budget

The capital budget is a budget reflecting expenses related to the purchase of major capital items such as plant and equipment. These items require major expenditures that must be anticipated and financed. Since a whole chapter of this text (Chapter 13) is devoted to capital budgeting, let it suffice here to say that the capital budget is usually a long-term budget, the current portions of which are reflected in the operating and cash budgets. An example of a minimal capital budget can be found in Table 8-4.

The Financial Statements

In addition to these four budgets, many health care organizations produce pro forma income statements, balance sheets, statements of cash flows, and selected ratios. Examples of these statements can be found in Tables 8-5 through 8-7.

Budget Preparation: An Example

To those who have never prepared one, the actual preparation of a budget may seem somewhat mystical and quite complex. In fact, although there are often numerous compo-

Table 8-3 Community Clinic Cash Budget for 19X2.

	Jan	Feb	Mar	Apr	May	Jun	Jul	Aug	Sep	Oct	Nov	Dec
Beginning Balance	$9,462	$11,000	$11,000	$11,000	$11,000	$11,000	$11,000	$11,000	$11,000	$11,000	$11,000	$11,000
Cash Collections	33,078	43,197	60,383	66,810	57,910	63,077	55,282	54,095	65,415	63,970	64,868	69,111
Less Expenditures	61,931	44,199	48,923	73,977	46,429	44,374	69,481	53,362	55,347	73,819	52,070	49,756
Cash Available Before Borrowing	-$19,391	$9,998	$22,460	$3,833	$22,481	$29,703	-$3,199	$11,733	$21,068	$1,151	$23,798	$30,355
Cash Requirement	11,000	11,000	11,000	11,000	11,000	11,000	11,000	11,000	11,000	11,000	11,000	11,000
Cash Shortage or Excess	-$30,391	-$1,002	$11,460	-$7,167	$11,481	$18,703	-$14,199	$733	$10,068	-$9,849	$12,798	$19,355
From Investments	30,391	1,002	0	7,167	0	0	14,199	0	0	9,849	0	0
Remaining Deficit	0	0	0	0	0	0	0	0	0	0	0	0
From Additional Debt	0	0	0	0	0	0	0	0	0	0	0	0
Cash From All Sources	11,000	11,000	22,460	11,000	22,481	29,703	11,000	11,733	21,068	11,000	23,798	30,355
Less: Transfer of Excess to Investments	0	0	11,460	0	11,481	18,703	0	733	10,068	0	12,798	19,355
Less: Repayment of Line of Credit	0	0	0	0	0	0	0	0	0	0	0	0
Ending Balance	$11,000	$11,000	$11,000	$11,000	$11,000	$11,000	$11,000	$11,000	$11,000	$11,000	$11,000	$11,000

Table 8-4 Community Clinic Capital Budget for 19X2.

Purchases	Purchase Price	Date of Purchase	Down Payment	Amt. of Loan	Interest Rate (%)	Financing Life (Years)	Monthly Payment	Balance of Principal	No. Pmts. Left	Source of Financing
Anticipated Purchases for 19X2										
Computer	$8,000	4/1/X2	$8,000	0						
Lab Equipment	3,000	7/1/X2	3,000	0						
Purchases from Prior Years										
X-Ray Equipment	30,000	1/1/X0	3,000	27,000	Variable	8	Variable	22,723	72	Commercial debt
Children's Waiting Room	15,000	6/1/X0	7,000	8,000	12	5	363	3,559	41	Commercial debt
Office Furniture	27,000	7/1/X1	2,700	24,300	8	5	422	24,335	54	Commercial debt

Table 8-5   Community Clinic Pro Forma Income Statement for 19X2.

Unrestricted revenues, gains and other support:	
Net patient revenue	$695,932
Other revenue	31,654
Total revenue, gains and other support	727,586
Expenses:	
Labor	384,062
Supplies	103,336
Interest	11,075
Penalties	129
Depreciation	9,427
Utilities	14,500
Rent	48,000
Cleaning	3,600
Telephone	4,200
Travel	804
Insurance	81,000
Maintenance	1,020
Provision for bad debts	19,667
Other	1,164
Total expenses	681,984
Excess of revenues over expenses	45,602
Extraordinary items	0
Increase in unrestricted net assets	$45,602

nents, the actual preparation of a budget is relatively simple when broken down into its component parts. A good place to begin is to look at the end products of the budgeting process and then determine how they were derived. As discussed previously, there are two standard outcomes of the budgeting process: budgets and pro forma financial statements. There are four budgets: the statistics budget, the operating budget, the cash budget, and the capital budget. The pro forma financial statements are the income statement, the balance sheet, and the statement of cash flows (Figure 8-2). Examples of these budgets and financial statements are found in Tables 8-1 through 8-6. These documents represent the end products of the budgeting process for Community Clinic, a hypothetical not-for-profit organization, which will be

Table 8-6 Community Clinic Pro Forma Balance Sheet for December 31, 19X2.

Assets		Liabilities and Equities	
Current Assets		**Current Liabilities**	
Cash	$11,000	Current debt on capital	$6,873
Short-term investments	13,000	Accounts payable	50,027
		Salaries payable	0
Accounts Receivable	51,914	Short-term loan payable	0
Less: Uncollectables	(4,860)		
		Total current liabilities	$56,900
Net Receivables	$47,054		
Inventory	8,592		
Prepaid Assets	585		
Total Current Assets	$80,231		
Noncurrent Assets		**Noncurrent Liabilities**	
Equipment (at cost)	73,000	Long-Term Debt	99,097
Less: Accumulated	(23,618)		
Depreciation	49,382		
Long-Term Investments	428,427	Total Liabilities	$155,997
Total Noncurrent Assets	$477,809	Net Assets	402,043
Total Assets	$558,040	Total Liabilities and Equities	$558,040

Table 8-7 Community Clinic Selected Pro Forma Ratios for Year Ending 12/31/X2.

Liquidity	
Current ratio	1.40
Quick ratio	1.25
Turnover	
Total asset turnover	1.30
Average collection period	24.68 days
Accounts payable period	176.70 days
Profitability	
Operating margin	6.27%
Return on assets	8.20%
Return on equity	11.30%
Capitalization	
Long-term debt to total assets	0.18
Times interest earned	5.12

used in this section to illustrate the process of budget preparation. The budget development process described here is generic, and any particular organization will likely have its own idiosyncrasies.

The Statistics Budget

The first budget document to be prepared is the statistics budget (Table 8-1). The statistics budget is a forecast of the amount of activity, or volume, that can be expected during the period for which the budget is being prepared.

Developing volume projections is considered by many to be the most crucial step in budget preparation, because estimates of volume will lead to estimates of the amount of services that will be provided. Eventually, the service estimates are converted into estimates of (1) the dollars in revenue that can be expected as a result of service delivery, and (2) the amounts of resources needed to provide services and their associated expenses and expenditures.

For providers of health care services, the initial step in developing volume estimates is to develop initial patient volume estimates by payer type. Payer organizations develop estimates of the number and type of enrollees and their expected utilization of services. For ambulatory care organizations such as Community Clinic, volume is initially estimated in terms of the number of visits that can be expected. Many organizations will refine these estimates by categorizing visits by level of intensity or go still one step further by converting estimates of visit by intensity into relative value units.

Estimating visits for the next year (Table 8-8) is typically accomplished by reviewing the amounts and types of services the organization delivered last year and modifying last year's statistics based upon management's environmental assessment and the organization's plans for the coming years(s).

For those desiring more precision, the next step is to adjust these estimates for their intensity. This step recognizes that not all visits will require the same number of resources. For instance, in an ambulatory setting it may take very few resources, including time, to take out stitches or to treat a flu patient, whereas a considerable amount of resources may be needed for a full physical. Community Clinic categorizes its patients into three levels of intensity: those requiring a brief visit, those requiring a routine visit, and those requiring a complex visit. To convert its estimated visit statistics (Table 8-8) into visits by level of intensity (Table 8-9), Community Clinic merely has to multiply its estimated visits in any payer category by the expected percentage of those visits that it expects in each level of intensity.

Example: For the month of January, Community Clinic estimates it will have 483 visits by patients who pay charges (Table 8-9). Of these visits, it forecasts that approximately 7% will be brief visits, 54% will be routine visits, and 39% will be complex visits. With this information, Community Clinic estimates the number of visits by level of intensity as follows:

Table 8-8 Community Clinic Projected Number of Visits by Type of Payer for 19X2.

Payer Type	Jan	Feb	Mar	Apr	May	Jun	Jul	Aug	Sep	Oct	Nov	Dec	Total
Charge-based	483	646	869	795	754	659	546	564	715	780	658	565	8,034
Cost-based	153	192	242	183	217	204	190	226	220	211	194	197	2,429
Flat fee	55	55	55	55	55	55	55	132	121	55	55	55	803
Calculation of capitated visits													
19X2 enrollment	2050	2091	2133	2176	2220	2263	2830	2972	3120	3276	3440	3612	32,183
% making visit	3%	4%	4.97%	6%	4%	5.04%	10%	15%	15%	12%	10%	9.97%	
Capitated visits	62	84	106	131	89	114	283	446	468	393	344	360	2,881
Total visits	753	977	1,272	1,164	1,115	1,032	1,074	1,368	1,524	1,440	1,251	1,177	14,147

1. Visits in January by charge-based patients: 483   483   483

2. Percentage of visits by level of intensity:
   A. Brief   7%
   B. Routine   54%
   C. Complex   39%

3. Charge-based visits by intensity in January.   34   261   188

Although estimates have now been derived of the number of visits by intensity, no estimate has been made of the relative amount of effort it will take to provide service for a brief visit versus routine and complex visits. In our example, assume that Community Clinic estimates that a brief visit takes approximately 15 minutes, a half-hour for a routine visit, and one hour for a complex visit. Thus, the ratio among these three types of visits is 1:2:4, respectively. The unit of measurement by which the relative amount of resources is measured is called a **relative value unit** (RVU). In this example, one relative value unit equals 15 minutes of time.

To convert its estimates of number of visits by intensity (Table 8-9) into RVUs (Table 8-10), Community Clinic merely multiplies the number of expected visits in each level of intensity by its corresponding relative value weight.

Example: For the month of January, Community Clinic estimates it will have 34 brief visits, 261 routine visits, and 188 complex visits by its charge-based patients (Table 8-9). The clinic uses a relative value scale where one RVU equals 15 minutes, and the ratio of brief to routine to complex visits in RVUs is 1:2:4. Community Clinic converts its estimated visits by intensity into estimates of RVUs needed next year as follows:

		Visit Type		
		Brief	Routine	Complex
1.	Number of visits by type	34	261	188
2.	Relative value weight of visit	1	2	4
3.	Number of RVUs for charge-based payers in January (Table 8-10)	34	522	752

Tables 8-8 through 8-10 present Community Clinic's estimate of its 19X2 number of visits by payer type, number of visits by intensity and payer type, and RVU by payer type, respectively. Depending upon how precise an organization makes its budget estimates and the types of services involved (not all services can be readily converted into RVUs), any of these three estimates might serve as the statistics budget for the rest of the budgeting process. For the example presented here, we will use the RVU estimate as the statistics budget for Community Clinic.

Table 8-9 Community Clinic Visits by Level of Intensity Projected for 19X2.

Payer Type	Jan	Feb	Mar	Apr	May	Jun	Jul	Aug	Sep	Oct	Nov	Dec	Total
Charge-based													
Brief	34	45	61	56	53	46	38	39	50	55	46	40	563
Routine	261	349	469	429	407	356	295	305	386	421	355	305	4,338
Complex	188	252	339	310	294	257	213	220	279	304	257	220	3,133
Total	483	646	869	795	754	659	546	564	715	780	658	565	8,034
Cost-based													
Brief	15	19	24	18	22	20	19	23	22	21	19	20	242
Routine	101	127	160	121	143	135	125	149	145	139	128	130	1,603
Complex	37	46	58	44	52	49	46	54	53	51	47	47	584
Total	153	192	242	183	217	204	190	226	220	211	194	197	2,429
Flat fee													
Brief	6	6	6	6	6	6	6	16	15	6	6	6	91
Routine	40	40	40	40	40	40	40	95	87	40	40	40	582
Complex	9	9	9	9	9	9	9	21	19	9	9	9	130
Total	55	55	55	55	55	55	55	132	121	55	55	55	803
Capitation													
Brief	4	6	7	9	6	8	20	31	33	28	24	25	201
Routine	36	49	62	76	52	66	164	259	271	228	200	209	1,672
Complex	22	29	37	46	31	40	99	156	164	138	120	126	1,008
Total	62	84	106	131	89	114	283	446	468	394	344	360	2,881
Total visits	753	977	1,272	1,164	1,115	1,032	1,074	1,368	1,524	1,440	1,251	1,177	14,147

Table 8-10 Community Relative Value Units of Service Projected for 19X2.

Payer Type	Jan	Feb	Mar	Apr	May	Jun	Jul	Aug	Sep	Oct	Nov	Dec	Total
Charge-based													
Brief	34	45	61	56	53	46	38	39	50	55	46	40	563
Routine	522	698	938	858	814	712	590	610	772	842	710	610	8,676
Complex	752	1,008	1,356	1,240	1,176	1,028	852	880	1,116	1,216	1,028	880	12,532
Total	1,308	1,751	2,355	2,154	2,043	1,786	1,480	1,529	1,938	2,113	1,784	1,530	21,771
Cost-based													
Brief	15	19	24	18	22	20	19	23	22	21	19	20	242
Routine	202	254	320	242	286	270	250	298	290	278	256	260	3,206
Complex	148	184	232	176	208	196	184	216	212	204	188	188	2,336
Total	365	457	576	436	516	486	453	537	524	503	463	468	5,784
Flat fee													
Brief	6	6	6	6	6	6	6	16	15	6	6	6	91
Routine	80	80	80	80	80	80	80	190	174	80	80	80	1,164
Complex	36	36	36	36	36	36	36	84	76	36	36	36	520
Total	122	122	122	122	122	122	122	290	265	122	122	122	1,775
Capitation													
Brief	4	6	7	9	6	8	20	31	33	28	24	25	201
Routine	72	98	124	152	104	132	328	518	542	456	400	418	3,344
Complex	88	116	148	184	124	160	396	624	656	552	480	504	4,032
Total	164	220	279	345	234	300	744	1,173	1,231	1,036	904	947	7,577
Total RVUs	1,959	2,550	3,332	3,057	2,915	2,694	2,799	3,529	3,958	3,774	3,273	3,067	36,907

The Operating and Cash Budgets

Once the statistical budget has been developed, it becomes possible to develop the operating and cash budgets. These budgets are parallel in form. The major difference between the two is that the operating budget is prepared on the accrual basis of accounting, whereas the cash budget is prepared on the cash basis of accounting. The two sections of the operating budget are *revenues* and *expenses* (Table 8-2). The two sections of the cash budget are *receipts* and *expenditures* (Table 8-3). Since the cash receipts projections are developed on the basis of the accrual revenue estimates, and the expenditure projections (cash) are derived from the expense budget (accrual), we will develop the revenue and receipts budgets and then develop the expense and expenditure budgets.

The Revenue Budget

Accrual Basis. There have traditionally been three major phases in developing the revenue budget for providers of health care services: (1) developing estimates of gross patient revenues; (2) developing estimates of net patient revenues; and (3) developing estimates of other revenues. The results of these three steps are then combined to develop the revenue budget. In the future as more payers move to flat fee or capitation payment, the first step will be eliminated.

Estimates of patient revenues are developed by applying a fee schedule to the projections made in the statistics budget. A fee schedule is a list of the full amounts an organization will charge for its various services. Hospitals may have literally thousands of chargeable items. On the other hand, a small clinic may group its charges into relatively few categories.

Let us assume that Community Clinic has three basic charges: professional fees per RVU, lab fees per RVU, and supply charges per RVU (Table 8-11). These charges are all based on charges per RVU of service.

A person making a brief visit to Community Clinic will be charged $17.75, a person receiving any type of visit classified as routine will be charged $35.50, and a person receiving services classified as a complex visit will be charged $71.00, regardless of the specific services received. Community Clinic merely has to apply its fee schedule to its service estimates

Table 8-11 Community Clinic Fee Schedule for 19X2.

Charge	Brief Visit	Routine Visit	Complex Visit
Professional fees	$11.50	$23.00	$46.00
Laboratory fees	3.00	6.00	12.00
Supply charges	3.25	6.50	13.00
Total charges/visit	$17.75	$35.50	$71.00

to develop a forecast of gross revenues (Table 8-12). The gross charges to charge-based payers in January for each of the three services (professional, laboratory, and supplies) would be calculated in the following example.

Example: For the month of January, Community Clinic charges $11.50 per RVU for each professional visit, $3.00 per RVU for laboratory services, and $3.25 per RVU for supplies. It expects to deliver 1,308 RVUs of service to its charge-based patients this month.

	Professional	Laboratory	Supplies	Summary
Estimated January RVUs (note 1)	1,308	1,308	1,308	1,308
Fees (note 2)	$11.50	$3.00	$3.25	$17.75
Gross charges for January (note 3)	$15,042	$3,924	$4,251	$23,217

Note 1. From statistics budget (Table 8-1).
Note 2. From fee schedule (Table 8-11).
Note 3. The summary figure is shown on the gross revenue schedule (Table 8-12).

Although the above method is appropriate for charge-based patients, a different method of calculating gross revenues may be used where contracts for HMO or preferred provider organization (PPO) services have been negotiated. Rather than report what the charges would have been had the services been cost- or charge-based, the organization records the actual negotiated price that a third party has agreed in advance to pay.

For instance, if Community Clinic had negotiated with a third party to provide physical examinations for $13.00 each, even though the examinations consumed one hour each, $13.00 would be recorded rather than the $71.00 that would have been recorded under the RVU method of charging. This approach is similar to that used by many health care organizations for budgeting for DRGs. However, instead of having just one item paid on a flat fee, over 400 would have to be taken into account. One of the major advantages of this method of recording and reporting transactions is that it more nearly reflects the fiscal realities of the situation. A major disadvantage is that it is more difficult to compute how much the organization is gaining or losing on this category of patients compared to normal charges.

The capitated visits are based upon the negotiated rate per each enrollee assigned to Community Clinic, not upon the estimated visits or RVUs for this category of payer. Thus, if Community Clinic has negotiated a fee of $7.50 per enrollee per month, regardless of the number of visits the enrollees make and the services they receive, it will record total revenues on the basis of $7.50 for each enrolled client.

Table 8-12 Community Clinic Gross Patient Revenues for 19X2.

Payer Type	Jan	Feb	Mar	Apr	May	Jun	Jul	Aug	Sep	Oct	Nov	Dec	Total
Charge-based	$23,217	$31,081	$41,802	$38,234	$36,264	$31,702	$26,270	$27,140	$34,400	$37,506	$31,666	$27,158	$386,440
Cost-based	6,479	8,112	10,224	7,739	9,159	8,627	8,041	9,532	9,301	8,929	8,219	8,307	102,669
Flat fee	715	715	715	715	715	715	715	1,716	1,573	715	715	715	10,439
Capitation	15,375	15,683	15,998	16,320	16,650	16,973	21,225	22,290	23,400	24,570	25,800	27,090	241,374
Total	$45,786	$55,591	$68,739	$63,008	$62,788	$58,017	$56,251	$60,678	$68,674	$71,720	$66,400	$63,270	$740,922

Table 8-13 Community Clinic Revenue Deductions and Allowances for 19X2.

Payer Type	Jan	Feb	Mar	Apr	May	Jun	Jul	Aug	Sep	Oct	Nov	Dec	Total
Charge-based	$1,161	$1,554	$2,090	$1,912	$1,813	$1,585	$1,314	$1,357	$1,720	$1,875	$1,583	$1,358	$19,322
Cost-based	1,620	2,028	2,556	1,935	2,290	2,157	2,010	2,383	2,325	2,232	2,055	2,077	25,668
Flat fee	0	0	0	0	0	0	0	0	0	0	0	0	0
Capitation	0	0	0	0	0	0	0	0	0	0	0	0	0
Total	$2,781	$3,582	$4,646	$3,847	$4,103	$3,742	$3,324	$3,740	$4,045	$4,107	$3,638	$3,435	$44,990

Example: Community Clinic has negotiated with the community to provide 55 physicals a month for $13.00 each. The clinic has also contracted with an HMO and has agreed to accept $7.50 per month per enrollee, regardless of services rendered. For the month of January, Community Clinic would compute its anticipated gross revenue for the flat-fee and capitated patients as follows:

Flat-fee charge per visit	$13	
Flat-fee visits	55	
Capitation per month		$7.50
Capitation enrollees	____	2,050
Total gross charges	$715	$15,375

The next step, developing estimates of revenue deductions and allowances, requires that the health care organization estimate the amount of its gross revenues that it will not be able to collect, called deductions and allowances, and then subtract this amount from gross revenues. There are two major categories of revenue deductions and allowances: contractual allowances and charity deductions. **Contractual allowances** are estimates of the difference between gross charges and the amount that third parties agree to pay. The **charity deduction** estimates the difference between the amount that a health care organization would normally charge for its services to charity patients and the amount that it expects to receive from those patients. Formerly, an allowance for bad debts was also included as a deduction. Now, however, the amount of charges not collected from those able to pay is an expense, which will be discussed later.

As with all forecasts in the budget, the amount of deductions and allowances is derived by reviewing the past history of the organization in this regard and making projections based upon assumptions derived in the planning process. One of the most common ways of developing estimates of deductions and allowances is to estimate what percentage of revenues earned this year will likely not be collected because of contractual and charity allowances. The percentage estimate is converted into a dollar amount by multiplying the percentage of deductions and allowances by the corresponding gross charges by payer category.

Example: Assume Community Clinic estimates that for its charge-based patients there will be 5% contractual allowances and 0% charity allowances in January. The dollar amount of deductions and allowances for this category of payer is figured as follows:

Charges	$23,217	(Table 8-12)
Deductions	x .05	
Total deductions and allowances	$ 1,161	(Table 8-13)

The deduction and allowance estimates for the other payer were derived in a similar manner (Table 8-13).

Once deductions and allowances have been computed, net operating revenues are determined by subtracting deductions and allowances from gross charges (Table 8-14). For example, the charge-based net revenue by payer category was calculated as follows:

Total gross charges	$23,217	(Table 8-12)
Deductions and allowances	– 1,161	(Table 8-13)
Net operating revenue	$22,056	(Table 8-14)

The net revenue estimates for the other payers are derived in a similar manner (Table 8-14).

The third step in developing the accrual revenue budget is to develop estimates of other operating revenues, gains or losses. A health care organization earns other operating revenues, gains or losses from activities other than delivering health care to patients or providing insurance coverage to enrollees. Examples include interest earned on investments, fees from educational programs, consulting contracts, and parking lot revenues. Community Clinic's estimates of its other operating revenues can be seen in Table 8-15, the revenue budget.

The last step in developing the revenue budget is to summarize the operating and other revenues (Table 8-15).

Example: For January, Community Clinic determines its net revenues for all payers as follows:

Gross patient revenues	$45,786	(Table 8-12)
Deductions and allowances	2,781	(Table 8-13)
Total	$43,005	(Table 8-14)
Other revenues	2,486	(Table 8-15)
Net revenues	$45,491	(Table 8-15)

Cash Basis. Once the accrual-based revenue budget has been developed, the cash basis revenue budget can be derived. This is accomplished by making a payment profile of each type of payer and applying that profile to this year's estimated revenues.

Example: Community Clinic is estimating that, of the amount billed charge-based payers in the month of January, $23,217 (Table 8-12), 31% will be collected in January, 51% will be collected in February, 6% will be collected in March, 3% will be collected in April, and the rest will not be collected. The 9% that will not be collected includes the 5% contractual allowance as well as 4% for bad debts. The clinic estimates its cash collections of January's charges as follows:

	Jan.	Feb.	Mar.	Apr.	Total
Total gross charges	$23,217				
Percent of January charges collected in various months	31%	51%	6%	3%	91%
Cash receipts	$7,197	$11,841	$1,393	$697	$21,127

These numbers can be found beginning with the number in the top left hand corner of the cash collections schedule, Table 8-16, and stairstepping down to the right in each successive month. The $21,127 that will be collected over the first 120 days from the date of service represents 91% of the charges. The other 9% is the amount attributed to deductions and allowances as well as to bad debts. A 4% bad debt rate is also assumed for cost based revenues but a 1% bad debt rate is expected for the fixed fee revenues.

In addition to the cash receipts from operations that have just been computed, cash receipts from other operating sources must be estimated in a similar manner. Once this information is developed, the cash receipts budget can be derived by aggregating the information for all payers and other operating items (Table 8-17).

The Expense and Expenditure Budgets. As with the revenues, the costs of the organization are estimated on both accrual and cash bases. The **expense budget** estimates the costs of the organization on the accrual basis, whereas the **expenditure budget** estimates them on a cash basis. Together, the accrual revenue budget and the expense budget will be brought together in the operating budget. The cash receipts budget and the expenditure budget are combined to make the cash budget of the organization.

Both the expense and the expenditure budget derive their information from four sources, each of which is a budget in and of itself: (1) the supplies budget, (2) the labor budget, (3) the administrative and general expense budget, and (4) the capital budget (Figure 8-3). Each of these budgets will be discussed in turn. Since the cash budgets can be derived directly from their accrual counterparts, both the accrual and the cash-based budget will be discussed together.

The Supplies Budget. There are two major steps in developing the supplies expense budget on the accrual basis (Table 8-18): estimating variable supplies expenses and estimating fixed supplies expenses.

The amount of variable supplies that will be needed each month is estimated by multiplying the number of units of services to be administered by the variable cost of each unit. In the case of Community Clinic, the number of units has been projected on the statistics budget. The cost per unit of variable supplies as well as the fixed cost per month is usually derived from past experience, modified for any major changes expected during the period for which the budget is being prepared.

Example: Assume Community Clinic estimates that its variable supply cost per RVU is $2.60. It has projected 1,959 RVUs in January. Furthermore, it estimates it will use $615 in fixed expenses each month. These consist mainly of office and miscellaneous supplies. Community Clinic would determine its cost of goods sold (COGS) for January as follows:

Supply cost per RVU	$ 2.60	Estimate
January RVUs	x 1,959	Statistics budget
January variable COGS	$ 5,093	
January fixed supplies usage	615	Estimate
January supplies expense	$ 5,708	Supplies budget (accrual basis) (Table 8-18)

Table 8-14 Community Clinic Net Patient Revenues for 19X2.

Payer Type	Jan	Feb	Mar	Apr	May	Jun	Jul	Aug	Sep	Oct	Nov	Dec	Total
Charge-based	$22,056	$29,527	$39,712	$36,322	$34,451	$30,117	$24,956	$25,783	$32,680	$35,631	$30,083	$25,800	$367,118
Cost-based	4,859	6,084	7,668	5,804	6,869	6,470	6,031	7,149	6,976	6,697	6,164	6,230	77,001
Flat fee	715	715	715	715	715	715	715	1,716	1,573	715	715	715	10,439
Capitation	15,375	15,683	15,998	16,320	16,650	16,973	21,225	22,290	23,400	24,570	25,800	27,090	241,374
Total	$43,005	$52,009	$64,093	$59,161	$58,685	$54,275	$52,927	$56,938	$64,629	$67,613	$62,762	$59,835	$695,932

Table 8-15 Community Clinic Revenue Budget for 19X2.

Revenue Type	Jan	Feb	Mar	Apr	May	Jun	Jul	Aug	Sep	Oct	Nov	Dec	Total
Gross patient revenues	$45,786	$55,591	$68,739	$63,008	$62,788	$58,017	$56,251	$60,678	$68,674	$71,720	$66,400	$63,270	$740,922
Less deductions & allowances	2,781	3,582	4,646	3,847	4,103	3,742	3,324	3,740	4,045	4,107	3,638	3,435	44,990
Net patient revenues	43,005	52,009	64,093	59,161	58,685	54,275	52,927	56,938	64,629	67,613	62,762	59,835	695,932
Other revenues	2,486	2,272	2,532	2,471	2,654	2,681	2,661	2,690	2,647	2,886	2,763	2,911	31,654
Total revenues	$45,491	$54,281	$66,625	$61,632	$61,339	$56,956	$55,588	$59,628	$67,276	$70,499	$65,525	$62,746	$727,586

Table 8-16   Community Clinic Cash Collection Schedule for 19X2.

Payer Type	Jan	Feb	Mar	Apr	May	Jun	Jul	Aug	Sep	Oct	Nov	Dec	Total
Charge-based													
Current month	$7,197	$9,635	$12,959	$11,852	$11,242	$9,827	$8,144	$8,413	$10,664	$11,627	$9,816	$8,419	$119,795
30-60 days	6,183	11,841	15,851	21,319	19,499	18,495	16,168	13,398	13,842	17,544	19,128	16,150	189,418
61-90 days	834	727	1,393	1,865	2,508	2,294	2,176	1,902	1,576	1,628	2,064	2,250	21,217
91-120 days	520	417	364	697	932	1,254	1,147	1,088	951	788	814	1,032	10,004
> 120 days	0	0	0	0	0	0	0	0	0	0	0	0	0
Total	$14,735	$22,620	$30,566	$35,733	$34,181	$31,870	$27,635	$24,801	$27,033	$31,587	$31,822	$27,851	$340,434
Cost-based													
Current month	1,166	1,460	1,840	1,393	1,649	1,553	1,447	1,716	1,674	1,607	1,479	1,495	18,479
30-60 days	766	1,620	2,028	10,450	1,935	2,290	2,157	2,010	2,383	2,325	2,232	2,055	32,251
61-90 days	797	797	1,685	2,109	2,658	2,012	2,381	2,243	2,091	2,478	2,418	2,321	23,991
91-120 days	70	61	61	130	162	204	155	183	173	161	191	186	1,736
>120 days	0	0	0	0	0	0	0	0	0	0	0	0	0
Total	$2,799	$3,938	$5,614	$14,082	$6,404	$6,059	$6,140	$6,152	$6,321	$6,571	$6,320	$6,057	$76,457
Flat fee													
Current month	179	179	179	179	179	179	179	429	393	179	179	179	2,612
30-60 days	501	250	250	250	250	250	250	250	601	551	250	250	3,903
61-90 days	501	501	250	250	250	250	250	250	250	601	551	250	4,154
91-120 days	57	57	57	29	29	29	29	29	29	29	69	63	506
>120 days	0	0	0	0	0	0	0	0	0	0	0	0	0
Total	$1,238	$987	$736	$708	$708	$708	$708	$958	$1,273	$1,360	$1,049	$742	$11,175
Capitation													
Current month	13,838	14,114	14,398	14,688	14,985	15,275	19,103	20,061	21,060	22,113	23,220	24,381	217,235
30-60 days	469	1,538	1,568	1,600	1,632	1,665	1,697	2,123	2,229	2,340	2,457	2,580	21,897
61-90 days	0	0	0	0	0	0	0	0	0	0	0	0	0
91-120 days	0	0	0	0	0	0	0	0	0	0	0	0	0
>120 days	0	0	0	0	0	0	0	0	0	0	0	0	0
Total	$14,306	$15,652	$15,966	$16,288	$16,617	$16,940	$20,800	$22,184	$23,289	$24,453	$25,677	$26,961	$239,132
Total	$33,078	$43,197	$52,883	$66,810	$57,910	$55,577	$55,283	$54,095	$57,916	$63,971	$64,868	$61,611	$667,198

Table 8-17 Community Clinic Cash Collections Budget for 19X2.

Revenue Type	Jan	Feb	Mar	Apr	May	Jun	Jul	Aug	Sep	Oct	Nov	Dec	Total
Patient	$33,078	$43,197	$52,883	$66,810	$57,910	$55,577	$55,282	$54,095	$57,915	$63,970	$64,868	$61,611	$667,196
Other	0	0	7,500	0	0	7,500	0	0	7,500	0	0	7,500	30,000
Total	$33,078	$43,197	$60,383	$66,810	$57,910	$63,077	$55,282	$54,095	$65,415	$63,970	$64,868	$69,111	$697,196

Table 8-18 Community Clinic Supplies Budget—Accrual Basis for 19X2.

Supplies	Jan	Feb	Mar	Apr	May	Jun	Jul	Aug	Sep	Oct	Nov	Dec	Total
Variable supplies	$5,093	$6,630	$8,663	$7,948	$7,579	$7,004	$7,277	$9,175	$10,291	$9,812	$8,510	$7,974	$95,956
Fixed supplies	615	615	615	615	615	615	615	615	615	615	615	615	7,380
Total supplies	$5,708	$7,245	$9,278	$8,563	$8,194	$7,619	$7,892	$9,790	$10,906	$10,427	$9,125	$8,589	$103,336

Figure 8-3   The Expense Budgets (on the cash basis these are referred to as expenditure budgets).

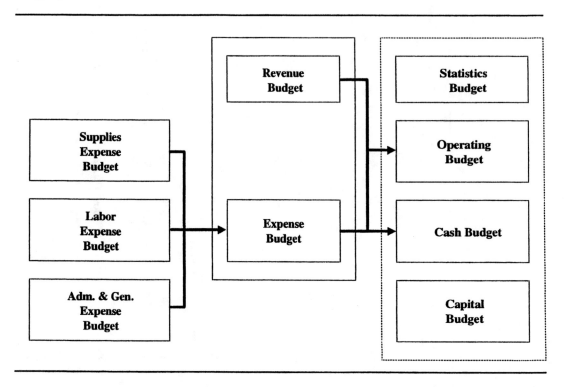

The amount reported on the supplies expenditure budget depends upon the amount of goods purchased and the payment schedule. The amount to be purchased in any month is dependent upon the amount of supplies on hand at the beginning of the month, the amount of supplies needed during the month, and the amount of supplies that needs to be available at the beginning of the next month. The costs of supplies used during the month can be derived as in the example just given, and a similar approach is used to determine the amount of goods that must remain in ending inventory. Once these are known, the amount of purchases needed each month can be estimated using the following formula:

Purchases   = Desired ending inventory
              + Estimated cost of supplies used
              – Beginning inventory

To determine the amount to be reported on the cash expenditure budget, the organization merely has to develop a payment schedule and apply it to the amount of purchases each month.

Example: Assume Community Clinic estimates that it must have goods on hand at the beginning of February equal to 115% of February's cost of goods sold. Community Clinic begins the year with $5,154 worth of goods, and will pay for any purchases in the month following the purchase. Variable supplies purchased in December 19x1 were $8,510. Fixed supplies purchased and used each month are $615. They are paid for in the next month. To estimate purchases in January, Community Clinic makes the following calculations:

Supply cost per RVU	$ 2.60	Given
February RVUs	x 2,550	Statistics budget
February COGS	$ 6,630	Calculated
Safety stock factor	x 115%	Given
January ending inventory	$ 7,625	Calculated
January COGS	5,093	Above example
Goods available	$12,718	Calculated
Jan. beginning inventory	- 5,154	Given
Variable purchases for January	7,564	Calculated
Fixed purchases for January	615	Given
Total purchases for January	$ 8,179	Calculated

Since Community Clinic assumes that it pays its supplies bills the month after goods are purchased, the $8,179 becomes the budget figure for the supplies cash budget in February (Table 8-19).

The Labor Budget. There are two major types of labor costs: fixed and variable. The preparation of the cash and accrual labor budgets entails preparing estimates of the costs for both types of labor as well as their accompanying benefits.

Estimating the salary and benefits of fixed labor is relatively straightforward. Records are usually kept either by person, position, or both, depending upon the sophistication of the organization's compensation and personnel policies. For positions that are presently filled, the current salary is carried forward into the budget year, with modifications made for expected raises and adjustments. Unfilled positions are similarly budgeted, with salaries beginning either at the beginning of the year, on the date the position is authorized to be filled, or when the position is actually expected to be filled. Choosing one of these alternatives depends upon the policies and procedures of the organization. The data needed to calculate Community Clinic's fixed labor budget (Table 8-21) are found in Table 8-20, which presents fixed labor payroll data.

Example: The following example for Physician B is drawn from the fixed labor payroll data given in Table 8-20. The results can be found in Table 8-21, which presents salaries and benefits data for full-time employees:

Table 8-19 Community Clinic Supplies Budget—Cash Basis for 19X2.

	Jan	Feb	Mar	Apr	May	Jun	Jul	Aug	Sep	Oct	Nov	Dec	Total
Variable supplies	$8,510	$7,564	$8,967	$7,841	$7,524	$6,918	$7,318	$9,459	$10,459	$9,740	$8,315	$7,893	$100,508
Fixed supplies	615	615	615	615	615	615	615	615	615	615	615	615	7380
Total supplies	$9,125	$8,179	$9,582	$8,456	$8,139	$7,533	$7,933	$10,074	$11,074	$10,355	$8,930	$8,508	$107,888

Table 8-21 Community Clinic Salaries and Benefits for Full-Time Employees.

Position	Jan	Feb	Mar	Apr	May	Jun	Jul	Aug	Sep	Oct	Nov	Dec	Total
Physician (A)	$6,985	$6,985	$6,985	$6,985	$6,985	$8,985	$8,985	$6,985	$8,985	$8,985	$8,985	$8,985	$83,823
Physician (B)	5,068	5,068	5,068	5,068	5,068	5,068	5,929	5,929	5,929	5,929	5,929	5,929	65,981
Nurse midwife	2,957	2,957	2,957	2,957	2,957	2,957	2,957	2,957	2,957	2,957	3,401	3,401	36,373
Registered nurse	2,530	2,530	2,530	2,530	2,530	2,530	2,530	2,530	2,530	2,530	2,530	2,530	30,359
LPN (A)	1,843	1,843	1,843	1,843	1,843	1,843	1,843	1,843	2,120	2,120	2,120	2,120	23,226
LPN (B)	1,675	1,926	1,926	1,926	1,926	1,926	1,926	1,926	1,926	1,926	1,926	1,926	22,861
Medical technician	1,930	1,930	1,930	1,930	1,930	1,930	2,219	2,219	2,219	2,219	2,219	2,219	24,897
Receptionist	1,337	1,337	1,337	1,337	1,337	1,337	1,337	1,337	1,337	1,337	1,337	1,337	16,044
Billing clerk (A)	1,213	1,213	1,213	1,359	1,359	1,359	1,359	1,359	1,359	1,359	1,359	1,359	15,868
Billing clerk (B)	0	0	1,114	1,114	1,114	1,114	1,114	1,114	1,114	1,114	1,114	1,114	11,137
Office manager	0	0	0	0	0	1,332	1,332	1,332	1,332	1,332	1,332	1,332	9,324
Total	$25,538	$25,789	$26,903	$27,049	$27,049	$28,381	$29,531	$29,531	$29,808	$29,808	$30,252	$30,252	$339,891

Table 8-20   Community Clinic Fixed Labor Payroll Data for 19X2.

Position	Current Salary	Benefit (%)	Date of next raise	Annual Raise* (%)
Physician (A)	$65,131	17	Jan/X2	10
Physician (B)	51,976	17	Jul/X2	17
Nurse midwife	30,857	15	Nov/X2	15
Registered nurse	23,571	15	Jan/X2	12
LPN (A)	19,235	15	Sep/X2	15
LPN (B)	17,476	15	Feb/X2	15
Medical technician	20,139	15	Jul/X2	15
Receptionist	13,643	12	Jan/X2	5
Billing clerk	12,998	12	Apr/X2	12
Billing clerk	11,932	12	Mar/X2	0
Office manager	14,271	12	Jun/X2	0

*Raise given on anniversary date of hire.

$ 4,331.33	Monthly salary before raise ($51,976 / 12)
736.33	Monthly benefits before raise
$ 5,068	Monthly salary and benefits before raise (after rounding)
$ 5,068	Monthly salary after raise
862	Monthly benefits after raise (rounded)
$ 5,929	Monthly salary and benefits after raise (after rounding)

Variable staffing is being used increasingly by health care providers in place of full-time or fixed staffing. The use of variable staffing allows the organization to staff according to the actual volume or need for staff, whereas with fixed staffing there tend to have either too many or too few staff to meet demand. Similarly, in many cases, variable labor is paid a flat rate per unit, receiving few if any benefits, as opposed to fixed labor whose benefits may be approximately 20% of salary. In the case of Community Clinic, the variable staffing is designed to allow temporary staff to fill in when the patient load becomes too great for its full-time licensed practical nurses (LPNs) to handle.

To derive how many variable staffing hours are needed, Community Clinic needs to make assumptions concerning (a) the number of full-time LPNs; (b) the number of RVUs each full-time LPN can service per day; (c) the pay rate per hour per LPN; (d) the workdays per month; and (e) the number of RVUs that temporary staff LPNs can provide per hour. This information, as it is compiled by Community Clinic, appears in Table 8-22 and is used in compiling the data in the variable staffing budget.

As is shown in Table 8-23, the computation of variable staffing needs begins with a listing of the number of workdays in the month. When this number is multiplied by the maximum number of RVUs per day per LPN, it yields the maximum number of RVUs per month per LPN:

Table 8-22 Community Clinic Variable Staffing Data for 19X2.

	Jan	Feb	Mar	Apr	May	Jun	Jul	Aug	Sep	Oct	Nov	Dec
Work days per month	20	20	22	22	20	22	23	21	21	22	19	20
Maximum RVUs per LPN per day	50	50	50	50	50	50	50	50	50	50	50	50
Full-Time LPNs	2	2	2	2	2	2	2	2	2	2	2	2
LPN pay rate per hour	$10	$10	$10	$10	$10	$10	$10	$10	$10	$10	$10	$10
RVUs per hour for temporary LPNs	2.66	2.66	2.66	2.66	2.66	2.66	2.66	2.66	2.66	2.66	2.66	2.66

Table 8-23   Community Clinic Variable Staffing Budget for 19X2.

	Jan	Feb	Mar	Apr	May	Jun	Jul	Aug	Sep	Oct	Nov	Dec	Total
Work days per month	20	20	22	22	20	22	23	21	21	22	19	20	252
Maximum RVUs per LPN per day	50	50	50	50	50	50	50	50	50	50	50	50	50
Monthly RVU capacity per LPN	1,000	1,000	1,100	1,100	1,000	1,100	1,150	1,050	1,050	1,100	950	1,000	12,600
Fixed full-time LPNs	2	2	2	2	2	2	2	2	2	2	2	2	2
Monthly fixed LPN capacity	2000	2000	2200	2200	2000	2200	2300	2100	2100	2200	1900	2000	
Budgeted RVUs for month	1,959	2,550	3,332	3,057	2,915	2,694	2,799	3,529	3,958	3,774	3,273	3,067	36,907
Understaffed RVUs	0	550	1,132	857	915	494	499	1,429	1,858	1,574	1,373	1,067	11,748
RVUs per hour for temporary LPNs	2.66	2.66	2.66	2.66	2.66	2.66	2.66	2.66	2.66	2.66	2.66	2.66	
LPN hours needed	0	207	426	322	344	186	188	537	698	592	516	401	4,417
LPN pay rate per hour	$10	$10	$10	$10	$10	$10	$10	$10	$10	$10	$10	$10	
Variable wages	$0	$2,070	$4,260	$3,220	$3,440	$1,860	$1,880	$5,370	$6,980	$5,920	$5,160	$4,010	$44,170

Days per month	20
Maximum RVUs per day per LPN	x 50
Maximum RVUs per month per LPN	1,000

The maximum number of RVUs per day per LPN is the number of RVUs of service provided by the clinic that can be serviced by an LPN in a single day. It should be noted that, for each RVU a patient is charged, the patient may in fact only be seen by the physician or the LPN for less than half that time. If only one RVU were being delivered at a time, and one RVU was equal to 15 minutes, and an LPN worked eight hours a day, then an LPN could deliver 32 RVUs per day (four RVUs per hour times eight hours). If the same LPN spends an average of 7.5 minutes per patient for each 15 minutes charged, the LPN could deliver 64 RVUs per day (eight RVUs per hour times eight hours). Community Clinic is assuming that its full-time LPNs can service about 50 RVUs per day.

When the maximum number of RVUs per month per LPN is multiplied by the number of full-time LPNs on staff, the result is the maximum number of RVUs per month that can be delivered by the full-time LPNs on staff.

Maximum RVUs per month per LPN	1,000
Number of LPNs on staff	x 2
Maximum RVUs that can be delivered this month	2,000

Subtracting the RVUs that will be delivered during this month from the maximum number of RVUs that can be delivered by the full-time LPNs during the month tells how many RVUs of service cannot be delivered by the existing full-time complement of LPNs. They are calculated as follows:

Maximum RVUs that can be delivered this month	2,000
RVUs expected this month	− 2,550
Excess RVUs being delivered this month	550

The extra number of LPN hours needed is based upon an estimate of the number of RVUs that a full-time LPN can provide in an average hour. Part-time help may not be as productive as full-time workers, perhaps because part-time help is less experienced or new to the system, or because the clinic cannot anticipate the patient flow precisely, so that there are times when part-time staff may be underutilized. For such reasons, Community Clinic has estimated that each temporary LPN can deliver 2.66 RVUs per hour. To determine the actual paid hours needed, the understaffed RVUs are divided by 2.66. For Community Clinic in February:

$$550 \text{ RVUs} / 2.66 \text{ RVUs per hour} = 207 \text{ hours.}$$

The final step in developing the variable staffing budget is to calculate the actual variable wages to be paid to the part-time LPNs who are hired. This is done by multiplying the paid hours needed by the hourly rate. For Community Clinic for February, the variable labor expense is:

$$\$10 \text{ per hour} \times 207 \text{ hours} = \$2070.$$

Once the fixed and variable labor budgets have been developed, the accrual and cash labor budgets can be drawn up. The accrual labor budget (Table 8-24) is merely a summary of the fixed and variable labor budgets. Since Community Clinic pays its wages twice a month and its second payment is made on the last day of the month, there are no accruals, and the cash labor budget is exactly the same as the accrual labor budget.

The Administrative and General Expense Budget. As the name implies, the administrative and general expense budget presents estimates of the administrative and general expenses for the next year. These expenses include such items as interest, depreciation, rent, and telephone. Community Clinic's administrative and general expense budget can be found in Table 8-25. Included in this budget is the provision for bad debts. Four percent of charge and cost based gross revenues are expected to be bad debts as well as one percent of fixed fee revenues. The actual payments for administrative and general expenses are reflected in Community Clinic's administrative and general expenditure budget, Table 8-26. Since the bad debts are excluded from the cash collections budget, they are not shown in the expenditure budget.

The Expense and Expenditure Budget. The information from the supplies, labor, and administrative and general expense budgets, together with information on the capital budget, is summarized in the expense and expenditure budget. The expense budget (Table 8-27) is the accrual analogue to the cash expenditure budget (Table 8-28).

Preparing the Operating and Cash Budgets. The operating budget is the accrual budget for the organization (Table 8-2). All the information necessary to prepare the operating budget has already been developed. The revenues for this budget come from the accrual revenue budget (Table 8-15), whereas the expenses were computed in the expense budget (Table 8-27). The only amount that needs to be computed is the excess of revenues over expenses, or net income, which is the difference between net revenues and net expenses.

The cash budget (Table 8-3) is the cash basis analogue to the operating budget. The revenues are those presented in the cash-based receipts or collections budget (Table 8-17) whereas the expenditures are taken directly from the expenditure budget (Table 8-28). However, in addition to the budget information that has already been developed, the cash budget requires some additional calculations in regard to what the organization plans to do if it has cash shortages or cash overages in any particular month.

The cash budget begins with a beginning balance, which in January comes from the 19X1 balance sheet. In all other months, the beginning cash balance is the ending cash balance from the previous month. To find out how much cash is available at the end of the month, the month's cash collections are added to the beginning balance, and the expenditures are sub-

Table 8-24 Community Clinic Labor Budget for 19X2—Accrual Basis.

Expenses	Jan	Feb	Mar	Apr	May	Jun	Jul	Aug	Sep	Oct	Nov	Dec	Total
Fixed salaries	$22,087	$22,305	$23,300	$23,430	$23,430	$24,619	$25,608	$25,608	$25,848	$25,848	$26,234	$26,234	$294,551
Fixed benefits	3,451	3,484	3,603	3,619	3,619	3,761	3,924	3,924	3,960	3,960	4,018	4,018	45,341
Subtotal	$25,538	$25,789	$26,903	$27,049	$27,049	$28,380	$29,532	$29,532	$29,808	$29,808	$30,252	$30,252	$339,892
Variable wages	0	2,070	4,260	3,220	3,440	1,860	1,880	5,370	6,980	5,920	5,160	4,010	44,170
Total	$25,538	$27,859	$31,163	$30,269	$30,489	$30,240	$31,412	$34,902	$36,788	$35,728	$35,412	$34,262	$384,062

Table 8-25 Community Clinic Administrative and General Expenses for 19X2—Accrual Basis.

Expense	Jan	Feb	Mar	Apr	May	Jun	Jul	Aug	Sep	Oct	Nov	Dec	Total
Interest	$891	$889	$887	$938	$934	$930	$945	$941	$936	$932	$928	$924	$11,075
Penalties	110	7	0	0	0	0	0	0	0	12	0	0	129
Depreciation	792	792	792	792	913	913	713	744	744	744	744	744	9,427
Utilities	1,500	1,500	1,100	1,000	700	900	1,500	1,500	1,500	800	1,000	1,500	14,500
Rent	4,000	4,000	4,000	4,000	4,000	4,000	4,000	4,000	4,000	4,000	4,000	4,000	48,000
Cleaning	300	300	300	300	300	300	300	300	300	300	300	300	3,600
Telephone	350	350	350	350	350	350	350	350	350	350	350	350	4,200
Travel	67	67	67	67	67	67	67	67	67	67	67	67	804
Insurance	6,750	6,750	6,750	6,750	6,750	6,750	6,750	6,750	6,750	6,750	6,750	6,750	81,000
Maintenance	85	85	85	85	85	85	85	85	85	85	85	85	1,020
Provision for bad debts	1,195	1,574	2,088	1,846	1,824	1,620	1,380	1,484	1,764	1,864	1,603	1,425	19,667
Other	97	97	97	97	97	97	97	97	97	97	97	97	1,164
Total	$16,137	$16,411	$16,516	$16,225	$16,020	$16,012	$16,187	$16,318	$16,593	$16,001	$15,924	$16,242	$194,586

Table 8-26 Community Clinic Administrative and General Expenditures for 19X2—Cash Basis.

Expenditure	Jan	Feb	Mar	Apr	May	Jun	Jul	Aug	Sep	Oct	Nov	Dec	Total
Principal	$245	$248	$250	$450	$453	$457	$527	$531	$535	$540	$544	$548	$5,328
Interest	891	889	887	938	934	930	945	941	936	932	928	924	11,075
Equipment Purchases	0	0	0	8,000	0	0	3,000	0	0	0	0	0	11,000
Penalties	0	110	7	0	0	0	0	0	0	0	12	0	129
Utilities	1,400	1,500	1,500	1,100	1,000	700	900	1,500	1,500	1,500	800	1,000	14,400
Rent	4,000	4,000	4,000	4,000	4,000	4,000	4,000	4,000	4,000	4,000	4,000	4,000	48,000
Cleaning	0	900	0	0	900	0	0	900	0	0	930	0	3,630
Telephone	340	350	350	350	350	350	350	350	350	350	350	350	4,190
Travel	45	67	67	67	67	67	67	67	67	67	67	67	782
Insurance	20,250	0	0	20,250	0	0	20,250	0	0	20,250	0	0	81,000
Maintenance	0	0	1,020	0	0	0	0	0	0	0	0	0	1,020
Other	97	97	97	97	97	97	97	97	97	97	97	97	1,164
Total	$27,268	$8,161	$8,178	$35,252	$7,801	$6,601	$30,136	$8,386	$7,485	$27,736	$7,728	$6,986	$181,718

Table 8-27   Community Clinic Expense Budget for 19X2—Accrual Basis.

Expense	Jan	Feb	Mar	Apr	May	Jun	Jul	Aug	Sep	Oct	Nov	Dec	Total
Labor	$25,538	$27,859	$31,163	$30,269	$30,489	$30,240	$31,412	$34,902	$36,788	$35,728	$35,412	$34,262	$384,062
Supplies	5,708	7,245	9,278	8,563	8,194	7,619	7,892	9,790	10,906	10,427	9,125	8,589	103,336
Interest	891	889	887	938	934	930	945	941	936	932	928	924	11,075
Penalties	110	7	0	0	0	0	0	0	0	12	0	0	129
Depreciation	792	792	792	792	913	913	713	744	744	744	744	744	9,427
Utilities	1,500	1,500	1,100	1,000	700	900	1,500	1,500	1,500	800	1,000	1,500	14,500
Rent	4,000	4,000	4,000	4,000	4,000	4,000	4,000	4,000	4,000	4,000	4,000	4,000	48,000
Cleaning	300	300	300	300	300	300	300	300	300	300	300	300	3,600
Telephone	350	350	350	350	350	350	350	350	350	350	350	350	4,200
Travel	67	67	67	67	67	67	67	67	67	67	67	67	804
Insurance	6,750	6,750	6,750	6,750	6,750	6,750	6,750	6,750	6,750	6,750	6,750	6,750	81,000
Maintenance	85	85	85	85	85	85	85	85	85	85	85	85	1,020
Provision for bad debts	1,195	1,574	2,088	1,846	1,824	1,620	1,380	1,484	1,764	1,864	1,603	1,425	19,667
Other	97	97	97	97	97	97	97	97	97	97	97	97	1,164
Total Expenses	$47,383	$51,515	$56,957	$55,057	$54,703	$53,871	$55,491	$61,010	$64,287	$62,156	$60,461	$59,093	$681,984

Table 8-28   Community Clinic Expenditure Budget for 19X2—Cash Basis.

Expenditure	Jan	Feb	Mar	Apr	May	Jun	Jul	Aug	Sep	Oct	Nov	Dec	Total
Labor	$25,538	$27,859	$31,163	$30,269	$30,489	$30,240	$31,412	$34,902	$36,788	$35,728	$35,412	$34,262	$384,062
Supplies	9,125	8,179	9,582	8,456	8,139	7,533	7,933	10,074	11,074	10,355	8,930	8,508	107,888
Administrative & General													
Principal	245	248	250	450	453	457	527	531	535	540	544	548	5,328
Interest	891	889	887	938	934	930	945	941	936	932	928	924	11,075
Equipment Purchases	0	0	0	8,000	0	0	3,000	0	0	0	0	0	11,000
Penalties	0	110	7	0	0	0	0	0	0	0	12	0	129
Utilities	1,400	1,500	1,500	1,100	1,000	700	900	1,500	1,500	1,500	800	1,000	14,400
Rent	4,000	4,000	4,000	4,000	4,000	4,000	4,000	4,000	4,000	4,000	4,000	4,000	48,000
Cleaning	0	900	0	0	900	0	0	900	0	0	930	0	3,630
Telephone	340	350	350	350	350	350	350	350	350	350	350	350	4,190
Travel	45	67	67	67	67	67	67	67	67	67	67	67	782
Insurance	20,250	0	0	20,250	0	0	20,250	0	0	20,250	0	0	81,000
Maintenance	0	0	1,020	0	0	0	0	0	0	0	0	0	1,020
Other	97	97	97	97	97	97	97	97	97	97	97	97	1,164
Total	$61,931	$44,199	$48,923	$73,977	$46,429	$44,374	$69,481	$53,362	$55,347	$73,819	$52,070	$49,756	$673,668

tracted. In January, there is a cash deficit of $19,391. This amount, called cash available before borrowing, is then compared with the cash requirements for the month.

Cash requirements refers to the amount of cash that an organization has deemed necessary to have on hand at the end of the month in order to begin operations the next month. An organization may estimate this number a variety of ways, two of the most common being as a flat amount, say $10,000, or as a percentage of next month's estimated need. Community Clinic has estimated its cash requirements as $11,000 per month, based on the relationship of cash needs and service to be rendered, taking the next month's cash inflows and outflows into account.

In comparing cash available before borrowing with the month's cash requirements, if the result is positive—that is, if there is more cash available before borrowing than the cash required for the month—then there is a cash excess. In the case of cash excesses, no money needs to be borrowed. In fact, excess cash should be invested.

If the cash available before borrowing is less than the cash requirements, there is a cash shortage. In such a case, Community Clinic has the choice of borrowing money and thus taking on additional debt, or taking money out of its investments. In deciding which of these options to choose, Community Clinic must carefully weigh the interest it must pay to borrow money with the interest it will lose by taking money out of its investments, should there be funds available in these accounts, and the associated penalties for doing so.

The cash generated from borrowing and/or taken out of investment accounts is added to the initial cash shortage to derive the cash from all sources. If the cash from all sources is greater than the cash requirements, the excess is transferred to investments, and the ending balance is equal to the cash available less the amount transferred. Cash and investment management are discussed more in Chapter 12.

The Capital Budget

The capital budget presents information concerning the major long-term investments of the organization proposed for this year. To help evaluate the proposed purchases, some organizations also list current capital obligations. Community Clinic's capital budget is presented in Table 8-4. The capital budgeting process is discussed in Chapter 13.

Pro Forma Financial Statements and Ratios

The Income Statement. Whereas actual financial statements are prepared at year-end (see Chapter 2), a pro forma income statement presents the forecasted revenues and expenses of an organization based on the accrual method of accounting (Table 8-5). This information has already been developed for Community Clinic in its operating budget (Table 8-2) and is summarized in the income statement.

The Balance Sheet. Most of the information necessary to develop the balance sheet (Table 8-6) has already been calculated. The only amounts that remain to be developed are accounts receivable and prepaid accounts. A discussion of these two items is beyond the scope of this chapter.

Ratios. From the information presented in the income statement and the balance sheet, it is now possible to calculate various ratios for Community Clinic (Table 8-7). In the past few years, boards of directors have broadened the scope of their budget review. Whereas some boards still primarily focus upon the cash budgets of the organization, there is a growing awareness of the importance of accrual-based financial statements and the added insight that ratios derived from these statements provide. A complete discussion of ratio analysis is included in Chapter 3.

Summary

This chapter began by emphasizing the interdependence of budgeting and planning and the use of the budget in program implementation and control. The end product of the planning process is the statistics budget, which in turn is used to estimate resource needs and revenues. The operating budget estimates revenue and expenses with the accrual basis of accounting, while the cash budget estimates associated cash flows. The capital budget is used to project expenses for large projects. Pro forma budgets can be summarized as financial statements. We concluded with a lengthy example of the preparation of a budget.

Bibliography

Cook, D. "Strategic Plan Creates a Blueprint for Budgeting" *Healthcare Financial Management* (May): 21-27, 1990.

Hilton, R.W. *Managerial Accounting.* New York: McGraw-Hill, Inc., 1991.

Kerschner, M.I. and J.M. Rooney. "Utilizing Cost Accounting Information for Budgeting" *Topics in Health Care Financing* 13(4): 56-66, 1987.

Ward, D.L. "Operational Finance and Budgeting" in Kongstvedt, P.R. *The Managed Care Handbook, Second Edition.* Gaithersburg, MD: Aspen, 1993.

Washburn, E.R. "Budgeting for a More Likely Future" *Medical Group Management Journal* (July/August): 74-78, 1995.

Terms and Concepts

authoritarian approach
budget preparation
budget schedules
budget timelines
capital budget
cash budget
charity deduction
contractual allowance
environmental assessment
external environment
expense budget
expenditure budget

goals
internal environment
objectives
operating budget
participatory approach
planning
programming
relative value units
responsibility management
revenue budget
rolling budgets
top-down approach

Questions and Problems

8-1 What is the purpose of a budget?

8-2 List the three stages of planning and briefly describe each.

8-3 Contrast the "authoritarian/top down" approach and the "participatory" approach with regard to budgeting. What are the advantages and disadvantages of each? Which approach would be more suitable for a small organization?

8-4 What are "rolling budgets"?

8-5 Name the four general types of budgets.

8-6 How do operating and cash budgets differ?

8-7 What is a fee schedule?

8-8 Table 8-16 reports collections from patients. What would be the advantages if all collections could be obtained within two months of the time from when services were rendered?

8-9 Tables 8-20 through 8-24 focus on expenses associated with salaries and other fringe benefits. Notice that there is a distinction between the way full-time and part-time employees are treated. Discuss major advantages and disadvantages of employing workers on a full-time versus a part-time basis.

8-10 Define RVUs (relative value units) as defined by Community Clinic. Why are RVUs employed?

8-11 List and briefly describe the three major phases in developing the revenue budget.

8-12 How would the revenue budget for a payer organization differ from that of a provider organization?

8-13 Assume Community Clinic wants to compare its current projections (Table 8-9) with projections based on the following assumptions: intensity levels for charge-based patients are 15% for brief visits, 25% for routine, and 60% for complex. Using Table 8-9 as a guide, calculate the new projection of visit level by intensity for charge-based patients. Would such changes in intensity be of consequence at the organizational level? How?

8-14 Given Community Clinic's supplies budget, assume that the price of syringes and paper gowns increased. This results in a supply cost per relative value unit increasing from the given $2.60 to $3.20. Show the new supplies budget on the accrual basis, assuming that the fixed supplies usage is $615 for each month.

8-15 Community Clinic estimates (see 8-14) that it needs to have enough goods on hand (at a cost of $3.20 per unit) at the beginning of the month of February equal to 125% of February's cost of goods sold. This 125% is the safety stock factor. The clinic starts the year with $5154 worth of goods, and will pay for any purchases the month after the purchase. Fixed supplies purchased and used each month are $615. They are paid for in the following month. Calculate the January purchases for the clinic.

8-16 According to the gross revenue budget in Table 8-12, approximately how many HMO enrollee visits are expected each month? For the entire year?

8-17 Suppose that the administration of Community Clinic determines that it needs to make a 5% charitable deduction allowance for charge-based patients. Determine the new monthly deductions and allowances for charge-based patients.

8-18 Calculate the cash collection for January charges if you expect the following collection schedule:

During month	35%
Following month	50%
Second month following	5%
Third month following	1%

8-19 Because of a nursing shortage, Community Clinic has had to raise RN salaries to $24,000 and benefits to 16%. Maintaining the same raise schedule and raise percentage, what is the effect on salaries and benefits for full-time employees (Table 8-21)?

8-20 If Community Clinic determined that the actual maximum RVUs per day per LPN were 55 rather than the previously calculated 50, how would this affect the variable staffing budget for January through March?

8-21 Richmond HMO, Inc. has asked you to prepare its operating budget for the upcoming quarter using the following information.

Expected number of:	July	August	September
Members	35,000	35,000	40,000
Hospital days per 1000 (per year)	250	245	260
Single member contracts	13,750	13,750	16,200
Family contracts	5,000	5,000	5,600
Prescriptions per 1000 (annualized)	3,982	4,000	4,100

- Premiums for single member contracts are $250 per month. For family contracts, which average 4.25 members, the premium is $425 per month.
- Hospital services are reimbursed at a rate of $1200 for an all-inclusive per diem rate.
- The average cost per member per month for specialty physician services is $31.05.
- Primary care physicians are paid $10 per member per month. However, if hospital utilization drops below 240 per 1000, they will be paid 25% of the difference between the projected and actual cost.
- Interest income is expected to be $2,500,000 per month.
- Outpatient services average $15 pmpm.
- Reinsurance premiums are $1.50 pmpm.
- The average cost of each prescription after copays is $30.
- ER and Out of Area Use average $10 pmpm.
- Income taxes are expected to equal 34% of Earnings Before Taxes.
- Administrative costs are $15.42 pmpm based upon 31,777 member months.
- Depreciation on the building and equipment is $49,000 per month.
- An interest expense of $25,000 is charged each month.

a. Formulate the operating budget for Richmond HMO, Inc. with the data provided.

b. Formulate the operating budget for the HMO if the number of hospital days is 230 per 1000 on an annualized basis during each month of the quarter.

8-22 Since some HMOs have experienced cash flow problems in the past, Bob's HMO, Inc. has asked you to prepare its cash budget for the upcoming quarter using the following information. The quarterly operating budget is as follows.

	July	August	Sept	Total
Net Revenues				
Premiums				
Employer1	$140,000	$115,000	$125,000	$380,000
Employer2	30,000	50,000	47,000	127,000
Coinsurance	20,000	23,000	22,000	65,000
Interest Income	5,000	5,000	5,000	15,000
Total	$195,000	$193,000	$199,000	$587,000
Expenses				
Hospital Svcs	$110,000	$105,000	$100,000	$315,000
MD Svcs	60,000	65,000	70,000	195,000
Administration	25,000	27,000	26,000	78,000
Interest	1,000	1,000	1,200	3,200
Total	$196,000	$198,000	$197,200	$591,200
Net Income	$ (1,000)	$ (5,000)	$ 1,800	$ (4,200)

Revenues from Employer1 and Employer2 are received in cash on the first day of the month for which services will be provided. Half of the coinsurance revenue is paid during the month that it is recorded as revenue; 40 percent is paid during the following month; ten percent is never received. The interest income is paid quarterly. It will be paid in September.

The HMO will pay for some new furniture, in the amount of $35,000, in cash in September. Payment for 90 percent of the amount of hospital services rendered to enrollees is made in the month after it is expensed. Ten percent of the hospital services expense is Incurred But Not Reported. This amount is expected to be paid during the next quarter. MD Services are paid in the month during which they are expensed. Administrative expenses are paid during the month they are expensed and include $10,000 depreciation expense per month. Interest for the previous six month period is due on October 15. A principal payment of $55,000 is also due on October 15.

The interest rate for short-term borrowing is 6 % per year. Payments are made during the month following the borrowing. (Assume that the amount is borrowed for an entire month.) There is currently no outstanding short-term borrowing.

A minimum cash balance of $25,000 must be maintained at the end of August and September. Assume that the beginning balance for August is only $20,000, however.

Formulate the cash budget for both August and September.

9 Standard Costs and Variance Analysis

One effective way to control and monitor health care costs is through the establishment of **standard costs** and a system for implementing them. A standard cost is a planned or allowable cost. It can be viewed as the amount budgeted for an hour of labor or per unit of services provided. Under a standard cost system, work is recorded at its standard cost, not at its actual cost. A **standard cost system** has three major goals:

1. to determine the resources that should be used to provide the service under consideration,
2. to determine the cost of those resources, and
3. to compare the actual and standard costs and explain and evaluate the resulting variance.

Once the input resources have been identified and costed, at standard, then the standard cost of a specific product or service can be calculated. Standard costs, expressed on a per-unit basis, are one of the most important managerial tools available. Monitoring per-unit costs, on an actual versus budget basis, is one of the most important tools necessary to manage under a capitated or fixed price system. Using actual and budgeted per unit costs, the manager can better understand the various factors influencing costs. Cost "drivers" become more obvious and the reasons for changes in costs become more clear. Under this approach departmental profits should be de-emphasized and managers should focus more attention on cost comparisons.

It is most important to stress that a standard cost approach is used to develop estimates for what a product or service should cost given desired levels of quality of care and efficient use of resources. Typically, the word "standard" is used when a single procedure, test, or service is being costed. It should be noted that a budget can also be considered a standard. However, a budget is really a group of standards, and that distinction will be continued in this text. It should be stressed that a thorough understanding of cost behavior is crucial for the development of standard costs.

Once standard costs have been developed and recorded, they can be compared to the **actual costs** incurred, and the resulting differences, called **variances,** can be used in evaluating performance. The major focus of this chapter is on understanding these two concepts. Figure 9-1 illustrates some of the relationships between standards and budgets and variances. Budgets and standards are set first. Variance analysis is then conducted after the operating results are known. Variance analysis does not provide answers; it only helps in framing the questions.

Figure 9-1 Variance Analysis Flow Diagram.

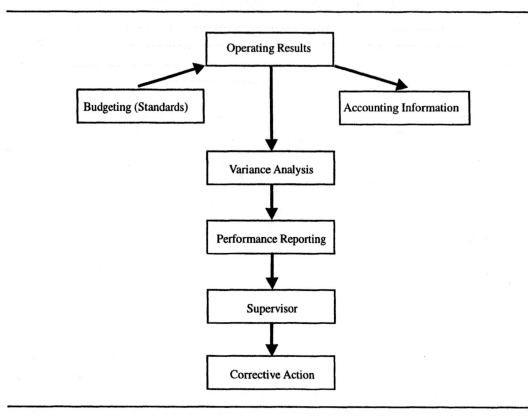

The reader should also note that the standard costs in this chapter are based on the cost allocation methods discussed in Chapter 6 and many of the same output costing techniques described in Chapter 7. The major additional concepts in this chapter extend all of the previous discussions, which were based on actual costs, to include both actual and standard costs in the manager's repertoire.

This chapter first describes standard costs and suggests ways to determine standard costs. Note that standard costs pertain to individual units of service provided to patients or clients. Standard costing for managed care organizations is not developed here. The majority of the chapter discusses variance analysis which focuses on budget line items. While the examples in this chapter focus on providers, the same techniques can be used by payers and other health care organizations. Since most cost accounting books also discuss variance analysis, we do not provide examples that also pertain to payers. Where appropriate standards can be determined, then the variance analysis techniques will apply equally to both providers and payers.

Standard Costs _____

Standard costing has been used successfully in manufacturing organizations for many years. Two major activities are needed: identifying **resource requirements** and costing those resources. As a first step in developing standard costs, knowledgeable individuals estimate the amount of resources required to provide a quality outcome. In a health care provider organization, the health professional or care-giver is usually the most appropriate individual to determine the required resources. Assistance can be obtained from management engineers and medical records personnel, but the importance of quality factors dictates that a care-giver should have the ultimate responsibility. In an HMO or managed care organization, health care professionals should still have the ultimate responsibility for determining standards that will be used to assess (and contract) patient care services.

The second step in developing standard costs is to estimate the cost of the specific resources. This estimation involves an understanding of fixed and variable costs, direct and indirect costs, and cost allocation techniques. In other words, all of the techniques already discussed in this book are necessary to understand and implement standard costing. Usually, financial management personnel are best qualified for this function, although increasingly physicians and nurses are becoming more proficient in these techniques. Table 9-1 summarizes the responsibilities of the different participants in a provider organization in the standard costing process.

The standard costing process is useful for direct patient care services as well as for indirect services such as admissions, accounting, and housekeeping. In an HMO or other managed care organization, direct services will concern the membership or the enrolled client base. Much of the "value-added" services under managed care concern patient management and patient records. Many of the record-keeping functions in a patient care organization, that are usually considered indirect services, are the major focus of managed care firms and are their direct services. As we have seen before, direct patient care services are provided in revenue centers and services that are not provided directly to patients are provided by service centers or non-revenue centers.

Although the techniques for estimating standard costs are well known, there is a large subjective component. In the next section, we illustrate these concepts with an example of how a **standard cost profile** for a nursing service could be developed.

Development of a Standard Cost Profile

One of the major costs of providing patient care is the cost of nursing services. The cost of nursing care depends on the type and level of care provided. This sections illustrates the the development of standard costs for one component of nursing services for one particular type of patient (under a particular Diagnosis Related Group). For example, responsible nursing supervisors determine nursing requirements for patients classified according to how much nursing care is required:

Patient Acuity	Nursing Hours Necessary
Nursing Care Level 1	1.5 nursing hours per shift
Nursing Care Level 2	2.2 nursing hours per shift
Nursing Care Level 3	3.5 nursing hours per shift

The amount of care at each of the nursing care levels has to be costed separately to determine the total cost of nursing care for each DRG or other patient category. Table 9-2 illustrates the standard cost computation for a day-shift of nursing care under DRG 201, Nursing Care Level 3. Only the "day-shift" is shown in this example. Overhead costs may be added to each shift, or just to one shift. In this case, assume that all overhead costs are "loaded" onto the day-shift. Note how the overhead costs "dominate" this particular set of standard costs. In most cases, the direct costs should be more prominent and overhead costs should not be lumped into a single category. More precision could be obtained in this example by constructing the standard costs for each shift separately.

The estimates of nursing care required are fairly straightforward and should be made by health care professionals. The data in Table 9-2 were developed in the following manner:

1. The required number of direct nursing hours for the day shift under DRG 201 (variable cost) was estimated by the appropriate nursing staff personnel. The quantity of each professional's time would be based on the intensity of care provided. The type of health care provided and the experience of the nurse, along with professional management engineering studies could provide additional input. For example, on the average 0.63 hours of registered nurse (RN) time was typically used for level 3 care in the past. The cost per hour, $6.92, is the estimate of the average hourly wage paid to RN's who are involved in providing level 3 care to patients classified under DRG 201. The finance department should have this information. The total variable cost of $11.59 is calculated by multiplying the two factors, quantity and wage rate, for RN care and for each of the other hourly nursing care categories and summing them together.

2. The computation of direct nursing hours (fixed cost) is based on the judgment of the senior nursing staff as to how much of their time is spent on DRG 201. The fringe benefit costs are determined by the finance department along with the average hourly wages for the supervisory and administrative staff.

3. The allocation of department overhead presents the most challenging computations. Because overhead costs, for such costs as depreciation and other indirect costs, are not direct costs of level 3 nursing care, they are typically allocated by an averaging technique using a projected total overhead cost and an appropriate activity base. For example, the total amount of depreciation expense for all equipment required for level 3 nursing care was caclulated by dividing the total depreciation of $27,000 by the total number of variable nursing hours required for all

Table 9-1   Traditional Responsibilities for the Standard Costing Process.

Resource category	Responsibility of the health professional	Responsibility of the financial professional
Labor	Time and type	Per unit costs
Supplies and materials	Amount and type	Per unit costs
Equipment	Type	Depreciation technique
Overhead		Allocation process

Table 9-2   Standard Cost Computation for Nursing Care Level 3, DRG 201.

Cost category	Quantity (hours)	Input cost	Per-unit cost
Direct nursing hours (variable cost)			
RN	0.63	$6.92	$4.36
LPN	0.83	6.01	4.99
Nursing assistant	0.11	5.15	.57
Unit aide	0.33	5.05	1.67
Total	1.90		
Total Variable Labor Cost			$11.59
Direct nursing hours (fixed cost)			
Supervisory	0.01	9.64	.10
Administration	0.03	8.10	.24
Secretarial	0.86	6.82	5.87
Total	0.90		
Total fixed labor cost			$6.21
Departmental overhead allocated			
Equipment depreciation			3.15
Indirect department overhead allocated			
Total standard costs for day-shift, DRC 201			
			125.00
			$145.95

Source: Adapted from a presentation of Ernst & Whinney's Standard Cost Manager System, Denver, Colorado, 1985.

level 3 care to be provided during the period of the time covered by the depreciation expense must be estimated (at 16,875 hours). This calculation provides the per hour equipment depreciation cost of $1.60 per variable nursing hour ($27,000/16,875 = $1.60). The estimated number of variable nursing hours on the day shift (1.9) times the estimated hourly rate ($1.60) equals the amount of depreciation expense ($3.15) to be allocated to DRG 201 level 3 nursing care (1.9 x $1.60 = $3.04). In a similar manner, the indirect departmental overhead costs would be estimated as follows if fixed nursing hours are used as the allocation base:

Estimated indirect department overhead costs	$88,960
Estimated fixed nursing hours	640
Estimated per unit costs for each nursing hour	($88,960/640) = $139
Indirect department overhead costs assigned to Level 3 Nursing Care	(.9 x 139) = $125

Standard costs would also be determined for nursing care levels 1 and 2 and incorporated into the determination of the unit cost of providing nursing service for DRG 201.

When the service being performed requires expensive equipment and supplies or materials, an expanded approach is needed to determine the standard costs. For example, in determining the standard costs for a radiology procedure, the resource requirements must first be estimated. Assume the radiology technician provides the estimates shown in Exhibit 9-1 for completing a Barium examination of the lower intestine. Restating these data in a standard cost format results in the standard cost model shown in Exhibit 9-2.

The depreciation costs for equipment and furnishings were determined in Exhibit 9-2 using the following computations:

Total costs of x-ray machine	$75,000
Estimated hours of use	2,143 hours
Cost per hour	$35
Total cost of other radiology furnishings	$150,000
Estimated hours of use	2,000 hours
Cost per hour	$75

The allocation of equipment cost, departmental overhead, and hospital indirect costs is the most difficult part in determining the cost per examination. For example, the depreciation expense for the x-ray machine was allocated on an hourly basis, which indicates that the hours of equipment usage was the activity measure. The same approach was used for the other radiology furnishings. The department overhead and the hospital indirect costs were allocated on a per-examination basis. The cost per examination for the overhead factors would be determined in the manner illustrated in Exhibit 9-2.

Exhibit 9-1   Resource Requirements for Barium Examination.

Radiology Technician Time	0.4 hours @ $11.50 per hour
Supplies (film, fluids, etc.)	8 units of film @ $2.00 per film
	9 ounces of fluids @ $1.25 per ounce
	development supplies @ $1.50 per exam
Equipment Required	
X-ray machine (original cost)	$ 75,000
Other radiology furnishings	$150,000
Department Indirect Costs for	
Supervision and Administration	$150,000
Hospital Indirect Expenses	
Allocated to Radiology Department	$200,000

Exhibit 9-2   Standard Cost Computation-Radiology Procedure: Lower Intestine.

Variable costs			
Labor:	Radiology technician	0.4 hours @ $11.50 =	$4.60
Supplies:			
	Film:	8 @ $2.00 each =	16.00
	Fluids:	9 oz. @ $1.25 =	11.25
	Development supplies:	$1.50 per examination =	1.50
Total direct variable expenses			$ 33.35
Fixed costs			
Equipment:	x-ray machine:	0.4 hours @ $35.00 per hour =	14.00
	other radiology furnishings:	0.4 hours @ $75.00 per hour =	30.00
			$ 44.00
Department overhead rate		$50.00 per examination =	50.00
Total department direct costs per exam			$127.35
Hospital indirect allocation per exam			25.00
Total standard cost per exam			$152.35

Clearly these allocation decisions will impact the cost determination. Management must be aware that other activity measures could be used, such as revenue dollars or square footage. Other difficulties in choosing the appropriate denominator (allocation base) will be discussed in greater detail later in this chapter.

Checklist for Standard Costs in Health Care Organizations

1. Standards should be developed for the primary patient care activities and major support activities.
2. Fixed and variable, and controllable and uncontrollable costs must be considered.
3. Standards should be accurate enough to meet management needs but not overly elaborate. The costs of developing and using the standards must be considered and weighed against the benefits.
4. Standards must reflect quality as well as quantity and time.
5. Management and health professionals must accept the standards and ensure that they are periodically evaluated and revised.

Establishing Standards

There are several potential sources of information for establishing standard costs for health care services including the following:

1. The medical staff and other health professionals are always important in providing information on how they typically perform the procedure, examination, or service. Individual biases and faulty recall are a problem when this approach is used.
2. Medical records can provide information on what resources were used in the past for specific procedures. However, in many cases, the records are not complete or were collected for another reason, and the data are not always accurate. Other sources must be used to supplement or verify this information.
3. Professional organizations such as professional review organizations (PRO), Blue Cross, and local health departments; medical and hospital associations; and professional groups such as the Medical Group Management Association, the American Medical Association, and nursing associations maintain numerous data bases, relative value tables, average length of stay indicators, and HCFA's guides for treatment protocols.
4. Special studies conducted by management engineers, consultants, and cost accountants can be used to supplement the basic data from the other sources.
5. Statistical data describing typical practice patterns.

The objective is to develop realistic standards that reflect how medical care is provided in each health care organization. Standard setting can also be categorized by how rigorous the standards are supposed to be. For example, resource requirement standards can be developed under the following guidelines:

1. Average performance based on historical data
2. Target performance for normal operating conditions
3. Target performance for optimum operating conditions.

Table 9-3 summarizes the strengths and weaknesses of each approach. One could conclude from this table that normal operating conditions should form the basis under which standards are determined. Only in this manner can performance be fairly evaluated and the results communicated to those responsible.

Table 9-3 Analysis of Standard Setting Approaches.

Type of standards	Strengths	Weaknesses
Based on historical average	Actual performance data easy to determine	Incorporates past inefficiencies Employees will work at less than full efficiency if they know it will be used to judge performance in future
Based on normal operating conditions	Reflects current performance Past inefficiencies not automatically included	Requires detailed analysis Required compromise on what is considered normal conditions
Based on optimum conditions	No inefficiencies built in to standard Established lowest cost	Impossible level of performance to sustain Impossible standards can harm personnel motivation

Most cost accounting systems should start with a "ground-up" approach, building standards for each procedure within a cost center. That is, procedures and fixed and variable costs form the building blocks for all other costing methods. Many of the other costing components discussed earlier are also used; for example, a standard cost system might be built on the following per-unit cost components, *all at standard*:

Variable labor	Fixed direct labor
Variable supplies	Fixed direct equipment
Variable other direct costs	Fixed direct facilities
Variable indirect costs	Fixed indirect costs

Procedure-based standard costs will aggregate some or all of these fixed and variable per-unit costs by filling in some or all of the cells in the table shown below, such that costs may be viewed as rows in a table and procedures (using x-ray films as an example) can be viewed as the columns:

	Knee	Ankle	X-ray Procedures Chest-acute	Chest-physical	Patient

Per-unit Standard Costs
  Variable labor
  Variable supplies
  Variable other direct costs
  Variable indirect costs
  Fixed direct labor
  Fixed direct equipment
  Fixed direct facilities
  Fixed indirect costs

Another example of such an approach can be based on cost center per-unit costs per visit established for each acuity level:

Acuity level	Minutes per visit	Direct Costs per visit	Indirect Costs per visit	Total Costs per visit
1	10	$ 5.00	$ 3.75	$ 8.75
2	20	10.00	7.50	17.50
3	30	15.00	11.75	26.75
4	40	20.00	15.00	35.00
etc.				

Note that the Direct Costs per Minute were $.50 per minute and the Indirect Costs per Minute were $.375 per minute. This example, based on acuity levels, shows how direct and indirect costs per unit can be built-up to arrive at the total costs of a particular kind of ambulatory visit. Similar results could be achieved under any type of patient classification system. The major point here is that different types of patients will use different resources, stated here in units of time. Each of these different sets of resources can be accumulated by using the per-unit direct and indirect costs which are then totaled for patients at each level of care provided.

Under any standard costing system, fixed costs are the most troublesome component. Building on the cost allocation concepts developed in Chapter 6, fixed costs and indirect costs are generally allocated first to cost centers, as described previously, and then to procedures or patients within revenue centers. Therefore, fixed costs and indirect costs are allocated first to revenue centers and then the costs per procedure or patient are determined within the revenue centers. The impact of fixed costs on per unit costs often present the most troublesome and confusing issues for managerial decision making. Our primary recommendation is to keep the fixed and variable costs per unit separated as much as possible.

Variance Analysis _____

An important benefit of a standard cost system is the ability to monitor activities during the operating cycle and take corrective action when necessary. **Variance analysis** involves the comparison of actual costs, from the firm's accounting system, with standard costs. The purpose of variance analysis is to identify areas for further investigation. This technique is illustrated in Figure 9-1.

A variance is any difference between a standard or expected amount and the actual results. It could be a variance in revenues. It could be a variance between standard costs per unit and actual costs per unit. For our purposes, to illustrate a typical variance analysis, we will look at the difference between costs estimated in the plan (the budget or standard) and the actual costs incurred. If the plan is realistic, these variances can provide useful information. In the remainder of this chapter we focus on the computation of variances and how they can be used.

Budget Variances

Variance analysis starts with the approved budget which shows estimated costs and revenues or standard costs on a per-unit basis. In Table 9-4 the budget for a hospital emergency room is illustrated. Several key features should be noted. First, a **flexible budget** approach is used, which indicates that fixed and variable cost components have been computed. Second, the number of visits used for the budget calculation is indicated. In many organizations, only the total budget figures would be shown, which can severely limit the usefulness of variance analysis. In Table 9-5, the actual costs for the month of January are shown.

In evaluating the financial performance of the emergency room, the initial step is to compute the various **budget variances**, using the following formula:

$$\text{Budget variance} = \text{Approved budget} - \text{Actual costs.}$$

The sum of the variances for the various items is the total budget variance for the emergency room. A static budget variance is one in which the approved budget has not been adjusted for differences between planned and actual volume of services provided. A flexible budget variance is one in which the approved budget has been adjusted for volume changes. Thus, it more realistically projects and communicates expected costs. Table 9-6 shows the individual and total static variances computed from the data in Tables 9-4 and 9-5. This analysis indicates that the emergency room experienced an unfavorable total variance of $1,119, or about 3%. But what about the reduction in visits from 1,500 to 1,400? Does this have an impact?

To compute the flexible budget variances, we would need to adjust the planned budget for 1,400 visits. Based on our discussion of cost behavior in earlier chapters, we would expect only the variable costs to change if the reduced number of examinations (100) is in the relevant range for the planned fixed costs. This seems to be a realistic assumption, as one would not expect the budgeted fixed costs to be changed for this relatively small reduction in num-

Table 9-4   Emergency Room Flexible Budget for the Month of January 19X8.

Cost category	Budget formula		Approved budget total
	Total fixed costs	Variable costs per unit	
Wage expense	$ 0	$2.00	$ 3,000
Salary expense	12,000		12,000
Employee benefits	9,000	0	9,000
Professional fees	0	2.67	4,000
Drug expense	0	0.70	1,050
General supplies	0	3.00	4,500
Repairs and maintenance	60	0	60
Telephone	18	0	18
Miscellaneous expenses	0	1.00	1,500
Total fixed and variable cost budget			$35,128
Expected volume (number of visits)			1,500 visits
Budgeted minutes (per visit)			10 min
Total budgeted minutes			15,000 min

Table 9-5   Actual Costs for January.

Cost category	Actual costs
Wage expense (variable)	$ 3,000
Salary expense (fixed)	13,000
Employee benefits	9,600
Professional fees	4,000
Drug expense	952
General supplies	4,200
Repairs and maintenance	70
Telephone	25
Miscellaneous expenses	1,400
Total costs	$36,247
Actual volume (number of visits)	1,400
Actual visits (minutes)	13,600

ber of visits. The flexible budget variances are calculated in Table 9-7, to yield a total unfavorable variance of $2,056 ($34,191 – $36,247) or 6%.

Which variance is right? The flexible variance approach provides more useful information to management, as this approach uses the fixed and variable cost information more effectively and provides more detailed management information. Table 9-8 provides a combined comparison of the static and flexible approaches by line item. The flexible budget variance analysis provides more detail on which costs are more likely to be controllable by management. That is, assuming that variable costs are controllable, then flexible budgeting provides the tools to help assess which costs are too high or too low.

As noted in the introduction, variance analysis should also help managers decide which variances to investigate further. In other words, not all variances should receive equal attention. Managers must choose from at least three possible explanations associated with any variance:

1. the performance was really quite exceptional, or quite poor;
2. the standards are out-of-date and must be revised; or
3. some random, non-recurring event is responsible (such as a flu epidemic among employees, union strike, or a hurricane).

Managers must also focus attention on large variances, either positive or negative. Large variances should be defined as a percentage of budgeted departmental costs, or other appropriate basis for comparison. "Large" must be defined in both absolute and relative terms. Managers must not focus on just the labels "favorable" or "unfavorable" because favorable does not always equate with "good"; nor is unfavorable always "bad." Managers must "get behind" the numbers and conduct an in-depth analysis of the large variances. Managers must

Table 9-6   Static Budget Variance.

Cost category	Approved budget	Actual costs	Variance
Wage expense	$ 3,000	$ 3,000	0
Salary expense	12,000	13,000	1,000U
Employee benefits	9,000	9,600	600U
Professional fees	4,000	4,000	0
Drug expense	1,050	952	98F
General supplies	4,500	4,200	300F
Repairs and maintenance	60	70	10U
Telephone	18	25	7U
Miscellaneous expenses	1,500	1,400	100F
Total costs	$35,128	$36,247	$1,119U
Volume (number of visits)	1,500	1,400	100

Table 9-7   Flexible Budget Variances.

Cost category	Approved budget	Actual costs	Variance
Wage expense (1,400 x $2.00)	$ 2,800	$ 3,000	$ 200U
Salary expense	12,000	13,000	1,000U
Employee benefits	9,000	9,600	600U
Professional fees (1,400 x $2.67)	3,738	4,000	262U
Drug expense (1,400 x $.70)	980	952	28F
General supplies (1,400 x $3.00)	4,200	4,200	0
Repairs and maintenance	60	70	10U
Telephone	18	25	7U
Miscellaneous expenses (1,400 x $1.00)	1,400	1,400	0
Total costs	$34,196	$36,247	$2,051U
Volume (number of visits)	1,400	1,400	0

Table 9-8   Variance Analysis.

Cost category	Actual costs	Planned budget (1,500 visits)	Budget variance	Flexible budget (1,400 visits)	Flexible variance	Difference in variances
Wage expense (variable)	$ 3,000	$ 3,000	0	$2,800	$ 200U	$ 200U
Salary expense	13,000	12,000	1,000U	12,000	1,000U	0
Employee benefits	9,600	9,000	600U	9,000	600U	0
Professional fees (variable)	4,000	4,000	0	3,733	267U	267U
Drug expense (variable)	952	1,050	98F	980	28F	70U
General supplies (variable)	4,200	4,500	300F	4,200	0	300U
Repairs and maintenance	70	60	10U	60	10U	0
Telephone	25	18	7U	18	7U	0
Miscellaneous expenses (variable)	1,400	1,500	100F	1,400	0	100U
Total costs	$36,247	$35,128	$1,119U	$34,191	$2,056U	$937U
Volume (number of visits)	1,400	1,500	100	1,400	0	100

also be concerned with trends in variances which may indicate an increasingly positive or negative impact on future expectations. In summary, managers must look more closely at large variances to understand why they occur and they must use the available data to make predictions about future costs and future variances.

In-Depth Variable Cost Variance Analysis

Where information is available, it is possible to perform an in-depth variance analysis, which provides more information to management and allows for appropriate corrective action. In-depth variance analysis can be accomplished for the fixed and variable components, but they require different approaches.

All variable costs are composed of a quantity and a price component. For example, the labor cost of an emergency room visit is comprised of a variable rate per hour and a measure of the time charged while the patient is being treated. The variance in wages could be caused by a price-per-hour variance or a difference in the quantity of hours required, or both. The price-per-hour variance is called a **price variance**. For labor costs, the variance based on time is called an efficiency variance. These formulas for computing variances are shown in Exhibit 9-3.

Determining at least two variances is useful because the price-per-hour and quantity of time factors could be the responsibility of different supervisors. For example, the hourly wage might be the responsibility of the personnel director or depend on union contracts, whereas the department supervisor might really only control the amount of time spent on the task.

In the emergency room example presented in Table 9-4, the standard wage cost was $2.00 [ten minutes per visit x $.20 per minute ($2.00 / 10 minute)]. The actual cost per minute was $.22 ($3000 / 13,600) (see table 9-5). Using the formula from Exhibit 9-3, the following price variance is calculated:

Standard cost per minute is: $.20 ($3000 / 15,000) (Table 9-4)
Actual cost per minute is: $.22 ($3000 / 13,600) (Table 9-5)

Price Variance = (.20 − .22) x 13,600 = $272 unfavorable (U)

Exhibit 9-3   Variance Analysis of Variable Costs.

Price Variance = Change in Price x Actual Units of Service
where Change in Price = Standard Price − Actual Price

Efficiency Variance = Change in Quantity x Standard Price
where Change in Quantity = Standard Quantity Required − Actual Quantity Used

In this case, the price variance is considered unfavorable because the actual cost per minute (.22) exceeded the standard cost per minute (.20). Any case where the actual cost exceeds the standard cost will be noted as unfavorable (U). Similarly, any variance where actual costs are less than standard costs will be noted as favorable (F). The $272 variance would be considered significant at 9% ($272/$3000) of the total cost.

The efficiency variance computation requires information about the actual amount of time spent to accomplish the examination. For example, if ten minutes were the standard, the total expected amount of time to complete 1,400 exams would be 14,000 minutes (1,400 x 10). If the actual amount of time used was 13,600 minutes, a favorable efficiency variance would be $80 calculated as follows.

> Standard minutes to be used is 14,000 (10 minutes x 1400) (Table 9-9)
> Actual minutes used is 13,600 (Table 9-5)
>
> Efficiency variance = (14,000 - 13,600) x .2 = $80F

As discussed above, the efficiency variance is considered favorable because the actual time was less than the standard time allowed. Since it is less than 3% of total wage costs ($80/$3000), it would not be significant in absolute or relative terms and would probably not be investigated further. However, if favorable labor efficiency variances do recur, this finding would be recognized when the standards were next revised or when new processes were considered.

The **net variance** for the wage component would be:

Price variance	$272U
Efficiency variance	80F
Net variance	$192U

Table 9-9   Variable Cost Variance Analysis.

A Actual quantity used per unit	B Actual wage per unit	C Actual output	D Budgeted wage per unit	E Budgeted quantity per unit
(9.71 min)	($12.20)	(1,400)	($12.00)	(10)

Price variance = (D – B) (C)
Usage variance = (E – A) (C) (D)
Total variance = Price + Usage variances

If the departmental supervisor was unable to control the wage rates of the employees, the supervisor really achieved a favorable variance of $80, not the unfavorable total variance of $192 (as shown above).

Material or supplies variances are computed in the same fashion as labor variances. For example, there would be a price and quantity standard for material variances. These standards would give rise to price and usage variances. In our emergency room budget, the budgeted cost of general supplies per patient visit was $3.00 (Table 9-4). The standard cost for 1,400 visits would be 1,400 times $3, or $4,200. Actual costs were $4,200 (Table 9-5). Therefore the total variance is zero ($4,200 budget minus $4,200 actual).

A total variance of zero does not necessarily mean the supply expense is being effectively managed. There may be offsetting variances; for example, the price per unit of the supplies may have been less than budgeted and the quantity used per unit of service more than budgeted. Information is necessary on the budgeted price to be paid and budgeted quantities to be used per unit of service.

Let us assume that the standard supply expense per visit was calculated as one paper bed cover, one tongue depressor, and two sheets of paper for medical records per visit, for a per unit cost of $3.00. If the actual cost of these units was $3.10, but the total variance was zero, then an unfavorable price variance must have been offset by a favorable usage variance. The calculations could be completed as follows:

$$1,400 \times (\$3.00 - \$3.10) = \$140 \text{ unfavorable price variance.}$$

This would indicate that the supplies usage variance was $140F, since the total variance of zero must equal the sum of the price variance ($140U) plus the usage variance ($140F). The supervisor must have used fewer supplies than planned to achieve the total variance reported. A favorable quantity variance of $140 would indicate that the supervisor only used 1,353.33 units of general supplies rather than the 1,400 units expected for 1,400 visits. Favorable usage or price variances may be inappropriate for health care organizations if quality of care is compromised. Managers of health care organizations must be careful not to assume that favorable cost variances are always desirable. Quality standards may not have been met and the favorable cost variance may just be an illusion. A favorable price variance could indicate that inferior supplies had been purchased or that inexperienced staff (paid at a lower rate) had been assigned to a particular department or activity. Similar calculations can be done for all the variable overhead cost factors if the appropriate information is available.

In-Depth Fixed Cost Variance Analysis

Fixed cost variances present a different set of issues than do **variable cost variances**, because by definition fixed costs do not vary with volume changes. Therefore, the efficiency computation cannot be done. Exhibit 9-4 identifies two types of fixed cost variance: **spending variance** and **overhead variance**.

The most straightforward fixed cost variance is the budget or spending variance. The budget or spending variance compares actual expenses with the budgeted amount. Because

Exhibit 9-4   Variance Analysis of Fixed Costs.

Spending Variance = Actual Fixed Costs – Budgeted Fixed Costs

Overhead Variance = Budgeted Fixed Cost per unit of service x
Number of Services Provided – Budgeted Fixed Costs

fixed costs do not vary with volume changes, the fixed costs are the same for both static and flexible budget comparisons.

In our emergency room example, the fixed cost budget is $21,078 ($12,000 + $9,000 + $60 + $18). The actual amount spent was $22,695 ($13,000 + $9,600 + $70 + $25). The spending variance was therefore $1,617 (unfavorable). This variance seems to be significant in absolute and relative terms (7.7% = 1617/21078).

This total variance should have been controllable by the supervisor, but it is still important to do a line-by-line analysis to determine just what areas were out of control. Table 9-10 illustrates the line-by-line spending variance computations for the fixed costs.

Table 9-10   Fixed Cost Spending Variance.

Cost Category	Actual	Budgeted	Variance
Wage	$13,000	$12,000	$1,000U
Benefits	9,600	9,000	600U
Repairs and maintenance	70	60	10U
Telephone	25	18	7U
	$22,695	$21,078	$1,617U

In reviewing the variances, management needs to have information about why the various categories were overspent in every instance. For example, it may be that the initial budget was not realistic or that prices were increased by outside parties, or it may be that the supervisor just didn't control costs. Recall that variance analysis does not provide answers; it only helps in framing the questions.

A key fixed cost variance that can provide timely information to management is the overhead **volume variance**. This variance is an artifact of the allocation of fixed costs to the various services and procedures. It is created because of the necessity to allocate the indirect overhead costs to direct patient costs to determine the fair price to be charged. A fair share of the indirect costs must be predetermined to establish the price or charge before the service is offered. Most patients, except those under cost-based reimbursement, will not buy a product without knowing the price in advance. Only cost-based payers take this approach when purchasing health services.

The process is started by the development of an **overhead rate** by using the budgeted fixed overhead and the planned number of procedures. In our emergency room example, this would be the total fixed costs of $21,078 divided by 1,500 visits, or $14.05. Each visit would include $14.05 of the budgeted fixed overhead in the charge for the visit. If 1,500 visits occur, then $21,078 (1,500 x $14.05) would be collected to pay for the fixed overhead.

In our example, only 1,400 examinations were completed, and only $19,670 was collected through the billing process (1,400 x $14.05). This results in a shortage of $1,405 (100 x $14.05). By monitoring the difference between planned and actual volume, management can forecast the deficit or surplus that will occur as a result of the volume being less or greater than budgeted. Management can then decide to either raise prices, reduce expenses, or both.

In this case, if management knew that only 1,400 visits were going to be completed by the end of the month, and 1,500 had been planned, then the price must be raised to generate $1,405 of additional revenue, or expenses must be cut by $1,405, to balance the budget. Other increases in price or reductions in expenses would be necessary to cover the unfavorable variances identified in the variance reports in Tables 9-6 and 9-7. A complete summary of all the variances is illustrated in Figure 9-2 for our emergency room example.

Expanded Variance Presentation including Revenue Variances

Variance analysis can be conducted in a variety of dimensions, ranging from the basic two-way approach illustrated herein up to a four-way or five-way analysis. Exhibit 9-5 provides an illustration of how the results of a variety of variance analyses might be communicated, using summary tables and graphical displays. While the numerical bases of these tables and graphs are not presented, the reader should note how a variety of factors are displayed in a single graph. For example, note how the effects of charges per stay, length of stay, and admissions are all shown in a single bar graph (Panel 6 as shown in Exhibit 9-5). This exhibit also shows how variance analyses can be extended to include revenues as well as costs.

Summary

The well-trained manager will be able to apply variance analysis to both costs and revenues and will be able to use a variety of report formats to communicate these results to other managers. A critical skill is the ability to identify the variables that seem to have the most influence on the variances. A related skill is the ability to identify the controllable and non-controllable factors in a variance report; the essential skill is the ability to de-emphasize the non-controllable variances such that they do not "swamp" or overwhelm or bias the report in a way that misleads the reader.

The discussion of variances in this chapter was designed to highlight and illustrate the potential uses of variance analyses. Variance analyses can help in improving performance measurement and management decisions. It should be recognized that the material introduced in this chapter is primarily introductory in nature. Readers are encouraged to review the references in the bibliography for more complete coverage.

Figure 9-2   Summary of Cost Variance Analysis.

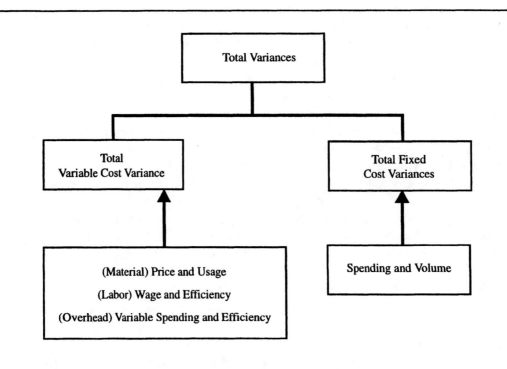

Exhibit 9-5   Examples of Two and Three-Way Variance Analysis

---

Panel 1: Factors in a two-way variance analysis

Planned admissions	1000
Actual admissions	954
Admissions variance	46
Planned revenue/case	$5,200
Actual revenue/case	$4,955
Price variance	($245)
Planned revenue	$5,200,000
Actual revenue	$4,727,070
Revenue variance	($472,930)

Panel 2: Findings of a two-way variance analysis

Admissions (volume) variance (actual – planned admissions) x planned
  price = (954 – 1,000) x $5,200   ($239,200)

Charge/admission (price) variance (actual – planned price) planned
  admissions = ($4,955 – $5,200) x 1000   ($245,000)

Price-volume interaction (actual – planned price) x (actual – planned
  admissions) = ($4,955 – $5,200) x (954 – 1,000) $11,270

Total variance   ($472,930)

Source: Dove, H.G. and T. Forthman. "Helping Financial Analysts Communicate Variance Analysis" *Healthcare Financial Management* (April): 53-54, 1995.

Exhibit 9-5   continued

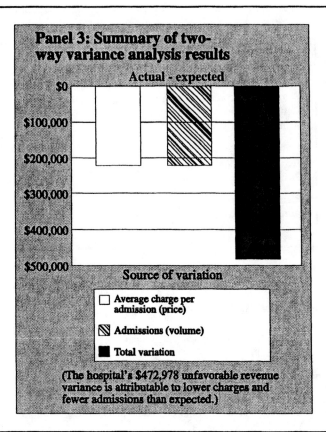

Panel 3: Summary of two-way variance analysis results

(The hospital's $472,978 unfavorable revenue variance is attributable to lower charges and fewer admissions than expected.)

Panel 4: Calculations involved in two-way variance analysis

	Average charge per admission (C)	Number of admissions (A)	Revenue
Planned	$5,200	1,000	$5,200,000
Actual	$4,995	954	$4,727,070
Actual – planned	($245)	($46)	($472,930)

		Absolute value	Allocation of C x A interaction	Allocations for Panel 3
Variation in charges per admission (C)	($245,000)	$245,000	$5,702	($239,298)
Number of admissions (A)	($239,200)	$239,200	$5,568	($233,632)
C x A interaction	$11,270		$11,270	
Total variance	($472,930)		($472,930)	

Exhibit 9-5   continued

Panel 5: Variables in a three-way analysis

	Planned	Actual	Variance
Average charges per day	$800	$693	($107)
Average length of stay	6.50	7.15	0.65
Number of admissions	1,000	954	46

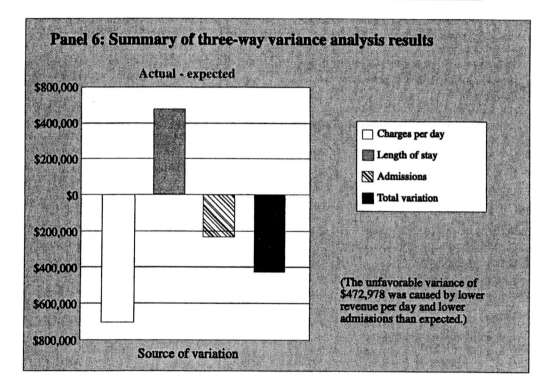

Panel 6: Summary of three-way variance analysis results

(The unfavorable variance of $472,978 was caused by lower revenue per day and lower admissions than expected.)

Panel 7: Possible variables used in a four-way variance analysis

	Planned	Actual	Variance
Average room and board charges per day	$500	$505	$5
Average ancillary charges per day	$300	$188	($112)
Average length of stay	6.50	7.15	0.65
Number of admissions	1,000	954	46

Bibliography

Awasthi, V.N. and L. Eldenburg. "Providing Cost Data to Physicians Helps Contain Costs" *Healthcare Financial Management* (April): 40-42, 1996.

Baker, J. J. "Activity-Based Costing for Integrated Delivery Systems" *Journal of Health Care Finance* (Winter): 57-61, 1995.

Canby IV, J.B. "Applying Activity-Based Costing to Healthcare Settings" *Healthcare Financial Management* (February): 50-56, 1995.

Carpenter, C.E., L.C. Weitzel, N.E. Johnson, and D.B. Nash. "Cost Accounting Supports Clinical Evaluations." *Healthcare Financial Management* (April): 40-44, 1994.

Dove, H.G. and T. Forthman. "Helping Financial Analysts Communicate Variance Analysis" *Healthcare Financial Management* (April): 52-54, 1995.

Granof, M.H., P.W. Bell, and B.R. Neumann. *Accounting for Managers and Investors*, Prentice Hall, Englewood Cliffs, NJ, 1993.

Karpiel, M.S. "Using Patient Classification Systems to Identify Ambulatory Care Costs" *Healthcare Financial Management* (November): 31-37, 1994.

Miller, T.R. and J.B.Ryan. "Analyzing Cost Variance in Capitated Contracts" *Healthcare Financial Management* (February): 22-23, 1995.

Ramsey, R.H. "Activity-Based Costing for Hospitals" *Hospital & Health Services Administration* (Fall): 385-396, 1994.

Ryan, J.B. and S.B. Clay. "Understanding the Law of Large Numbers" *Healthcare Financial Management* (October): 22-24, 1995.

Suver, J.D., B.R. Neumann, and K. Boles. *Management Accounting for Healthcare Organizations*, Pluribus Press, Oak Brook, IL: Hospital Financial Management Association, 1993.

Thorley Hill, N. and E. Loper Johns. "Adoption of Costing Systems by U.S. Hospitals" *Hospital & Health Services Administration* (Winter): 521-537, 1994.

Terms and Concepts

actual costs
budget variance
efficiency variance
fixed cost variances
flexible budget
net variance
overhead rate
price variance

resource requirements
spending variance
standard costs
standard cost system
standard cost profile
variable cost variances
variance
variance analysis
volume variance

Questions and Problems

9-1 Explain the standard costing process.

9-2 Explain why health professionals should determine the amount and type of resources needed to provide quality health care.

9-3 What are two major components in establishing a standard cost profile?

9-4 How are fixed costs, on a per unit basis, determined in the standard cost process?

9-5 What are the differences between direct and indirect costs in developing a standard cost per procedure?

9-6 A. What are the three approaches that can be used to establish standards?
B. What are the strengths and weaknesses of each?

9-7 A. Why is variance analysis important in performance measure?
B. Why are actual and standard costs both important to health care managers?
C. Discuss why revenue variances are as important as cost variances, or why they may be more important.

9-8 Name two types of variances that can be computed from routine cost reports.

9-9 Why does a flexible budget approach promote better information for performance evaluation?

9-10 Explain price, quantity, usage, and efficiency variances.

9-11 Explain the fixed cost spending variance.

9-12 Explain how the overhead volume variance is calculated.

9-13 How can the overhead volume variance be used in expenditure control or rate-setting decisions?

9-14 Define "standard costs."

9-15 The absolute minimum cost that would be possible under the best conceivable operating conditions is a description of which type of standard?

9-16 If a hospital follows a practice of isolating material variances at the earliest point in time, what would be the appropriate time to isolate and recognize a direct material price variance?
A. When material is issued to the department.
B. When material is purchased.
C. When material is used in providing patient care.
D. When the purchase order is signed.

9-17 The budget for a given volume during October 199X was $180,000. The actual cost for the month was $172,000. It can be said that the hospital administration did a better than expected job in controlling costs if:
  A. The costs were variable and actual patient days were 96% of planned patient days?
  B. The costs were variable and actual patient days equaled budgeted patient days?
  C. The costs were variable and actual patient days were 91% of budgeted patient days?
  D. The costs were fixed and actual patient days equaled budgeted patient days?

9-18 The budget for a given volume during November 199X was $195,000. The actual cost for the month was $176,000. It can be said that the hospital administration did a better than expected job in controlling costs if:
  A. The costs were variable and actual patient days were less than planned patient days?
  B. The costs were variable and actual patient days equaled budgeted patient days?
  C. The costs were variable and actual patient days were more than budgeted patient days?
  D. The costs were fixed and actual patient days equaled budgeted patient days?

9-19 Community Hospital uses a standard cost system. The raw materials used for x-ray procedures for the month of June were as follows:

Standard price per film	$1.60
Actual purchase price per film	$1.55
Actual quantity purchased	2,000 films
Actual quantity used	1,900 films
Standard film quantity allowed for actual patient tests	1,800 films

Assuming the direct material price variance is computed at the time of purchase, this variance would be:
  A. $95 favorable?
  B. $90 unfavorable?
  C. $100 favorable?
  D. $100 unfavorable?

9-20 Community Hospital uses a standard cost system. The raw materials used for x-ray procedures for the month of July were as follows:

Standard price per film	$1.70
Actual purchase price per film	$1.60
Actual quantity purchased	3,000 films
Actual quantity used	2,900 films
Standard film quantity allowed for actual patient tests	2,800 films

Assuming the direct material price variance is computed at the time of purchase, calculate this variance.

9-21 Bay Shore Community Hospital's direct material costs were:

Standard price per gram	$3.60
Actual grams purchased	1,600
Standard grams allowed for actual patient days	1,450
Material price variance favorable	$240

What was the actual purchase price per unit, rounded to the nearest cent?
A. $3.06
B. $3.11
C. $3.45
D. $3.75

9-22 Bay Shore Community Hospital's direct material costs were:

Standard price per gram	$4.65
Actual grams purchased	1,800
Standard grams allowed for actual patient days	1,676
Actual material purchase price variance	$4.15

Calculate the material purchase price variance.

9-23 The nursing supervisor at St. Joseph's Hospital was reviewing the following data:

Actual nursing hourly rate	$7.50
Standard nursing hours allowed for acuity levels provided by the ward	11,000
Actual nursing hours for the ward	10,000
Nursing hourly rate variance - favorable	$5,500

What was the standard nursing hourly rate in effect for the month of December?
A. $6.95
B. $7.00
C. $8.00
D. $8.05

9-24 Home Health Central uses a standard cost system based on the number of visits. Nursing cost information for home visits for the month of January is as follows:

Standard nursing rate	$16.00 per hour
Actual nursing rate paid	$16.10 per hour
Standard nursing hours allowed for actual number of visits	1,500 hours
Nursing hours efficiency variance	$600 unfavorable

What were the actual nursing hours worked?
A. 1,400
B. 1,462.5
C. 1,537.5
D. 1,600

9-25 Central Labs' technician salary costs for the month of January were as follows:

Actual direct labor hours	10,000
Standard direct labor hours	11,000
Direct labor rate variance - unfavorable	$3,000
Total payroll	$66,000

What was Central Labs' technician salary efficiency variance?
A. $6,000 favorable
B. $6,150 favorable
C. $6,300 favorable
D. $6,450 favorable

9-26 Central Labs' technician salary costs for the month of February were as follows:

Actual direct labor hours	11,000
Standard direct labor hours	11,500
Direct labor rate variance - unfavorable	$3,000
Total payroll	$68,000

What was Central Labs' technician salary efficiency variance?

9-27 The Visiting Nurses Association had nursing costs for the month of December as follows:

Actual nursing hours	134,500
Standard nursing hours	135,000
Total nursing payroll	$881,500
Nursing costs efficiency variance - favorable	$3,200

What was the nursing wage variance?
A. $17,250 unfavorable
B. $20,700 unfavorable
C. $21,000 unfavorable
D. $21,000 favorable

9-28 The Visiting Nurses Association had nursing costs for the month of November as follows:

Actual nursing hours	164,500
Standard nursing hours	166,000
Total nursing payroll	$791,500
Nursing costs efficiency variance - favorable	$3,200

What is the nursing wage variance?

9-29 Information on University Hospital's overhead costs was presented by the CFO to the director of nursing:

Actual variable nursing overhead	173,000
Actual fixed nursing overhead	117,000
Standard hours allowed for actual services	32,000
Budgeted overhead rate per direct nursing hour	$9.25

What is the total overhead variance?
A. $1,000 unfavorable
B. $6,000 favorable
C. $6,000 unfavorable
D. $7,000 favorable

9-30 Information on University Hospital's overhead costs was presented to the CFO by the director of nursing:

Actual variable nursing overhead	165,000
Actual fixed nursing overhead	234,000
Standard hours allowed for actual services	36,500
Budgeted overhead rate per direct nursing hour	$9.45

What is the total overhead variance?

9-31 City Hospital uses a standard cost system to determine overhead variances. For 199X, total overhead was budgeted at $780,000 based on a projected schedule of 320,000 paid nursing hours. Overhead is applied, or charged, to each patient day based on a standard of 4 nursing hours per patient day. The following information was obtained from the accounting records:

Number of patient days provided	79,500
Nursing hours paid	320,000
Actual overhead costs	$780,000

A. Determine the budgeted overhead rate per nursing hour.
B. Determine the amount of overhead applied.
C. What is the total overhead variance?

9-32 City Hospital uses a standard cost system to determine overhead variances. For 199X, total overhead was budgeted at $680,000 based on a projected schedule of 340,000 paid nursing hours. Overhead is applied, or charged, to each patient day based on a standard of 4 nursing hours per patient day. The following information was obtained from the accounting records:

Number of patient days provided	81,500
Nursing hours paid	320,000
Actual overhead costs	$696,000

A. Determine the budgeted overhead rate per nursing hour.
B. Determine the amount of overhead applied.
C. What is the total overhead variance?

9-33 Casper Hospital uses a flexible budget system and the board of directors approved the following budget for 199X:

	Percent of capacity	
	80%	90%
Direct nursing hours	24,000	27,000
Variable overhead	$156,000	$175,500
Fixed overhead	$708,000	$708,000
Total overhead rate per nursing hour	$36.00	$32.72

Casper Hospital operated at 80% of capacity during 199X but based its budgeted total overhead rate on 90% of capacity. Assuming that actual overhead was equal to the budgeted amount for the attained capacity, what is the total overhead variance for the year?
A. No variance
B. 19,500
C. $78,720
D. 98,160

9-34 Casper Hospital uses a flexible budget system and the board of directors approved the following budget for 199X:

	Percent of capacity	
	80%	90%
Direct nursing hours	24,000	27,000
Variable overhead	$156,000	$175,500
Fixed overhead	$708,000	$708,000
Total overhead rate per nursing hour	$36.00	$32.72

Casper Hospital operated at 80% of capacity during 199X and based its budgeted total overhead rate on 85% of capacity.

Assuming that actual overhead was equal to the budgeted amount for the attained capacity, what is the total overhead variance for the year?

9-35 As a new manager with STARTUP HMO INC, you are concerned about the cost of physician (specialist) services. You find that actual spending during the past year was $13,000,000 while the budget only authorized $12,000,000. The actual average amount paid to each physician for each visit was $80. On average, there were 3.25 visits per member during the year. The planned number of members was 54,054 and the expected rate for each physician visit was $74.

   a. Calculate the most useful variances that will help you evaluate specialist physician services at STARTUP HMO.

   b. Explain why the original budget data is not very useful for analyzing variances at the end of the year.

   c. Which variances would you investigate? Why?

   d. Identify the likely causes of the variances you decided to investigate. What types of implementation effects may result in the observed variances?

10 Pricing

Financial resources must be provided at the right time and in the right amounts to permit health care organizations to meet their commitments to their constituencies. We could claim that most organizations want to grow and prosper and they need the resources to accomplish these objectives. Most health care organizations want to continue to serve their patients or other clients and they certainly need financial resources to accomplish this objective. The American Hospital Association (AHA) has defined this objective under the term **total financial requirements (TFR)** as the resources necessary to meet both current and future community health care needs.[1] As the financial resources of most health care providers are derived chiefly from revenues received for providing health care services, it is essential that health care managers establish prices that will generate revenues sufficient to meet the organization's financial objectives. Similarly, a managed care organization must establish its prices in a way that will facilitate its long-run survival and success. This chapter looks at pricing primarily from the provider's perspective, but many of the techniques also apply to payers.

Current operating expenses are not the only factors in setting prices. Other considerations should also be included. For example, numerous regulatory constraints may be relevant. Competition and the relative prices among providers in the same community are becoming major factors. Some providers, such as various community-based not-for-profit health care organizations, that may not even charge for their services or may use a sliding fee scale, the establishment of prices can offer some estimate of the value of the services offered. These estimates can be effective inputs into budget determination and other management decisions for the allocation of resources.

This chapter concentrates on developing various pricing concepts and strategies designed to achieve a variety of goals. We develop pricing techniques to implement these strategies. Since many aspects of the health care sector are not yet market-driven, we also include reimbursement mechanisms where payment differs from the provider's price.

The five basic steps in any pricing model include the following steps:

1. Estimate the quantity of services that patients or clients will need. This quantity is not independent of the price that is ultimately selected. However, one logical starting point is an expert judgment on the scope and amount of services that are potentially needed in the community. Service quantities can be stated in terms of occupancy rates, dollar volume, number of procedures, or in some other fashion.

2. Determine the total and average costs based on the estimated volume.
3. Identify a proposed price and assess whether the volume estimates (from step 1) are reasonable and attainable under the proposed price.
4. Assess whether the organization's goals are achieved under the proposed prices.
5. Accept or revise the proposed prices, the volume estimates, and/or the cost estimates.

As part of step 1, the health care provider must explicitly or intuitively determine the basic relationship between price and demand for its services. That is, it must know approximately how sensitive the volume of services is to price. Emergency and surgical services are two examples where price is less important than such factors as quality or access, and therefore demand for these services is not as sensitive to changes in price as for other services. Elective procedures, such as plastic surgery, may be more sensitive to price.

Wherever services are sensitive to price, either the provider sets the price and the market sets the volume, or the provider establishes a volume target and the market determines the price necessary to achieve it. In such instances, the market signals a response to prices. Prices that are too low generate high demand that cannot be met with existing capacity. Prices that are too high create unused capacity. The best benchmark against which to evaluate prices is the market's perception of the value and benefit of the institution's services. This perception of value differs among patients, physicians, and other clients.

Most providers will be **price takers,** accepting a market or regulated price. Only a few fortunate providers will be **price setters** or **price leaders**, who are able to dictate the prices they receive for products and services. Those few price leaders are the ones who create market value and are perceived as offering products differentiated by quality levels. Price leaders are able to provide their desired quantities of services at the target price. Price takers may not be able to achieve their target prices or projected volume levels, and therefore may be unable to meet their financial goals. The next section discusses how a firm's financial goals form the basis for most pricing strategies.

Even though price often does not always affect individual patients' decisions to seek medical care, price does affect contracting for care with insurance companies, employers, HMOs, PPOs, and other large purchasers. Most of the impact of a health care provider's pricing strategies will be on these payers who will have a significant impact on the provider's ability to meet its financial objectives, especially as these payers attempt to improve their own bottom-line profitability while impeding or constraining that of the health care provider. Of course, the bargaining power of the respective parties (e.g., number of members in an HMO, being the sole provider in town) will have a major impact on contract prices.

As step 5 implies, price determination is an iterative process that is repeated until the organization's goals are achieved, the prices are satisfactory, and the organization's objectives for meeting community needs are likely to be achieved.

Financial Goals

The financial goals for any health care organization depend on the nature of the services provided, the environment in which the institution operates, and the specific characteristics of the institution. Consequently, no single or universal formula exists to specify or model the firm's goals. Each firm must develop its own financial goals and frequently adjust them as conditions change.

Generally, basing the determination of financial goals solely on information obtained from the accounting system is not sufficient. Some costs are not recognized under generally accepted accounting principles or third-party reimbursement regulations. Such items as replacement costs of assets, debt repayment, and new technology requirements are not generally considered expenses in the accounting records. In addition, third-party regulations may not permit payment for charity care requirements and other uncompensated services that must be considered in determining one's financial goals.

One important determinant of any firm's financial goals includes the **costs of doing business**. This is related to the primary purpose of the institution: What services does the institution provide, and what are the primary environmental characteristics involved in providing those services? One important set of financial resources concerns direct patient care expenses which is normally derived from data in the accounting system and consists of salaries, supplies, and utilities. Education and research expenses are very much a part of the health care process. Although managers may contend that these are necessary costs, various payers may question just how necessary such costs are to the actual provision of health care. Other costs will meet with varying levels of acceptance by payers or purchasers of health care. For example, some major payers will not pay for charity care or bad debts incurred by other clients. However, to the health care provider, these expenses represent financial requirements that must be covered.

Financial resources are also necessary to acquire and operate facilities and to cover the long lead times in collecting revenues from a variety of payers or clients. Health care organizations typically expect to become permanent fixtures in the community; therefore, they must have the resources necessary to replace their assets and incorporate new technology as it becomes available.

Financial resources are also needed to cover the **costs of changing business**. Health care organizations must meet changing requirements and competitive conditions. They must be prepared to change existing services or to offer new ones when new community needs are identified. For instance, wellness programs and home health services are emerging as a response to community needs and to competitive factors.

All organizations that provide services use capital resources, and these capital resources have a cost. Capital cannot exist without some return or yield. Firms must identify sources of capital and earn appropriate returns as demanded by providers of capital. Not-for-profit community health care providers have received capital from community sources in the form of tax exemptions, appropriations, donations, and revenue-generating activities. Not-for-profit providers can use any excess resources to provide community services such as outreach programs, neighborhood health centers, education programs, and other health-related activities. Similarly, commercial firms (for-profit) also must obtain capital resources and use them appropriately. The capital markets facing such firms are usually more well-organized and more disciplined, some would say more "efficient." The returns necessary for commercial firms to thrive and succeed are usually dictated by these external markets.

All economic organizations operate in an uncertain environment. They face **costs of uncertainty** which are not explicitly recognized under generally accepted accounting principles and therefore are not usually entered in the accounting records. Yet the prudent manager must make allowances for each and allocate appropriate resources to meet unforeseen demands. For instance, contingency allowances and political contributions must be included in the planning process and in the pricing structure, even though they cannot be publicized, nor are they appropriately charged to most payers.

Because of the vital impact that financial resources have on the determination of prices, it is important that management recognize and make a "best possible" estimate of all types of financial needs. Several methods can be used to estimate the yields or returns above operating expenses that might be required. One method is to develop an overall estimated rate of return on total assets that would return sufficient capital to the organization's goals. Individual rates under this method would be set to provide this overall return. Hugh Long[2] estimated that a return of approximately 15% would be appropriate to meet the goals of typical health care provider. Dick Furst[3] developed an approach that concentrates on determining goals for various types of financial resources. Using pro forma financial statements, an estimate is made for each major financial resource and prices are established accordingly.

A complete discussion of these techniques is beyond the scope of this book; however, the reader is encouraged to review the references cited above for greater detail. It is important to stress that most health care providers are, at best, only meeting 25% to 50% of the returns that Furst and Long have estimated as required to remain financially viable. The required returns, or appropriate returns, are contentious issues which are difficult to answer precisely. In many cases, government regulation and intervention will be the dominant factors affecting pricing and the returns that health care organizations are allowed to retain. The seriousness of this problem, and its effect on pricing, indicates that strategies to meet financial goals must be a prime concern of health care managers. The next section concentrates on a discussion of appropriate pricing strategies.

Pricing Strategies _____

Both for-profit and not-for-profit providers should develop pricing strategies, since both provide services that recognize the quasi-regulatory nature of the health care sector as well as the market forces that result from competition with each other. Such strategies (e.g., always meeting the competition's price, being the low-cost provider in the community, or, conversely, being the price leader) can provide the resources necessary to meet the firm's financial goals. However, these decisions should be rational choices by management, not ad hoc approaches to crisis events. This section focuses on developing the tools necessary to aid in this decision process.

There are three major approaches for establishing prices for health care services:

- Cost-based
- Negotiated
- Market-driven

These approaches are not mutually exclusive and are used in various combinations. The nature of the services, the type of provider, the competitive conditions, and the primary third-party payer all interact to determine the best approach for any single provider.

The Cost-Based Approach

The **cost-based approach** is the starting point for many pricing strategies. It is used either as a basis for establishing cost plus prices or for reimbursement. Third-party payers may require a determination of the allowable cost of providing services to their clients. The allowable cost has usually been determined on a retrospective or after-the-fact basis and requires that external auditors verify the actual costs incurred.

Most cost-based approaches for pricing are based on average costs where the full costs of the service are divided by the number of units of service provided. The full cost of any service consists of direct costs and a share of the indirect costs realized by a provider. As discussed in Chapter 6, a cost allocation technique such as the step-down or reciprocal method can be used to allocate indirect costs.

While we have discussed these methods in Chapter 7, Exhibit 10-1 reviews two necessary calculations to cost-based prices. In the first part of Exhibit 10-1, only direct costs are used. In the second part, direct costs plus allocated costs are used. Both calculations could be conducted on a prospective or a retrospective basis, with varying degrees of accuracy and estimation bias.

However, one new variation of a cost-based approach to pricing is based on "activity-based" costs, sometimes called ABC costing. This approach is another variation of full-costing, where the methods used to determine the overhead allocations are much more accurate. Under ABC, cost "drivers" are identified, and then overhead costs are assigned based on many different cost drivers. ABC uses an expanded set of cost drivers, rather than the more typical limited set of activities on which to allocate overhead costs. In other words, ABC is more accurate because the overhead costs are traced more finely to the services that are provided to each patient. Whenever overhead costs are lumped together into an average cost, there is less precision and less variability in the relationship between overhead costs and services performed. Full costs based on ABC techniques are often viewed as more accurate than would full costs determined under the more traditional approaches.

Exhibit 10-1   Two Examples of Cost-Based Pricing.

<u>Direct Costs</u>

Outpatient Clinic Departmental Estimated Costs	$1,284,000
Projected Number of Clinic Visits	85,600
Projected Cost per Visit	$15.00

If one assumes a markup of 50% (or 1.5 x direct costs), then the proposed price will be $22.50.

<u>Direct Costs Plus Allocated Costs</u>

Outpatient Clinic Departmental Estimated Costs	$1,284,000
Allocated Administrative and other Overhead Costs	<u>856,000</u>
Total Clinic Costs	$2,140,000
Projected Number of Clinic Visits	85,600
Projected Cost per Visit	$25.00

If one assumes a markup of 50% (or 1.5 x direct costs), then the proposed price will be $37.50.

The Negotiated and Market Approaches

The **negotiation approach** is usually used with major nongovernmental third-party payers such as Blue Cross, or health maintenance organizations. Allowances, deductions, or discounts from full prices are negotiated on the basis of cost-saving factors such as prompt payment, absence of bad debts, desired volume of patients or efficiency incentives. In many of these negotiations, the ability of individual providers to negotiate successfully is questionable because of the sheer power and size of the third-party payer. In some areas, the providers form consortiums or alliances in an attempt to negotiate area-wide contracts. Much of the impetus for consolidations and mergers might be due to pricing pressures.

Another negotiated approach occurs whenever payers set target prices and contract to pay at (or below) those levels. These dictated prices are becoming more common. Little research has been conducted in this area and not much is known about the methods under which payers set such contract prices. Little is also known about provider responses to dictated prices.

The **market approach** generally implies the presence of competitive providers. Consumers, be they patients, physicians, employers, or payers, are assumed to be sensitive to the price differences between quality providers. Under the market approach, market forces set the price.

It is important to realize that the negotiation and market approaches are closely related to the cost-based approach. For instance, assume that the prices necessary to cover the firm's financial goals have been established. Then assume that the possible negotiated or market-based prices are less than those under the cost-based approach. The organization now has several choices: It must either (1) decrease its costs, (2) increase its volume (assuming that the service has a positive contribution margin), or (3) increase its prices on some other services (assuming everything else remains constant). In other words, market prices will usually dominate cost-based prices. In cases where market or negotiated prices may be lower than cost-based prices, those cost-based prices may not be used.

The next section focuses on specific pricing methods that can be used to implement pricing strategies that have been selected by management.

Pricing Parameters

Any pricing approach that is comprehensive and responsive to changing market conditions must include a financial model of the organization. We illustrate a simple financial model later in this chapter. Pricing decisions must also consider various dimensions of case mix or other descriptors of patients, as well as considering the effects of various levels of patient volume or departmental activities. Before discussing different pricing methods, we will discuss several basic input factors that must also be used in setting prices for health care organizations.

Output Definitions

Defining or choosing the unit of output has a major influence on pricing. Prices are always related to some unit of service or product. The provider, or the market, must define the unit of service that will be used as the basis for pricing. Prices are always tied to a unit of service. Several alternative output measures currently in use are:

1. Per procedure: payment is based on services provided.
2. Per diem: payment is based on price per day.
3. Per admission: payment is based on admission, not type of service.
4. Per discharge: payment is based on discharge, not type of service.
5. Per diagnosis: payment is based on diagnosis at either time of admission or discharge.
6. Capitation: payment is made in advance per individual (per capita, or per head), or per member per month (pmpm) as in HMOs and other managed care contracts, regardless of whether services are utilized.

All of these payment bases have been used at one time or another in various combinations and by various payers. All have their strengths and weaknesses in influencing desired behavior in providing service. The ideal is to ensure a high quality of care, encourage the most efficient use of resources, while maintaining appropriate quality of care. The exact impact of presence of substantial complications and/or comorbidities. The splitting process is illustrated in Figure 10-2. The complete list of MDCs is shown in Table10-2, and the DRGs for MDC01 are listed in Table 10-3. Note that in 1995, there were 490 different DRGs.

Implementing a DRG-based Pricing System

On October 1, 1983, a prospective DRG system was implemented that established a fixed price per DRG for operating costs of services for Medicare inpatients. This payment system was originally phased in over several years using national and regional DRG "blended" rates for each hospital. After the initial phase-in period, a national rate (per DRG) was established annually for Medicare payments to health care providers for inpatient care. Approved medical education programs and capital-related costs such as depreciation, interest, amortization, and leasing were originally excluded from the DRG rate and paid for separately. Capital costs are now reimbursed in a parallel prospective payment system, again on a phased basis. Medical education costs are still treated separately.

The Health Care Financing Administration (HCFA) has developed two payment methods for capital under PPS—the "hold harmless" method and the "fully prospective method." Any providers with a capital rate *below* the adjusted Federal rate are paid on the fully prospective method. Most, more than 70%, providers are expected to be paid under this method. However, since there are two alternative methods, providers must keep track of "old capital" versus "new capital" in their HCFA-2552 cost reporting forms. Old capital covers capital costs incurred or put into service prior to 1990, while new capital covers any subsequent capital costs. The implication of these differences is that pricing may be adjusted, or "gamed," in certain circumstances where a provider may have discretion in determining some of its capital costs. This example is meant to illustrate that pricing, even under a fairly definitive PPS system, still includes many areas where subjectivity and judgment may preclude precise answers.[4]

Although DRG-based rates have become quite standard, and accepted norm for Medicare payments to health care providers, there have been frequent adjustments ("fine-tuning") in many of the detailed rules governing both the capital and operating portions of DRG rates.

Similar concepts have also been developed for ambulatory health care. Service indicators, analogous to DRGs, have been designated as ambulatory visit groups (AVGs). These AVGs are being used to determine prospective prices for visits to medical clinics, physicians, etc. Physicians have now been subjected to another pricing method based on resource-based relative value units (RBRVS). These service indicators are designed to standardize measures of physician services, while AVGs are designed to capture both the physician and non-physician components of ambulatory services.

The importance of the major shift in reimbursement from a retrospective, cost-based system to a prospective, fixed-rate-per-DRG system should not be underestimated. Health care providers have the opportunity and the challenge to provide services at less than Medicare's fixed rate, because they then get to keep the difference. However, providers are also at risk for expenses that exceed the fixed rate. Some hospitals are certainly better off under DRG-based prices. For instance, many hospitals with aging physical plants or a less severe case mix of

Figure 10-2   Major Diagnostic Category 16: Diseases and Disorders of the Blood and Blood-Forming Organs and Immunological Disorders. Source: Ernst & Whiney. "The Revised DRGs: Their Importance in Medicare Payments to Hospitals," 1983.

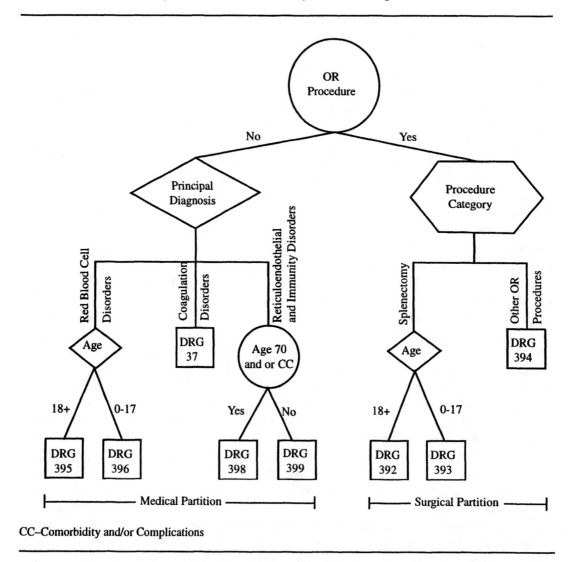

CC–Comorbidity and/or Complications

patients have experienced higher profit rates under the DRG-based prospective payment system (PPS). However, some providers have suffered losses greater than those incurred prior to DRG-based pricing. In particular, many small rural hospitals have been negatively affected under PPS.

Managerial Responses to DRGs _____

Managerial decision-making under DRGs has been difficult for several reasons:

1. Uncertainty over how capital costs are to be treated.
2. The use of blended and weighted rates (national versus specific facility) on varying fiscal periods.
3. The necessity to revise cost accounting systems and procedures to reflect new product and service definitions.
4. The uncertain effects of DRGs on volume, quality, and access.

Managerial performance reports typically generated under new DRG-based, or AVG-based, systems have often been confusing and misleading. They are often biased by faulty cost allocations or an emphasis on product profitability that is often uncontrollable given the provider's mission statement and objectives.

Management analysis and pricing by individual DRGs, or AVGs, can be very cumbersome and confusing, especially when both direct and indirect costs are considered. We recommend that the unit of analysis be established at a more highly-aggregated level of major diagnostic categories (MDC) or strategic product-line groupings (SPG).

SPGs are categories of products or services that are consistent with the provider's strategic plan. MDCs are one example of how SPGs might be defined. Other bases for categorizing products and services might be severity of illness, length of stay, or the organizational unit (department) providing care.

It is not the profitability of each DRG, or AVG, that is manageable or controllable. Instead, it is the profitability for related groups of services or procedures that can be monitored and influenced. Health care managers often cannot reduce or modify the kinds of tests or care provided to an individual patient. However, they can modify, by working with clinical professionals, the modal care patterns provided for whole groups of patients. The organizational structures, the capital-labor mix, and other factors can be changed for groups of patients and for entire departments, but not for individual patients or for individual DRGs or AVGs. Managers should focus attention on revenues, contribution margins, and profits for each MDC or SPG. Definition and management of SPGs should be distinct at each institution and should include clusters of similar services (based on DRGs or AVGs) performed by the same medical staff or service units. In many institutions, a few DRGs (50 or so) account for 98% of all patient days. If so, managerial attention should focus on that limited subset rather than generate long computer printouts of unprofitable DRGs that only have one or two cases each year. Those rare procedures will have little effect on overall profits and institutional fiscal health. It is the relatively few categories of services in which particular medical staff and departments have specialized that will have the greatest impact on long-run returns and survival.

Examples of possible SPGs include:

	DRG
Cardiology	121-127
Hematology	395-404
Obstetrics	376-381
Rehabilitative medicine	461-467

As indicated above, these SPGs will vary for each health care provider. Similar clusters can be defined for ancillary service departments and ambulatory care services. In each case, managerial attention should focus on the total revenue of each cluster rather than on individual prices and profits. The following sections indicate ways to set individual prices; however, managers should not fall into the trap of comparing unit prices and average costs; remember the impact of volume on average fixed costs. Instead, managerial attention should be devoted to total revenues and contribution margins generated by each category of services and procedures.

Current Issues in Pricing

Relative Value Units

Other approaches to developing an intensity-of-care approach have been used primarily in ancillary services. As indicated above, RBRVSs have been developed for most physician services. **Relative value units** (RVUs) have also been developed for laboratory procedures by the American College of Pathology and for the radiology departments by the American College of Radiology. The relative value approach depends upon developing some common element of resources required. Each procedure or test is then expressed in terms of this common factor. The total quantity of each procedure is multiplied by the weighted value to obtain the total weighted units to be performed. Dividing the financial goals for the department by the total weighted unit gives an average cost for each common factor. Multiplying the average common factor cost by the number of factors in each procedure gives the price to be charged for specific examinations. Table 10-4 illustrates this approach for a laboratory department.

The fairness and usefulness of the pricing information from the weighted and unweighted approaches illustrated in Table 10-4 depend upon the viewpoint of the service recipient and the manner. Clearly, some cost shifting was being done between examinations if the weighting of the individual examinations was a reasonably accurate assessment of the resources required. For example, a patient receiving test 5 would require 10 times as many resources as a patient receiving test 1, yet would pay the same price of $250 under the average cost calculations rather than a price of $862 under the weighted factor approach.

Surcharge Techniques

Several other techniques are commonly used to determine prices when certain conditions exist. One of these techniques is based on **surcharges** which is similar to mark-ups in a retail

Table 10-4 Development of a Weighted Factor Approach.

General information

Total tests to be performed =	10,000	Average cost per
Total financial requirements =	$2,500,000	exam = $250.00

Types of tests	Weighting index (common factors required)*	x	Unweighted no. of tests	=	Weighted no. of tests
1	1		5,000		5,000
2	2		1,000		2,000
3	4		2,000		8,000
4	6		1,500		9,000
5	10		500		5,000
			10,000		29,000

$$\text{Average common Factor cost} = \frac{\text{Total financial requirements}}{\text{Total weighted no. of tests}} = \frac{\$2,500,000}{29,000} = \$86.21$$

Based on these data, the rates for the exams would be established as follows:

Type of exam	Weighting index	Average cost per factor	Weighted rate to be charged
1	1	$86.21	$ 86.21
2	2	86.21	172.42
3	4	86.21	344.84
4	6	86.21	517.26
5	10	86.21	862.10

*The weighting index may be based on RVUs or on labor time necessary to perform each test.

store. For example, in a pharmacy or central supply setting where many low-cost individual units are issued or dispensed, the development of individual prices would be very time-consuming. In this type of setting, the surcharge or average mark-up approach is used to accomplish the goals of recovering costs, while minimizing the impact of record keeping. In the surcharge method, the goals of the department are divided through by some common element of cost that is routinely kept. In a pharmacy, this element of cost could be the cost of drugs, whereas in central supply pricing it could be the cost of supplies issued. Exhibit 10-2 illustrates this pricing approach.

Time-Based Techniques

When the major determinant of cost is the time factor involved, an hourly or per-minute rate approach can be developed. For example, in an operating room, most of the costs are relatively fixed for most surgical procedures. Dividing the financial goal of the operating room by the number of hours or minutes available gives the average charge **per unit of time**. Multiplying this average charge by the units of time for specific procedures gives the operating room charge to be established for individual procedures. Exhibit 10-3 presents an example of this approach. Using the data in Exhibit 10-3, a procedure requiring 38 minutes would be billed at $775.96 (38 minutes x 20.42 = $775.96).

Contribution Margin Techniques

Another pricing method that is simple to use, but often under-utilized, is based on contribution margins. The health care provider may use the contribution margin ratio from its income statement, or it may set a target contribution margin (e.g. 40%), such that a guideline for the expected contribution margin for each service or department is established. The departmental variable costs for each service or procedure are simply divided by the variable cost ratio (or 1.0 - the target contribution margin ratio to determine the budget price Table 10-5).

If the total fixed costs for this group of procedures and its financial requirements are $145,000, then the proposed prices will meet the organization's financial needs. If, however, the financial goals are $350,000, then the proposed prices are well off the mark.

Exhibit 10-2   The Surcharge Approach to Pricing.

$$\frac{\text{Total Financial Requirements}}{\text{Total Cost of Drugs Used}} = \frac{2,500,000}{1,250,000} = 2$$

The cost of each drug issued would be multiplied by a factor of 2 to obtain the rate to be charged.

For example, for a drug costing $20.00:

Drug Cost	$20.00
Rate To Be Charged	$40.00

Exhibit 10-3   Per-Unit-of-Time Approach to Pricing.

Total Financial Requirements	$2,500,000
Number of Hours Available (or Scheduled)	2,040
Number of Minutes Available (or Scheduled)	122,400
Rate per hour	$1,225.49
Rate per minute	$20.42

Table 10-5 Contribution Margin Pricing Example.

Procedure	Variable cost per unit	1 – Target Contribution margin ratio	Target price	Projected Volume	Projected Revenues	Variable Costs	Projected Contribution Margin
1	$120	0.60	$200	100	$20,000	$12,000	$8,000
2	240	0.60	400	200	80,000	48,000	32,000
3	300	0.60	500	300	150,000	90,000	60,000
Total					$250,000	$150,000	$100,000

Target CMR = .40

Target Price = V.C. /1-Target CMR

The contribution margin-based pricing model is easy to implement and easy to understand. It does not require complex cost allocation, and it is not biased by the costs of services in other departments. It is easily integrated with the most financial planning models, as well as with the paragon pricing model described below. The contribution margin pricing model is easy to use because it is based solely on the direct or variable costs of a service or procedure. Such data can be easily understood and communicated by departmental managers, and they are very reliable and not usually sensitive to changes in volume. In other words, as occupancy or utilization levels change, the contribution margin ratio does not usually change significantly. Therefore, prices will be more stable and more directly related to overall institutional goals. Even though contribution margins may vary by department, their impact on institutional profitability can be conveniently modeled, and "what-if" analyses can be conducted to fine tune proposed prices. A brief example of such modeling techniques is shown in the next section.

Inclusive Versus Individual Prices

Up to now, the approaches described in this chapter have concentrated on developing individualized prices. This approach is consistent with current payment schemes encountered by most health care providers. However, another school of thought encourages the use of an **all-inclusive approach** to billing and reimbursement. We believe that the administrators of a health care provider need to know individual costs and prices. However, they do not need to bill patients on an itemized approach. The all-inclusive approach offers several advantages and disadvantages as indicated in Exhibit 10-4.

The arguments presented in Exhibit 10-4 may become irrelevant, as it appears that many government and other contract purchasers of health care are proceeding toward an all-inclusive or flat-rate system of prospective payments under the DRG method. Whether the disadvantages of the prospective payment system will outweigh the advantages remains to be seen. As an extreme example of inclusive pricing, consider the concept of global pricing described in the next section.

Exhibit 10-4 Advantages and Disadvantages of Inclusive Prices.

<u>Advantages</u>

Ease of billing and reduction in administrative costs.

Patients know total cost before the service is provided and can plan accordingly.

Amount of medical care given is driven by quality requirements, not reimbursement implications.

<u>Disadvantages</u>

Patients pay whether they receive all the services or not.

Intensity of services provided is increased since no additional cost to the patients exists.

Patients may not receive adequate quality care since the bill remains the same regardless of actual care provided

---

Global Pricing

Global pricing represents an approach to risk sharing between the physician and the organizational unit providing care. Global pricing requires that a price be set for a particular service that includes both the physician component and the institutional (hospital, home care, clinic, etc.) component. Under global pricing, three categories of payments could be established in order to compensate providers for various services and risks:

- a risk pool to be used for outliers,
- a physician compensation pool, and an
- institutional payment rate.

Payments to the risk pool are usually taken "off the top" and paid first; for example, at a pre-specified rate of 25%. The providing institution then receives a fixed percentage of the global price, say 65%, while physicians are eligible to receive most of the remainder. For a surgical case, each surgeon, anesthetist, etc. might receive a pre-specified percentage of this remainder. Part of the remainder might be put into other incentive pools that relate to length of stay, ambulatory ability, patient satisfaction, etc.

One example of such an approach is shown in Table 10-6 which relates to heart bypass surgeries. In this case, 20% of the fixed payment of $30,000 goes into the risk pool for outliers. The hospital receives 70% of the remainder (= $24,000 = 80% of $30,000). The hospital portion could have been shown simply as 56% of the total payment (56% of $30,000 = $16,800). Note in this table that physicians seem to absorb most of the risk as the risk pool and the hospital portion are all paid at fixed rates. However, the physicians also have the greatest incentive to control length of stay as they will receive a transfer payment from the hospital under the two types of per diem incentives shown at the bottom of the table. In other words, the physicians will tend to gain the most when lengths of stay are controlled, and they will tend to lose under circumstances where many cost outliers occur and where the risk pool for outliers is over-extended.

Table 10-6 Allocation of Payment.

Payee	Standard amount	Percent of payment
Hospital	$16,800	70.0%
Surgeon	3,360	14.0
Anesthesia	1,680	7.0
Invasive cardiologist (catherterization)	1,320	5.5
Attending cardiologist	840	3.5
Physician subtotal	7,200	30.0
Total payments	$24,000	100.0%
Per diem incentive for each day below the corridor (less than 8 days)	$500 goes from hospital to physician pool	
Per diem incentive for each day below the corridor (greater than 12 days)	$300 goes from hospital to physician pool	

Source: Kelly, Margo P. "How Global Pricing Works." *Healthcare Financial Management* (December) 1995, p.18.

Other incentives could be created such that the hospital shares in the risk pool for outliers. Surgeons could have different incentives than consultants, etc. Any global pricing scheme exposes all providers to different risks than would have been experienced under cost-based reimbursement (CBR). Such risks certainly include length of stay, as noted above, as well as the risks due to severity of care and physician treatment preferences. The advantages of global pricing suggest that all providers must cooperate and share in all the risks, rather than subjecting hospitals to risks that may conflict with risks incurred by physicians and patients.

Another variation of global pricing under a risk sharing approach might put part of the fixed price into a patient-related pool that would be shared (returned) to patients who engaged in preventive measures, who followed their drug protocols, and who sought appropriate and timely treatment. In other words, rather than leaving patients out of this equation, a global pricing scheme should include patient behaviors to the same extent that physician and institutional factors are considered.

Medicare Risk Contracting

Many hospital providers are now considering how to develop **capitated prices** for some or all of their patient populations. This trend has been most extensive for Medicare patients enrolled in health maintenance organizations (HMO's). Medicare publishes its capitation rates for every U.S. county at a pre-set rate based on adjusted average per capita costs (AAPCC). These rates are adjusted to reflect differences in HMO location, members' age, sex and ambulatory status, and other factors. HMO's are paid at a percentage (e.g., 95%) of the AAPCC.

An example of how to calculate hospital payments under a Medicare risk contract are shown in Exhibit 10-5. These calculations are driven by the hospital's expected market share of the total Medicare population served in the region. The AAPCC is simply multiplied by the

Exhibit 10-5   Sample Calculation of Hospital Payments Under a Medicare Risk Contract.

Hospital Location	Atlanta, Georgia (Fulton County)
Number of Medicare admissions	3,000
Estimated size of Medicare population served	15,000
AAPCC for Part A, Fulton County, Georgia	$257.94
Total Part A budget per year	(257.94 x 12 months) x 15,000 = $46,429,200
Estimated hospital share	90%
Estimated hospital capitation budget per year	$46,429,200 x .90 = $41,786,280
Estimated hospital budget per inpatient admission per year	46,429,200/3,000 = 15,476.4 x .90 (hospital portion) = $13,929 (rounded)

Source: Kolb, D.S. and J.L. Horowitz. "Managing the Transition to Capitation" *Healthcare Financial Management* (February) 1995, p. 65.

expected number of Medicare enrollees on an annual basis. This revenue stream is then converted to a per admission rate which can then be compared with average costs, using the techniques described earlier in this text.

More sophisticated analyses would include using type of case served, average length of stay, proportion of inpatient vs. outpatient care, etc. Using gross averages, as in Exhibit 10-5, would not give managers a sufficient basis on which to decide how to improve care treatment patterns or how to negotiate with an HMO that might propose capitation rates lower than the AAPCC rates. In other words, managers need more prices and costs that reflect both fixed and variable elements as well as other patient attributes and conditions.

Another element that must be considered under risk-sharing agreements is the level of risk relative to the level of control that must be exercised. Figure 10-3 shows how level of risk is almost perfectly correlated with the level of control that is necessary under capitated risk-sharing schemes. In other words, the provider must develop and implement fairly tough controls that affect physicians, patients and internal systems in order to survive under capitated risk-sharing schemes. These controls include:

Figure 10-3 Risk-Control Continuum.

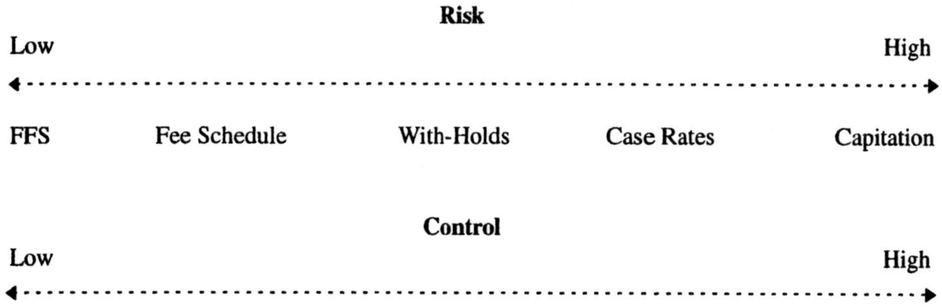

Risk

Low   High

◄┄┄►

FFS   Fee Schedule   With-Holds   Case Rates   Capitation

Control

Low   High

◄┄┄►

Adapted from: Coyne, J.S., "Is Your Organization Ready to Share Financial Risk with HMOs?" *Healthcare Financial Management* August, 1994, p. 31.

- utilization review and case management programs,
- quality assurance programs,
- physician credentialing programs,
- provider and facility selection criteria,
- patient education and patient wellness programs, and
- comprehensive, "real-time" managed care MIS.

Our main point in including this brief discussion of the controls necessary under risk-sharing schemes is to emphasize that pricing is no longer an isolated management decision. It must interface with many other parts of the patient care and management process. Pricing under capitation and risk sharing requires a full integration of all management systems.

Prospective Versus Retrospective Reimbursement

The retrospective cost-based reimbursement system whereby payment is based on actual costs of the service has been subject to considerable criticism in recent years. It has been claimed that the payment of actual costs provides little incentive for providers to control expenditures; in fact, it seems to encourage just the opposite. Reimbursement increases as costs increase. The practice of auditing costs after the service has been provided can also lead to denial of payment for services already provided, leaving the institution saddled with after-the-fact, uncollectible bills.

Prospective reimbursement is one attempt to provide proper incentives to the health care provider to contain health care costs. Under a prospective system, the provider agrees in advance to provide services for an established price. This amount can be based on a total budget with unlimited services (an HMO approach) or an individualized flat-rate service approach (such as DRGs). Any of the methods of reimbursement illustrated earlier can be used; the major difference is that the provider is now at risk. If the costs for providing the service are greater than budgeted, the provider loses. If the costs are less, the provider gains. Prospective pricing can also appeal to regulators, because under a total budget approach they can limit or at least know their resource requirements in advance.

The shift of risks will mandate that health care providers obtain access to better cost and utilization information. Once prices have been negotiated, the provider must be prepared to make adjustments to nongovernment patients or adjust expenses accordingly when conditions change from the plan.

Cost Shifting

The impact of "discount" payers on the pricing process has been receiving considerable attention from major purchasers of health insurance who pay full or discounted charges. The shifting of costs not reimbursed by the cost-based or other payers to the charge-based payers has become a primary method by which health care providers meet their financial objectives.

As health care costs have escalated, many private insurance carriers and self-insured employer groups have been forced to reconsider their routine acceptance of the cost shifting process. The magnitude of cost shifting is indicated in Exhibit 10-6. From a fair share of $2,100, the charge to the charge-based payer must increase to $3,500 to meet the firm's financial goals. This is clearly an unrealistic expectation which only ensures that the institution's financial goals are not met.

Price Adjustments

The heavy fixed costs of most health care providers make individual prices extremely sensitive to changes in mix and volume of services offered. Many health care providers now only adjust their prices on an annual basis. We believe that this annual adjustment is usually insufficient for proper management of the financial resources of the organization. For example, more frequent price adjustments would mean a smaller percentage increase each time rather than a single adjustment each year. The advantages of frequent price increases, especially from a political perspective but also from a fairness and financial perspective, should be seriously considered. If prices should be higher than currently charged, the private-pay patient is not being properly charged for the interim period. Also, if a prospective pricing system is in operation for cost-based payers, the relative seriousness of inadequate charges must be quickly determined and renegotiations started. Even if the price increase cannot be implemented immediately because of either an internal political problem or the requirements of a state review process, the administrator can manage more effectively if the revenue shortages are known in advance.

Under managed care, with a strong emphasis on negotiations and discounted prices, adjustments in prices occur on a monthly or very frequent basis. In fact, an entire chapter would be required to describe the process of pricing under managed care. In such cases, risk-based contracts are established between the provider and the purchaser. Based on preliminary estimates of volumes, patients' acuity, estimates of hospital versus ambulatory services, and estimates of preventive versus acute services, a contract price is established on a "per capita" or capitated basis. This capitated price is usually in effect for a fairly long period, a year or more. However,

Exhibit 10-6 The Cost Shifting Process.

Mix of Patients			Payment Method	
40% Blue Cross			costs + 10%	
30% Medicare			$2,000	
15% Medicaid			90% of costs	
10% self-pay			charges	
5% charity, bad debts			0	
Total costs (100 patients)			$200,000	
Desired margin			$ 10,000	
Total financial requirements			$210,000	

Fair Share Average	=	$210,000/100	=	$2,100 per patient
Cost Per Patient	=	$200,000/100	=	$2,000
Medicaid Cost	=	(.9)x(2,000)	=	$1,800
Fair Share Average Price		=		$2,100

Subsidies or Cost Shifts		$2,100
Charity, bad debt	[(5 patients x 2,100)/95 patients]	= + 111
	= New Fair Share Avg. Price	= $2,211
Medicare	[(2,211 – 2,000) x 30 patients)/65 patients]	= + 97
	= New Fair Share Avg. Price	= $2,308
Medicaid	[(2,308 - 1,800) x 15 patients)/50 patients]	= + 152
	= New Fair Share Avg. Price	= $2,460
Blue Cross	[(2,460 – 2,200) x 40 patients)/10 patients]	= +1,040
	Charge to Self-Pay	= $3,500

Source: Adapted from a presentation by Hugh Long, at the meeting of the American Academy of Medical Directors, Tulane University, Phoenix, AZ, 1982.

when the next purchase or bid request is made, the provider may adjust the prices on each component of service. It is this frequent adjustment, and the differing prices, depending on other contract terms, that typifies the new environment of managed care contracting and pricing.

Paragon Pricing

Paragon pricing is a new term describing a method for basing an institution's prices on a long-run perspective. Under paragon pricing, financial policies are set for the desired pricing structure necessary to achieve the firm's financial goals. The paragon price is what the institution would like to be able to charge for a particular service.[5] It is the yardstick against which actual prices are evaluated. The health care manager determines a paragon price for all major diagnostic categories and ambulatory services. Trends in actual prices are then monitored and compared with the paragon price.

It will be impossible to meet or exceed the paragon price for all services. However, in deciding whether to expand or contract a particular service, the historical variances between paragon and actual prices will be a useful signal of the desirability of expansion or contraction. Deviations below paragon prices will also be a signal to try to increase actual prices wherever possible.

The issue of paragon pricing becomes one of setting a paragon price and then deciding if the market price should be higher or lower. Alternatively, the manager's decision process becomes one of deciding what steps are necessary to achieve the paragon price.

The paragon price is often calculated to cover service delivery costs plus a margin in excess of costs, which is set by policy to provide an adequate return on capital. It is a long-term benchmark upon which to evaluate monthly or annual price (or service) adjustments.

Because it is a long-term concept, capacity levels and utilization capacity do not vary wildly in monthly recalculations as does volume of services. Cost accounting procedures typically suggest that overhead and other indirect costs be allocated or averaged on the basis of the estimated volume of services. This estimate is usually based on next year's forecast. However, paragon pricing is based on the less frequently used concept of "normal volume," which is a long-run (three to five years) estimate of capacity utilization that smooths the seasonal and annual variability in patient services. For example, consider the case of hospital with the following occupancy projections:

Year		
	1	60%
	2	70%
	3	55%
	4	75%
	5	65%
Average		65%

The long-run average of 65% would be used to set the paragon price for each of the five years. In other words, the denominator level of activity in each year would be based on the 65% long-run average level. Use of this long-run normal volume would then imply that prices would not drop precipitously when occupancy rises to 70%, nor would prices rise sharply the next year when occupancy falls to 55%. In each case, use of the normal, long-run volume dampens the pricing swings and helps to achieve a consistent and stable profit margin and return on capital.

Because of these volume-related effects, paragon pricing sidesteps some of the traps in cost accounting that may lead to erroneous price adjustments due to overhead allocation and volume estimates. It provides a signal to managers regarding which services to expand and regarding the impact of future strategies on profitability and survival.

Market Sensitivity

Even though pricing is important to health care managers, it may not always be very important to consumers, particularly those who are insulated from the bill by insurance or government payment programs, although pricing certainly has some impact on elective procedures and many wellness programs. In fact, only about 10% of patients choose a physician on the basis of fees, and a much smaller proportion use of out-of-pocket costs as the most important criterion in choosing a hospital. The major factor in making a choice is the physician's reputation (40%), whereas previous experience as a patient and location are given by about 30% each as the major criterion for choosing a physician.[6] As noted earlier, prices often do not affect individual patients' decisions when payments are through insurance companies, employers, HMOs, PPOs, and other large purchasers. Consumers are not very sensitive to price when the majority of charges are paid by other entities.

Financial Modeling

The use of a basic financial model to evaluate individual prices was first presented in Chapter 5. Using the financial modeling approach, an estimate of various price structures under varying cost or demand scenarios can quickly be determined. The use of a microcomputer can be most helpful here as the basic model can be programmed easily with little expertise. Most spreadsheet software packages available today offer some form of financial modeling.

The basic model for evaluating prices was discussed in Chapter 5. At the most basic level, prices can be viewed in the context of a cost-volume-profit model:

$$\text{Revenues} = \text{Fixed Costs} + \text{Variable Costs} + \text{Other Financial Objectives}$$

$$\text{Price} \times \text{Quantity} = \text{Fixed Costs} + (\text{Variable Cost per Unit} \times \text{Quantity}) + \text{Other Financial Objectives}$$

$$P \times Q = FC + (VCU \times Q) + \text{Other Financial Objectives}$$

For example:

$$FC = \$1,000,000$$
$$CU = \$15$$
$$\text{Other Financial Objectives} = \$250,000$$
$$Q = 20,000$$
$$P = ?$$

Substituting these data into the cost model, the following price (P) is determined:

$$P(20,000) = \$1,000,000 + \$15(20,000) + \$250,000$$
$$20,000(P) = \$1,550,000$$
$$P = \$77.50$$

As noted in Chapter 5, various scenarios can be simulated using a financial modeling approach. For example, volume, fixed costs, variable costs per unit, or other financial requirements can be varied to estimate the impact of alternative prices. The calculated prices can then be compared with competitors' prices or community service goals in order to judge their feasibility. The flexibility of the model can be especially important when frequent price adjustments must be made. The ability to compare actual revenues with budgeted revenues is also dependent on the accuracy of volume estimates. Note that the financial models described in the budgeting chapter can also be used to attain these same objectives.

Summary

Pricing is a vital management function for most health care providers. The lack of adequate information bases, the external restrictions, and the political nature of setting prices make the process difficult and challenging. The shift to prospective payment systems and managed care contracts only makes the need to establish viable and realistic prices more pressing. The use of financial modeling and computer-assisted decision techniques may offer the best approach in meeting future pricing needs.

Notes

1. From the American Hospital Association statement "Financial Requirements of Health Care Institutions and Services," 1979.
2. See Long, H. W. and J.B. Silvers. "Medicare Reimbursement Is Federal Taxation of Tax-Exempt Providers." *Health Care Management Review* 1(4): 31-47, 1976.
3. Furst, R.W., *Financial Management for Health Care Institutions*. Boston: Allyn & Bacon, 1981.
4. S. R. Coffey provides a set of worksheets and examples that may help a provider decide how to establish its capital prices under PPS ("Retroactive Reimbursement Under HCFA's PPS for Capital." *Healthcare Financial Management* (October): 60-66, 1993.)
5. Pearson, J.A. "Paragon Pricing." *Management Accounting* 67(12): 41-42, 1986.
6. Graham, J. (ed.) "Providers Not Picked by Price." *Modern Health Care* 16(16): 23, 1986.

Bibliography

Block, L.F. and C.E. Press. "Product Line Development by DRG Builds Market Strength." *Healthcare Financial Management* 39(12):50-52, 1985.

Borok, L.S. "The Use of Relational Databases in Health Care Information Systems." *Journal of Health Care Finance* (Summer): 6-12, 1995.

Brandeau, M. L., and D.S. Hopkins. "A Patient Mix Model for Hospital Financial Planning." *Inquiry*, 21(1):32-44, 1984.

Brewster, A.C., R.C. Bradbury and C.M. Jacobs. "Measuring the Effect of Illness Severity on Revenue under DRG's." *Healthcare Financial Management* 39(7): 52-60, 1985.

Bridges, M.J. and P. Jacobs. "Obtaining Estimates of Marginal Cost by DRG." *Healthcare Financial Management* 40(10): 40-46, 1986.

Coffey, R.S. "Retroactive Reimbursement Under HCFA's PPS for Capital." *Healthcare Financial Management* (October): 60-66, 1993.

Coyne, J.S. "Is Your Organization Ready to Share Financial Risk with HMOs?" *Healthcare Financial Management* (August): 31, 1994.

Czarnecki, M.T. "Benchmarking Can Add Up for Healthcare Accounting" *Healthcare Financial Management* (September): 62-67, 1994.

Eastaugh, S.R. "Differential Cost Analysis: Judging a PPO's Feasibility." *Healthcare Financial Management* 40(5): 44-51, 1986.

Eastaugh, S.R. and J.A. Eastaugh. "Prospective Payment Systems: Steps to Enhance Quality, Efficiency, and Regionalization" *Health Care Management Review* 11(4): 37-52, 1986.

Graham, J. (ed.), "Providers Not Picked by Price." *Modern Health Care* 16 (16): 23, 1986.

Jacobs, P. and C.R. Franz. "Developing Pricing Policies by Diagnostic Groupings." *Healthcare Financial Management* (January): 50-52, 1985.

Kelly, M.P. "How Global Pricing Works." *Healthcare Financial Management* (December): 18, 1995.

Kolb, D.S. and J.L. Horowitz. "Managing the Transition to Capitation" *Healthcare Financial Management* (February): 65, 1995.

Kongstvedt, P.R. *Essentials of Managed Health Care.* Gaithersburg, Maryland: Aspen Publishers, Inc., 1995.

Long, H. W., and J.B. Silvers. "Medicare Reimbursement Is Federal Taxation of Tax-Exempt Providers." *Health Care Management Review* 1(1): 9-23,1976.

Pearson, J.A., "Paragon Pricing." *Management Accounting* 67(12): 41-42, 1986.

Reif, R.A., P.A. Bickett, and D.E. Halberstadt. "Case Study: Analyzing the Market Using DRGs and MDCs." *Healthcare Financial Management* 39(12): 44-47, 1985.

Ross, E. "Making Money with Proactive Pricing" *Harvard Business Review* 62(6): 145-155, 1984.

Suver, J.D., W.P. Jessee, and W.N. Zelman. "Financial Management and DRG's" *Hospital and Health Services Administration* 31(1): 75—85, 1986.

Terms and Concepts

all-inclusive approach
capitated prices
case mix
cost-based approach
cost shifting
costs of doing business
costs of changing business
cost of uncertainty
diagnosis related group (DRG)

global pricing
market approach
negotiation approach
per-unit-of-time approach
price setter
pricing strategies
price taker
relative value unit
surcharge approach
total financial requirements

Questions and Problems _____

10-1 Define the major categories in the determination of total financial requirements.

10-2 What is meant by "costs of uncertainty," and why are they important to consider?

10-3 Why is proper pricing vital for a health care provider?

10-4 Does your answer differ if the health care provider is an investor-owned, for-profit organization rather than a not-for-profit organization?

10-5 Explain the three basic pricing strategies available to a health care provider.

10-6 Under what circumstances would each of the strategies be used by a provider?

10-7 Explain the basic cost model and its components.

10-8 What are activity bases? Explain the major activity bases used by health care providers in determining prices.

10-9 Why is the intensity-of-care approach useful in setting prices? Explain the advantages and disadvantages of establishing many different price categories.

10-10 What are diagnosis-related groups?

10-11 What are DRGs based on?

10-12 Describe what a relative value unit is, and what it is used for.

10-13 Explain the surcharge and unit-of-time approaches to developing prices.

10-14 Explain the advantages and disadvantages of all-inclusive prices.

10-15 Explain how cost shifting has led to higher charges to self-pay patients.

10-16 Who should review the prices set by health care organizations? Why?

10-17 Explain the major arguments against continuing to use the retrospective reimbursement system for health care.

10-18 What effect will prospective reimbursement have on the need to establish realistic prices?

10-19 The data in the accompanying table were collected for the Mission Medical Center to determine prices for routine inpatient care:
   A. Determine the existing charges for each of the revenue-producing departments.
   B. The number of patient days is expected to increase by 5% in the medical/surgery nursing departments and by 10% in the remaining areas. What is the total profit if all other factors remain the same?
   C. Variable costs are expected to increase by 13% and fixed costs by 10% during the next year. What prices should be established to break even if the number of patient days in B is anticipated?
   D. Mission Medical Center wishes to make an extra 10% profit on the services it provides. Given the cost increases above, what prices should be established for each patient care department if the number of patient days remains the same as last year?

10-20 The Sky Blue County Hospital Board of Trustees reviewed the data submitted by the administrator for the past year of operation. The primary concern of money trustees was to have each service pay for its own costs. Answer the following questions based on the submitted data which is presented in the accompanying table:
   A. Determine the existing prices for each service.
   B. By how much would existing prices have to be increased (decreased) in order to break even by individual service? (Determine dollars and percentages.)
   C. If financial goals are estimated to be $600,000 over the costs of providing the services, what prices would you change to make up the increase?
   D. Explain the justification for your answer to C.

10-21 The Pear County Hospital Board of Trustees recently changed the method of determining costs for patients seeking emergency room service. The current fee is $35 based on a flat rate scale. It does not include physician fees or medical supplies other than routine requirements. In 1982, there were 27,737 visits to the emergency room. The proposed method will replace the flat fee with a scale based on the amount of time spent in emergency room treatment. Only time spent in treatment, not waiting time, will be counted. A one-month survey of the emergency room patients showed that 49% were in the shortest visit category, 39% were in the 16 to 60 minute category, 4% were in the 61 to 120 minute category, 6% in the 121 to 240 minute category and the remainder in the more than 240 minute category. The proposed rates are:

   $27 for 15 minutes or less,
   $35 for 16 to 60 minutes,
   $70 for 61 to 120 minutes,
   $140 for 121 to 240 minutes,
   $245 for more than 240 minutes.

A. Determine the impact on the revenues of the emergency room if the same number of visits occur with the same relative distribution during the next year.

B. If existing emergency rooms in the area charge from $35 to $75, what do you anticipate could happen to the relative mix of the type of patients seen by Pear County Hospital?

10-22 Given the following data, develop recommended prices using the contribution margin method and a target contribution margin of 40%. Develop two sets of prices, one set at an average rate of 40% for all departments and one set at 40% for each.

Dept.	V.C./unit	Quantity
A	10	1,000
B	20	500
C	40	400

10-23 Identify the environmental conditions and type of healthcare organizations that would justify the use of paragon pricing.

10-24 The Greeley Public Health Department has the following budget for next year:

	Division A	B	C	Total
Revenues	$120,000	$80,000	$50,000	$250,000
Variable Costs	96,000	56,000	35,000	187,000
Fixed Costs	11,000	6,000	4,000	21,000
Total Costs	107,000	62,000	39,000	208,000
Net Income	$13,000	$18,000	$11,000	$42,000

A new service is being considered. This service will require new equipment costing $18,000 with a three-year life and no salvage value. Service revenues of $25,000 are expected in the first year, and $30,000 per year after that. Variable costs will be 60% of revenues. No new facilities will be required.

Should the new service be introduced? What return on investment would this service provide? How should fixed costs be allocated to this service? How do fixed costs affect return on investment?

10-25 The Orange County Clinic anticipates the following service quantities at each of the listed prices:

Price	Estimated Quantity
$60.00	100,000
50.00	150,000
40.00	180,000
30.00	200,000
20.00	400,000

Its variable costs are $12.00 per unit and its separable fixed costs are $280,000 per year.

A. What price should be charged? Why?
B. How would your recommendation change if insurance costs were estimated at $7.00 per unit? Why?
C. How would your recommendation in A change if allocated fixed costs were estimated at $500,000 per year? Why?

11 Working Capital Management

Working capital management is the management of the firm's current assets and current liabilities. The term **working capital** refers to current assets. The term **net working capital** refers to current assets less current liabilities. Current assets consist of those assets that will be converted into cash within one year. As noted in Chapter 2, current assets include cash, accounts receivable, short-term investments, inventories, and prepaid assets. Current liabilities are obligations due within one year. They typically include such accounts as wages payable, accounts payable, taxes payable, and current maturities on long-term debt.

Current assets and liabilities are important because they are the vehicles by which the fixed capacity of the organization, plant, property, and equipment, is converted into services. For example, current assets permit personnel to be hired and paid and supplies to be purchased. Current liabilities accrue as personnel earn wages and supplies are delivered to the firm. Thus, working capital permits the use of people and materials, along with the fixed assets necessary to provide health care services or to contract with providers for services for enrollees.

Goals of Working Capital Management

As with all of the resources of the organization, current assets and liabilities must be managed efficiently. The goal of working capital management is to balance the costs of holding current assets and liabilities with the costs of holding insufficient amounts of each. No more than the optimum amount of working capital should be maintained.

The cash conversion cycle in Figure 11-1 illustrates some of the aspects of working capital management. The figure shows the activities necessary to convert cash outflows for supplies, labor and provider contracts into cash inflows from patients, other payers, or enrollees. Payments from patients, third party payers, and enrollees in a health plan increase the firm's cash as do sources of long-term capital, debt, donations and equity. Payments to personnel, debtholders, suppliers and outside providers decrease the cash available.

Managers must determine the appropriate amount and type of working capital needed by the firm. The quantity and composition of the organization's investment in working capital are a function of a number of different factors which include the mix and type of health care services or products produced, length of the cash conversion cycle, level of revenues, inventory policies, credit policies, and preferences for liquidity and earnings (return). For example, an acute care hospital has a lower need for short-term investments than does a health maintenance organization. Each has a different length of cash conversion cycle as well. Revenues

Figure 11-1 Cash Conversion Cycle.

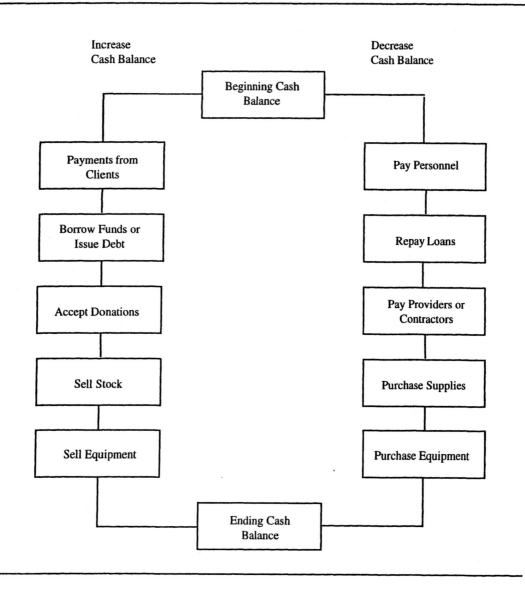

affect accounts receivable, as does the credit policy of the firm. Costs affect cash flow, inventory balances, and accounts payable balances.

Working capital management can be challenging because the level of each component changes continually. For example, supplies inventories are constantly being drawn down and replenished. A complete understanding of working capital flows requires study of the Statement of Cash Flows, which has been described in Chapter 2. More detailed working capital transactions are shown in Appendix 11A.

In addition to dealing with fluctuations in working capital accounts, managers must maintain adequate liquidity so that the firm's bills can be paid. **Liquidity** is the ability to convert assets into cash. Timing differences between transactions and the receipt or payment of cash in the cash conversion cycle make this challenging. The primary timing differences are related to cash paid for payable accounts and cash received for receivable accounts. For example, for providers and manufacturers, goods and services are delivered and accounts receivable are recognized 30 to 120 days before patients, third party payers or other clients pay in cash. In contrast, for payer organizations, premiums are typically received prior to the coverage period so accounts receivable are low and cash flows are relatively constant. Cash outflows for care provided by outside providers may be much more variable. As a result of the timing differences, there is usually an imbalance between cash outflows and inflows at any given time such that a buffer of current assets, or cash equivalents, must be maintained. This buffer is the organization's net working capital.

Finally, managers must determine how to finance the firm's investment in current assets. Both short-term and long-term sources can be used.

In the remainder of this chapter, we discuss decisions regarding the total amounts of current assets and liabilities to hold. First, we summarize the costs of holding current assets. Next we discuss policies concerning the total amount of current assets to hold and how current assets should be financed. In Chapter 12, we address management of various types of current assets. In Chapter 14, we describe short-term liabilities.

Costs and Working Capital Management

There are costs incurred both for maintaining an insufficient level of current assets and for maintaining too high a level of current assets. The manager must balance these two costs to minimize the cost of working capital.

Costs of maintaining insufficient current asset balances include costs of foregone investment opportunities and the costs of not being able to meet current payments on a timely basis. Firms that are not liquid cannot take advantage of investment opportunities and, therefore, forego the returns from these investments. They also cannot buy on credit, may have to negotiate with a banker about overdrawn accounts and bounced checks, and may have to pay in advance for certain purchases (e.g., utilities, telephone), all of which increase the costs of foregone investment. Liquidity also permits firms to take advantage of purchase discounts and to plan their borrowing for times when interest rates are low. Of special importance is the risk of default on either short-term or long-term debt. The smaller the level of net working capital, the greater the risk of default or delays in meeting financial obligations as they are due which may result in demands for payment in advance by suppliers or higher interest costs by lenders. At the extreme, an organization with extremely high risk cannot borrow at any interest rate and may be forced to close its doors because no working capital is available.

To maintain working capital balances, other costs are incurred. Some of these costs must be incurred for the firm to operate, but managers can minimize them by not holding too high levels of working capital. Thus, the firm should hold an **optimal level of working capital** that minimizes the costs of holding insufficient and too high levels of working capital. Costs of maintaining working capital balances include (1) administrative costs, (2) interest expenses associated with financing the current assets, and (3) foregone returns. Maintaining supplies inventories provides an example of the first type of costs. Transactions must occur for supplies to be purchased and used. Other costs of maintaining inventory include storage costs, and the costs of any wastage or spoilage.

The second type of cost is the interest cost associated with financing the current assets. The interest cost may be explicit as in the case of debt financing or implicit as with using accounts payable. The latter cost is discussed thoroughly in Chapter 14.

Finally, there is the cost of foregone profitability. A general premise in business finance is that the lower an asset's risk, the lower the expected earnings are from that asset. Current assets are normally less risky than fixed assets, since they can be more easily converted into cash. Therefore, current assets normally earn lower returns than fixed assets. As a result, an increased level of net working capital represents less risk, or more liquidity, and less return, whereas a lower level of working capital represents more risk and greater returns from alternative investments. These concepts can be expressed slightly differently as alternative current asset investment policies.

Current Asset Investment Policy

Figure 11-2 illustrates three different policies for working capital levels relative to revenues from health care services. It shows the level of net working capital or current assets when current liabilities are held constant at each revenue level.

Policy C is a conservative policy in which the health care firm holds a relatively high level of current assets at each revenue level. Policy A is an aggressive policy, holding smaller amounts of current assets, and thus has a lower level of net working capital. Finally, Policy B is more balanced and represents an intermediate position.

These three policies are represented in Table 11-1 by three different levels of current asset balances. Assume that the firm maintains either $60, $70, or $80 as current asset balances. The remaining data are held constant to show the effects of these different current asset options. The constant net income also reflects the lower return on current assets than on long-term assets.

The aggressive policy yields the largest return on total assets (12.5%), whereas the conservative policy yields the lowest return. As Table 11-1 indicates, because net income is constant across all three policies, the average return ratio (Net income/Total assets) goes

Figure 11-2   Three alternative working capital policies. An aggressive working capital policy (A) would hold lower amounts of net working capital (or current assets) at each revenue level. Conversely, the most conservative policy (C) would hold substantially higher net working capital balances at each level of activity.

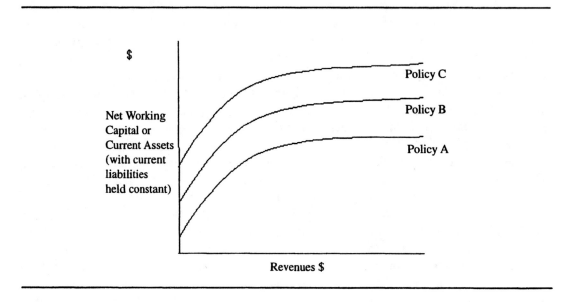

Table 11-1   Risk and Return of Three Alternative Working Capital Policies.

	Aggressive	Balanced	Conservative
Current assets (CA)	$ 60	$ 70	$ 80
Current liabilities (CL)			
(assumed constant)	30	30	30
Net working capital (CA-CL)	30	40	50
Fixed Assets (FA)	100	100	100
Total assets (TA = FA + CA)	160	170	180
Revenue	200	200	200
Net income (NI)	20	20	20
Expected return on			
total assets (NI/TA)	12.5%	11.8%	11.1%
Current ratio (CA/CL)	2.0	2.33	2.67

down as total assets increase. Risk is higher under the aggressive policy (net working capital of $30) than under the conservative policy (net working capital of $50). As more working capital is held, risk decreases. The current ratio also indicates the relative risk levels. The lower the current ratio, the higher the risk that the firm will be unable to pay its current liabilities.

These examples of alternative policies indicate the fundamental working capital dilemma. By increasing working capital, or liquidity, the firm has lower risk of being unable to meet short-term obligations but lower profit ratios. Conversely, by decreasing working capital, more risk is assumed, but higher profit rates are achieved. The board or other governing authority must decide the preference for risk, but it is the chief financial officer who will implement the board's policy and match risk and return preferences.

Current Asset Financing Policy

In addition to choosing the amount of current assets to hold, managers must determine how to finance them. Typically, managers are advised to match the length of the life of an asset with the maturity of its financing source. This is called **maturity matching**. For example, long-term assets are typically financed with long-term debt or equity. To apply the maturity matching concept to working capital management, an understanding of permanent and temporary current assets is necessary.

As noted previously, working capital inflows and outflows are tied to the provision of goods and services by the firm. As more goods and services are provided, more working capital is needed and vice versa. An **operating cycle** is usually viewed as a cash-to-cash cycle. Within each operating cycle, working capital needs typically fluctuate because of changes in the volume of goods and services provided. Demand for health care services changes as a result of seasonal patterns, holidays, and various events such as natural disasters, labor strikes, and changes in insurance coverage. These fluctuations can normally be directly correlated with subsequent fluctuations in working capital needs.

Permanent current assets do not fluctuate with seasonal or other demand changes. The amount of permanent current assets is constant if the volume of goods and services produced is steady. If the volume of output increases, permanent working capital needs also increase. **Temporary current assets** are needed to cover seasonal and other fluctuations in demand. Figure 11-3 graphically illustrates how to distinguish between permanent and temporary working capital. Permanent working capital is the quantity of working capital that, historically, represents the lowest average monthly requirement. Temporary working capital is that needed from time to time above the base level of permanent working capital.

In Figure 11-3, three alternative policies for financing permanent and temporary current assets are shown. For each of the three, the graphs show the fluctuations in temporary current assets over time. Permanent current assets increase as the firm grows and invests in more fixed assets.

The first financing policy, the moderate policy, follows maturity matching. It uses short-term debt financing for all temporary current assets. Both permanent current assets and fixed

Figure 11-3 Current Asset Financing Policies.

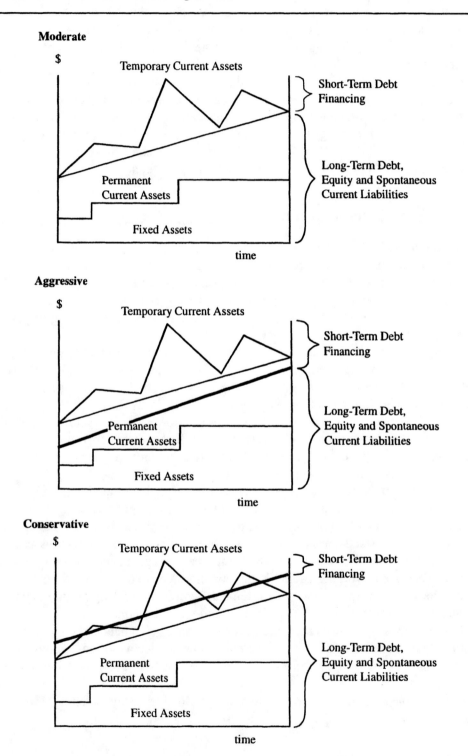

assets are financed with permanent sources, debt, equity and spontaneous current liabilities. Spontaneous current liabilities are payables and accruals that arise in the normal course of business operations and are, therefore, permanent sources of financing.

The goal of the aggressive policy is to increase profitability. With it, the firm uses more short-term than long-term debt. Because short-term debt is generally less costly than long-term debt, expenses are lower and expected profitability is higher. A consequence of the policy is that the firm has a lower level of net working capital. It faces more risk of not being able to meet its short-term obligations and incurring the associated costs. An additional risk associated with the aggressive policy is refinancing risk. It can be manifested in two ways. First, the firm may not be able to roll over its short-term debt when it matures. Second, even if the firm can roll over the short-term debt, it may face a higher interest rate than it previously paid.

With the conservative current asset financing policy, the firm uses more long-term financing sources and less short-term debt. It finances all of its fixed assets, permanent current assets and some of its temporary current assets with long-term debt, equity or spontaneous current liabilities. When excess funds are available, they are reinvested in short-term securities until the funds are needed. The firm's net working capital is higher with this policy than with the moderate or aggressive policies. Thus, it faces less risk of not being able to meet its short-term obligations. However, since long-term financing sources generally require higher rates of return than short-term debt, the firm's financing costs are also higher which lowers its expected profitability.

An Example of the Costs of Working Capital

Table 11-2 illustrates the costs of four working capital alternatives and shows how to compute the cost of holding various levels of working capital. The firm has determined that $422,000 of permanent working capital is needed along with at least $78,000 and up to $378,000 of temporary working capital. The costs shown are those from interest, forgone profitability and insufficient liquidity. In the example, short-term interest costs are projected to be 12% per year and the return on assets of the firm's long-term assets is 15%. Since the firm cannot take advantage of discounts on accounts payable, the cost of insufficient working capital is 36%. Determination of the cost of not taking discounts on accounts payable is shown in detail in Chapter 14.

The example clearly indicates that the goal of the firm should be to minimize the costs of maintaining insufficient or too high levels of working capital not simply to minimize working capital. When no working capital is held, substantial costs are incurred.

In this example, working capital costs are minimized at $500,000. Several other options could also be tested, but the driving factor in this example is the opportunity cost rate of 36%. If this rate had actually been significantly lower, then the other working capital options would have been estimated to have lower total costs.

Table 11-2 Costs of Holding Various Levels of Working Capital.

	Levels of working capital held			
Costs of working capital	$0	$422,000	$500,000	$1,000,000
Short-term credit @ 12%	0	$ 50,640	$60,000	$120,000
Return on assets if invested in operations or long-term investments @ 15%	0	63,300	75,000	150,000
Costs of insufficient working capital @ 36%	180,000*	28,080**	0	0
Total	$180,00	$142,020	$135,000	$270,000

*$500,000 x 0.36
**($500,000 - $422,000) x .036

Table 11-3 Effects of Inflation on Net Working Capital.

Working capital	Base case	Inflation at 10%
Cash	$ 300,000	$ 330,000
Accounts receivable	2,000,000	2,200,000
Supplies	1,000,000	1,100,000
Net current assets	$3,300,000	$3,630,000
Accounts payable	200,000	220,000
Short-term loan	1,100,000	1,210,000
Net current liabilities	$1,300,000	$1,430,000
Net working capital	$2,000,000	$2,200,000
Current ratio	2.54	2.54

In this example, inflation in all components of working capital is assumed to be 10%. Thus, to keep the current ratio constant, cash must also increase by 10%. The crucial managerial question is, what are the possible sources for the incremental cash necessary to keep up with inflation?

Effects of Inflation

Estimates of working capital needs are usually calculated on the basis of historical records. To the extent that inflation affects future supply and payroll costs, the calculation of working capital needs must recognize the inflationary impact. Managers must anticipate inflation and compensate for its effects in their contract prices and other rate schedules.

Inflationary effects on working capital will usually result in deterioration of the current ratio or cash balances. Almost all of the components of working capital are affected by inflation. As Table 11-3 illustrates, inflation affects all elements of working capital such that cash must also increase in inflationary periods in order for the current ratio to remain constant. This example shows the insidious effects of inflation on all elements of working capital. Of course, in real life situations, the current ratio probably would decrease, rather then be held constant, since additional sources of cash are usually limited.

Summary

Working capital management involves management of the firm's current assets and current liabilities. As with all of the resources of the organization, current assets and liabilities must be managed efficiently. The goal of working capital management is to balance the costs of holding current assets and liabilities with the costs of holding insufficient amounts of each. There are both costs of maintaining an insufficient level of current assets and costs of maintaining too high a level of current assets. Costs of maintaining insufficient current asset balances include costs of foregone investment opportunities and the costs of not being able to meet current payments on a timely basis. Costs of maintaining working capital include (1) administrative costs of maintaining current asset balances, (2) interest expenses associated with financing the current assets, and (3) foregone returns. Managers must balance these costs to maintain the optimum amount of working capital.

Bibliography

Black, C. "Use and Abuse of Net Working Capital" *Accountants' Journal* 72(3): 76-78, 1993.

Gallinger, G.W. and P.B. Healey. *Liquidity Analysis and Management*. Reading, MA: Addison-Wesley Publishing Co., 1987.

Nelson, B. "Improving Cash Flow Through Benchmarking" *Healthcare Financial Management* (September): 74-78, 1994.

Richman, T. "Performance Measurement" *Harvard Business Review* 73(4): 10-11, 1995.

Saccurato, F. "The Study of Working Capital" *Business Credit* 96(1): 36-37, 1994.

Soenen, L.A. "Cash Conversion Cycle and Corporate Profitability" *Journal of Cash Management* 13 (4): 53-57, 1993.

Sylvestre, J. and F.R. Urbanic. "Effective Methods for Cash Flow Analysis" *Healthcare Financial Management* (July): 62-72, 1994.

Terms and Concepts _____

liquidity   optimal level of working capital
maturity matching   permanent current assets
net working capital   temporary current assets
operating cycle   working capital

Questions and Problems _____

11-1   Define working capital in your own words (two sentences). State three examples of liabilities that are part of working capital. Why are these liabilities considered to be part of working capital?

11-2   Identify at least two problems that may be caused by too much working capital; by too little working capital.

11-3   Identify several circumstances that would lead to a zero balance of working capital. Why does a zero balance result in high costs?

11-4   What circumstances could lead to negative cash balances? Where would such balances be shown on the balance sheet? Why do you suppose that balance sheets rarely show negative cash balances?

11-5   Identify costs that may be incurred by poor working capital management.

11-6   Why does a health care organization need temporary working capital? Do you suppose that a visiting nurse service or a hospital would have a greater degree of variability in temporary working capital needs? Why?

11-7   The manager of a proprietary hospital once stated that the primary source of operating funds for his facility was depreciation. Was he correct? Explain.

11-8   What is the operating cycle and how does it influence working capital management?

11-9   Why does inflation have such insidious effects on working capital needs?

11-10 From the following data, graph permanent and temporary working capital needs for 19x2.

Month and Total Amount of Working Capital Needs ($ million)

Jan	1.0	Jul	1.75
Feb	1.5	Aug	1.5
Mar	1.75	Sep	1.25

Month and Total Amount of Working Capital Needs ($ million)(continued)

Apr	2.0	Oct	1.25
May	2.5	Nov	1.0
Jun	2.0	Dec	1.0

11-11 Recalculate or reformulate Table 11-2 using these new assumptions and the same levels of working capital held (0; $422,000; $500,000; and $1 million):

A. $800,000, as determined by management is the optimum quantity of working capital

B. Short-term credit costs are 16%

C. Operating assets earn only 9%

D. Opportunity costs of insufficient working capital are 30%

Appendix 11A

Working Capital Transactions

This appendix develops an accounting transaction and balance sheet approach to working capital. In a series of six steps, we show how working capital levels change with a variety of transactions. We also show, in the last step, how depreciation does **not** affect net working capital or cash flows. Note that we use the term "equities" to refer either to owners' equity for the investor owned firm or net assets for the not-for-profit firm.

1. Assume a health care organization begins the year with no assets. Its balance sheet would look like the one below:

Assets	$0
Liabilities and Equities	$0

2. In order to acquire assets, the organization issues bonds for $10 million. After this transaction, the organization will have increased its working capital by $10 million:

<u>Assets</u>	
Cash	<u>$10,000,000</u>
<u>Liabilities and Equities</u>	
Long-Term Debt	<u>$10,000,000</u>

   Net working capital is now $10 million.

3. Next, assume the organization acquires plant, property, and equipment with the proceeds of the bonds and receives a donation of $1 million. After these transactions, the organization will have only $1 million in working capital, as well as fixed assets and long-term debt.

<u>Assets</u>	
Cash	$ 1,000,000
Property, Plant, and Equipment	<u>$10,000,000</u>
Total Assets	$11,000,000

Liabilities and Equities
Long-Term Debt $10,000,000
Owner's Equity $ 1,000,000

Total Liabilities and Equities $11,000,000

4. Next, assume: (a) the organization provides patient services and bills patients for those services at $3 million; (b) $1.8 million is collected; (c) the costs of supplies, wages, and utilities amount to $2.5 million; and (d) $2 million is paid to vendors and employees.

	Cash	Accounts Receivable	Long-Term Assets	Liabilities	Equities
Beginning Balance	$1,000,000		$10,000,000	$10,000,000	$1,000,000
Transaction A		$3,000,000			3,000,000
Transaction B	1,800,000	(1,800,000)			
Transaction C				2,500,000	(2,500,000)
Transaction D	(2,000,000)			(2,000,000)	
Ending Balance	$ 800,000	$1,200,000	$10,000,000	$10,500,000	$1,500,000

The balance sheet now shows an increase in net working capital of $500,000. The reader should be very careful to understand why the working capital **change** is only $500,000. The increase occurs because of a $1 million increase in current assets ($200,000 decrease in cash, $1.2 million increase in receivables) and a $500,000 increase in current liabilities (accounts payable). Net working capital is now $1.5 million ($800,000 in cash + $1.2 million in receivables - $500,000 in accounts payable).

Assets
Cash $ 800,000
Accounts Receivable   1,200,000
Property, Plant, and Equipment   10,000,000

Total Assets $12,000,000

Liabilities and Equities
Accounts Payable $ 500,000
Long-term Debt   10,000,000
Equities   1,500,000

Total Liabilities and Equities $12,000,000

5. Now assume that a payment on long-term debt of $600,000 is due and paid. This transaction reduces current assets. The balance sheet now indicates that net working capital is $900,000; current assets are valued at $1.4 million, and current liabilities are $500,000.

Assets	
Cash	$ 200,000
Accounts Receivable	1,200,000
Property, Plant, and Equipment	10,000,000
Total Assets	$ 11,400,000
Liabilities and Equities	
Accounts Payable	$ 500,000
Long-term Debt	9,400,000
Equities	1,500,000
Total Liabilities and Equities	$ 11,400,000

6. Finally, assume that depreciation is recognized and recorded at $1 million. Note carefully that depreciation only affects noncurrent accounts and, by definition, cannot affect current assets or current liabilities. Net working capital is unchanged at $900,000.

Assets	
Cash	$ 200,000
Accounts Receivable	1,200,000
Property, Plant, and Equipment (Net)	9,000,000
Total Assets	$ 10,400,000
Liabilities and Equities	
Accounts Payable	$ 500,000
Long-term Debt	9,400,000
Equities	500,000
Total Liabilities and Equities	$ 10,400,000

12 Managing Current Assets

As discussed in Chapter 11, working capital management involves managing current assets and current liabilities. In that chapter, we discussed policies regarding the level of total current assets to hold relative to current liabilities. In this chapter, we address the management of three types of current assets: cash, marketable securities, and accounts receivable. These are typically the most active current assets in a health care organization. In addition, as noted in Chapter 2, these current assets affect the financial status of the service organization more significantly than other current assets such as inventories and prepaid items. As a result, the latter are not discussed in this chapter.

The general problem for managers is to balance the costs of holding a particular type of current asset with the costs of a shortage of the current asset. As is discussed in more detail below, holding costs include resources expended to manage an asset and opportunity costs. An **opportunity cost** is the lost return from the next best alternative course of action. For example, an opportunity cost of holding cash is the return lost from investing the funds in the stock market. Shortage costs are costs incurred when too little of the asset is held. An example is the financing cost incurred for borrowing when too little cash is available. The benefit of devoting resources to current asset management is the ability to minimize both the holding and shortage costs.

The chapter begins with a discussion of the reasons why cash is important to health care providers and payers and of the methods of cash management. It proceeds to a review of marketable securities as cash substitutes and as investments of excess cash. The final topic is management of accounts receivable. Here, we focus on the advantages and disadvantages of holding various levels of accounts receivable as well as on credit and collection policies.

Cash

Cash is needed for three very important reasons: (1) transactions, (2) buffer for uncertainty, and (3) speculation or investment. Each is discussed in turn.

Cash is needed for transactions to pay obligations as they arise or as they are due. No organization can survive for very long without paying its suppliers or employees, which are two of the most critical and recurring types of cash outflows. Banks and governmental entities may actually close the doors on a health care firm if their payment requirements are unmet. They can force bankruptcy when their loan covenants are not met. The Internal Revenue Service can force businesses to shut down when employee tax withholdings and other taxes are not remitted. These examples provide vivid evidence of the risks of not having sufficient cash for transactions.

Cash can also be used as a **buffer** to meet unexpected needs. In this sense, cash is like a safety valve which can be used to deal with contingencies. One of the most effective ways of dealing with uncertainty is to have cash available.

The third reason for holding cash relates to profitability because cash is a vehicle for investment in physical or financial assets. Economists term this a **"speculative motive"** in that the institution is speculating that it will earn a return commensurate with the risks involved with the investment.

Health care organizations must balance the benefits and costs of having cash on hand. Since cash earns no or low returns, managers should minimize the amount held while ensuring that there is sufficient cash to meet the transactions, buffer, and investment and speculative needs of the firm. The task is made more difficult because the cash conversion cycle, which was shown in Chapter 11, has delays in converting cash outflows into cash inflows. Cash requirements and availability may be different at any point in time. In addition, there are many uncertainties in the cash flow process. Cash collections can be different than planned, and cash outflows may be delayed or accelerated.

These are the essential problems of cash management: (1) to predict cash inflows and outflows and (2) to minimize the amount of cash balances. Accurate prediction of inflows and outflows ensures that payments can be made on a timely basis, the cost of borrowing can be minimized and excess cash can be invested efficiently. The firm seeks to minimize cash balances because cash tends to be an asset that earns either no or low returns. Primary methods of cash management involve cash flow synchronization, accelerating receipts, and controlling disbursements. Each is discussed below.

Cash Flow Synchronization

Cash flow synchronization involves synchronizing cash inflows and outflows. Cash budgeting and timing billing cycles to provide steady streams of cash are among the methods firms can use to synchronize cash inflows and outflows. Since cash budgeting is among the most important cash management techniques, it is discussed here and in greater detail in Chapter 8.

Cash Budgeting. The cash budget is used to project sources and uses of cash; it is used to identify where cash will be obtained and how it will be used. By looking separately at operating sources and uses of cash, the manager can ascertain how much cash is available for investments and how much must be borrowed or otherwise obtained from external sources.

Each health care firm must construct a cash flow budget that accurately reflects the sources and timing of its expected cash inflows and outflows. It is beyond the scope of this text to describe all types of cash receipts and disbursements and their attendant cash management problems. To demonstrate the different concerns of different types of health care firms, brief examples for a provider firm and for a payer firm are shown. A more complete cash budget example was provided in Chapter 8.

For most *providers*, one of the most challenging aspects of cash management is predicting the timing of collections of accounts receivable. By looking at sources of cash flow from operations and the time lags between the date of service and date of payment, the financial manager can develop a historical pattern of the inflow or collection side of the cash cycle. Four steps in this inflow pattern must be performed:

1. estimate future cash flow percentages by category of payer,
2. estimate average lag time between service and cash receipts,
3. calculate cash collection ratios, and
4. calculate expected cash collections by month.

Step 1. The first step in estimating cash flows from operations is to accumulate all the net revenues billed for the most recent 12 months by major category of payers. This information is available from collection records, and Table 12-1 illustrates its use. The percentage distribution of payment source is the most essential ingredient in selecting cash management strategies. For example, if only 14% of the firm's revenues are from self-paying patients and private insurance companies, then the majority of the cash management activities should not be directed toward this segment, unless of course the policies and procedures of the other payers are essentially too rigid to be influenced significantly.

Step 2. Once the percentage distribution of revenue is obtained, the next step is to determine the average time lag between date of service and date of collection. The recommended procedure is to establish the collection pattern within one, two, three, or more months after the date of service. For example, Table 12-2 shows that 23% of the Medicare billings may be received within one month after service, while 17% are received more than three months after service is delivered. This same data should be calculated for each payer category (Medicaid,

Table 12-1   Net Revenues Categorized by Payer.

Payer	Revenue	Percent
Medicare	$ 8,000,000	22.8
Medicaid	12,000,000	34.3
Blue Cross	10,000,000	28.6
Private Insurance and Self-Pay	5,000,000	14.3
Total	$35,000,000	100.0

Table 12-2   Summary of Time Lags Between Service and Payment Dates, by Payer.

	Percentage Paid				
Payer	Within 1 Mo.	Within 2 Mo.	Within 3 Mo.	More than 3 Mo.	Total
Medicare	23	29	31	17	100
Medicaid	5	25	40	30	100
Blue Cross	10	39	31	20	100
Private	60	30	8	2	100

Blue Cross, private pay, etc.). We recommend conducting separate analyses of the number of collections and the dollar amounts of collections. Collections and dollar amounts should then each be transformed into percentages. If great differences between the two exist, e.g., a considerable number of small collections in one time period, it may be fruitful to try to encourage that class of payer to accumulate payments into larger checks. This will help to minimize the firm's processing and accounting costs.

The output of these procedures will be distributions showing time lags for each payer category (Table 12-2). These distributions represent the cash collection cycle. They are used to transform projected revenues from patient services into projected cash inflows.

Step 3. The next step is to calculate the percent of total revenues received in cash in any one time period from each category of payer. These percentages are called **cash collection ratios**. The cash collection ratios are calculated by multiplying the percentage of revenues categorized by payer (Table 12-1) by the percentage of collections received in months subsequent to service (Table 12-2). For instance, the 5.24 figure in column one of Table 12-3 was derived by multiplying 22.8% (Table 12-1) by 23% (Table 12-2). Note that this example only calculates collection percentages for four months when in reality they should be calculated for an entire year.

The sum of the collection patterns by month will equal a weighted average estimate of the percentage of payments the organization will receive in any particular number of months after service, taking into account all payers. For instance, 18.4% of total service revenues is estimated to be received in cash within one month after service. Therefore, the cash collection ratio for one month is 18.4%. This ratio can be calculated on an annual basis, or it can be computed using a rolling average of the 12 most recent months.

Step 4. These cash collection ratios (bottom row in Table 12-3) are used to calculate cash inflows that are expected from each month's services. Assume for instance that the health care organization delivers $500,000 worth of service for four consecutive months as shown in Table 12-4. Collection percentages are depicted at the bottom of the figure. Therefore, 18.4% of billings will be collected in the first month of service, 30.63% within two months of service, and so on. Also note in the total column on the right that after four months (April) 89.92% or $899,150 of the total billings for January and February ($1,000,000) have been collected (Table 12-4). This total collected is comprised of all of January's revenues and all but 20.17% of February's revenues. In actuality, this process can be considerably more complicated as amounts of billings and collections vary from month to month. That is, it would be a rare case to find all billings collected with precision within four months. Note also that the example assumes no bad debts, which is not usually the case for most providers.

Once collection patterns are known and expenses are estimated, a pro forma cash budget can be constructed (Table 12-5). It combines the cash inflow projections with projected cash outflows such that a cash minimum balance is maintained.

In contrast to service providers, many *payer* firms face more uncertainty concerning cash outflows for accounts payable to service providers with whom they contract than concerning accounts receivable. Therefore, one of their major cash management tasks is to project cash outflows in a manner similar to the way providers project cash inflows.

Table 12-3 Cash Collection Ratios.

Payer	Within 1 month	2 months	3 months	More than 3 months	Total
Medicare	5.24*	6.61	7.07	3.88	22.8
Medicaid	1.72 +	8.58	13.72	10.29	34.3
Blue Cross	2.86	11.15	8.87	5.72	28.6
Private	8.58	4.29	1.14	0.29	14.3
Totals	18.40	30.63	30.80	20.17	100.0

*22.8% x 23% = 5.24% (see Tables 5-3 and 5-4)
+34.3% x 5% = 1.72%

Table 12-4 Cash Collections for the First Quarter of 19XX*.

	January	February	March	April	Total
Billings	$500,000	$500,000	$500,000	$500,000	
Cash collection					
January	92,000	153,150	154,000	100,850	500,000
February		92,000	153,150	154,000	399,150
March			92,000	153,150	245,150
April				92,000	92,000
Total	$92,000	$245,150	$399,150	$500,000	$1,236,300

Collection Percentages = 18.40% within 1 month after service
30.63% between 1 and 2 months after service
30.80% between 2 and 3 months after service
20.17% between 3 and 4 months after service

*This example assumes that January is the first month of service and that no uncollectables are incurred.

Table 12-5   A Hypothetical or Pro Forma Cash Budget.

	Month 1	Month 2	Summary
Cash inflows from operating activities			
Beginning balance	$200,000	$201,800	$200,000
Collections: current month	496,800	601,000	1,097,800
Collections: prior months	3,000,000	2,827,100	5,827,100
Other operating revenues	150,000	175,000	325,000
Cash available	$3,846,800	$3,804,900	$7,449,900
Cash outflows from operating activities			
Payment on account	$510,000	$620,000	$1,130,000
Payroll	2,000,000	2,200,000	4,200,000
Utilities	580,000	600,000	1,180,000
Repairs and Maintenance	400,000	395,000	795,000
Miscellaneous	185,000	189,000	374,000
Total outflows	$3,675,000	$4,004,000	$7,679,000
Cash provided by operating activities	$ 171,800	$(199,100)	$(229,100)
Loans	30,000	300,000	330,000
Fixed assets sales (purchases)	0	100,000	100,000
Transfer to (from) other funds	0	0	0
Ending balance*	$ 201,800	$ 200,900	$ 200,900

*Minimum cash balance required: $200,000.

Table 12-6   Cash Outflows for Payer Medical Care Expenses.

		Cash Outflows During				
Month	Expenses	Jan.	Feb.	March	April	May
Jan.	$75,000	$56,250	$9,375	$9,375	0	0
Feb.	85,000	0	63,750	10,625	10,625	0
March	80,000	0	0	60,000	10,000	10,000

75% of expenses are disbursed in the current month. 12.5% are disbursed in each of the following two months.

Table 12-6 illustrates how medical care expenses are translated into cash outflows for a payer, such as a health maintenance organization. Included in the expenses of any payer are **incurred but not reported** (IBNR) expenses. These are expenses that are estimated to have been incurred by enrollees but have not yet been reported to the payer by providers. To match expenses to revenues, which are premium revenues, these amounts are expensed in the month in which they are incurred. Naturally, they cannot be paid for in cash until they are billed by the provider. In the example in Table 12-6, we assume that 75% of medical care expenses are reported to the payer during the month in which they are incurred and that the payer pays them in that month. However, 12.5% of the expenses are reported and paid for in cash during each of the next two months. The cash outflow data in Table 12-6 would be combined with information regarding cash inflows to formulate a cash budget.

Accelerating Receipts

By accelerating collection of receipts, the health care firm has the use of cash sooner than it would otherwise. This acceleration can be accomplished through efficient billing practices and by minimizing some types of float as well as through other accounts receivable activities described more completely later in this chapter.

Efficient billing by health care providers is especially important. Cash collections from fee-for-service payers can be accelerated by collecting payer information prior to admission or utilization of services or requiring prepayment of deductibles, copayments or a deposit. In addition, providers can implement systems to collect information for all chargeable services and goods on a timely basis.

Float refers to the time during which money is in the process of changing hands. Cash flows can be measured by cash balances at the bank or by cash balances on the health care organization's books or financial records. Any difference between these figures is called the float. It is defined either as the length of the time taken to record a transaction in both places, or as the dollar difference in the cash balances as viewed from the perspectives of the two entities at a given time.

There are several types of float which are associated both with collections, where they are seen as types of **collection float**, and with disbursements, where they are types of **disbursement float**. **Mail float** is the delay during which checks are in the mail. There is also a **processing float**, which is the time it takes the payee to process a cash receipt and deposit the check in the bank. There is finally a **clearing float**, which is the time it takes for a check to clear the banking system once it is received so that the cash is available for other transactions. Of the kinds of floats, processing float is obviously the most controllable and the one most susceptible to managerial intervention.

Effective management of processing float tries to minimize the lag between the time when checks are first available to the provider and the time when the checks have been converted into "spendable" cash. Checks should not be unnecessarily held in-house awaiting internal processing or accounts receivable posting and updates. Checks should be taken to the bank and deposited at least daily. A **lockbox** system can be used whereby the checks are mailed by patients, third parties or employers to a post office box that is emptied hourly by the bank. In such cases, deposits are made almost instantaneously, with minimal time lags for processing. The bank then forwards the payment information to the institution for accounts receivable processing and reconciliation. Payer firms may find it useful to have employers transfer premium payments automatically from their bank accounts.

Large payments from third parties can be made on a tape-to-tape system. Patient claims data can now be sent electronically over telephone lines. Payment data from the third party's computer is then relayed electronically to the provider's computer. With no paper interface, the potential for delays or errors that paper processing might invoke is avoided.

Disbursement Control

Disbursement control involves methods to slow the availability of funds to suppliers, employees and others so that the firm has the use of the cash longer. Methods include not taking advantage of purchase discounts, maximizing disbursement float and using overdraft and zero-balance accounts.

Chapter 14 discusses the advantages and disadvantages of taking purchase discounts on accounts payable by paying bills within an available discount period. In the event that discounts are insignificant or unattractive, the prudent financial manager should ensure that bills are never paid until the end of the normal due period. This is not to say that bills should be held until they are overdue. Instead, it suggests that once a discount is lost, then no incentive to pay exists until some other kind of economic cost will be incurred for slow payment (e.g., poor vendor relations or cessation of credit). The financial manager must set up the payment system to take advantage of all the time available before an account is due. A firm can then obtain the maximum benefit from its investable funds. This technique is sometimes called "the check is in the mail" deferment plan.

Maximizing disbursement float is the opposite of minimizing collection float. Mail float may be maximized by strategic use of mailing points and time. For example, the firm may mail its payments at the end of the day if the supplier uses the postmark date to determine whether payment was made on time. Processing float may be maximized by writing checks against funds not yet deposited. Payroll checks can often be issued on Fridays, but corresponding deposits delayed until the following Mondays. Practiced on a recurring basis, this technique can earn significant interest every pay period. Finally, clearing float can also be maximized for disbursements if checks are drawn upon banks located far away from the supplier's bank. The success of the latter, however, may be limited since clearing float has been decreasing in the banking system.

Overdraft and zero-balance accounts minimize the cash that must be kept in low earning accounts. With **overdraft systems**, banks automatically issue loans to cover the amount of overdrafts on a bank accounts. Of course, the bank charges interest on the loans. **Zero-balance accounts** occur where zero balances are maintained until the bank notifies the firm of the total amount of checks presented against the account. The firm then transfers sufficient funds to cover the checks. For such a service, the bank charges a fee.

Costs and Benefits of Cash Management

The benefit of devoting resources to current asset management is the ability to minimize, or balance, the holding and shortage costs. Among the costs of a shortage of cash are poor relations with vendors and financing costs. Shortages of cash may result in slow payment to vendors and others. A consequence of slow payment may be unwillingness to grant credit in the future or to demand payment in advance. Financing costs may be higher than they would normally be if the firm must borrow hastily to meet its needs when it has cash shortages.

Holding costs for cash include opportunity costs incurred if the firm does not invest its cash in securities or the firm's physical assets. The returns on investment will be higher for the firm when interest rates are high or when many good alternative investments are available for the cash. Other holding costs include managerial time, the direct costs of lockbox systems, zero-balance accounts and the like. Cash management to accelerate inflows, decelerate out-flows and minimize cash balances will be more valuable when alternative opportunities have high returns. Thus, by spending more on management, the firm can lower its opportunity costs. Appendix 12A provides an example of an evaluation of the opportunity and financing costs of cash excesses and shortages.

Marketable Securities

So far, we have been discussing cash as though it were only currency. In reality, market-able securities, which are short-term interest bearing securities, are also an important part of the "cash" balances of the firm. They are often called **cash equivalents**. Financial managers use them for temporary investments of excess cash and as cash substitutes. Marketable securities are liquid and typically have low risk. When securities are first issued, we say they are sold in the **primary market**. When they are resold before they mature, or when they can be redeemed, they sell in **secondary markets**. If they can easily and quickly be sold in second-ary markets, the securities are highly liquid and have excellent marketability.

The primary benefit of purchasing marketable securities with excess cash is that, unlike for holding cash, a return is provided. On the down side, transaction costs of buying and holding the securities are incurred and the firm faces some added risk. Although it is typically small with these securities, there is some default risk. **Default risk** is the risk that the issuer will not be able to make interest or principal payments as promised. U.S. government securi-ties have no default risk, but securities issued by corporations have varying degrees of default risk. Another risk is **price risk**, which is relevant if the firm sells the security prior to its maturity. If interest rates change while the security is held, the price the firm can obtain for a security changes. If rates increase, the price decreases and vice versa. Finally, there may be **liquidity risk** because not all marketable securities can be resold easily. We would say that there is not a good secondary market for those securities.

In this section, we describe some of the most common types of marketable securities available. Table 12-7 summarizes the securities and some of their important characteristics.

Table 12-7   Types of Common Marketable Securities.

Security	Maturities When Issued	Minimum Denomination	Special Features
Treasury Bills	91 days, 182 days, 52 weeks	$10,000	No default risk, excellent marketability.
Federal Agency Issues	30 days to 1 year	$1,000	Low default risk, good marketability.
Negtiable Certificates of Deposit	30 days to 1 year	$100,000	Default risk varies, up to $100,000 insured by Federal Deposit Insurance Corporation (FDIC), good marketability.
Commercial Paper	30 to 270 days	$100,000	Default risk low but higher than other securities, poor to fair marketability.
Banker's Acceptances	30 to 180 days	$25,000	Default risk typically low, good marketability for acceptances issued by larger banks.
Eurodollar Deposits	Overnight to 360 days	$1,000,000	Default risk typically low, good marketability.
Money Market Mutual Funds	None	Varies	Low default risk, good marketability.
Repurchase Agreements	1 to 30 days	$500,000	Low default risk, poor marketability.

Treasury Bills

Treasury bills (T-bills) are issued by the U.S. government on a weekly basis in a variety of maturities (time period until redemption). 52 week securities are offered monthly. Purchases greater than $500,000 must be on a competitive bid basis. Purchases in lesser amounts can usually be made through local banks or investment houses. Since they are issued by the U.S. government, with its taxing authority, these securities have no default risk and can easily be resold in secondary markets.

T-bills are sold at a discount from the face value. For example, a $10,000 par (face) value at an annual yield of 10% in 90 days (maturity) could be purchased for $9,756.10. As discussed in Chapter 13, this amount is the present value of a future amount ($10,000), such that the $9,756.10 will accumulate $243.90 of interest (at 10% in 90 days) so that the T-bill can be redeemed at its face amount.

Federal Agency Issues

Some federal government agencies can issue debt on their own. Although these **Federal Agency Issue** securities are not backed by the U.S. Treasury, most investors assume they are implicitly guaranteed by the U.S. government. As a result, the risk of default is low and their marketability is good.

Certificates of Deposit

Certificates of deposit (CDs) are short-term promissory notes paying interest. They are issued by commercial banks in denominations of $500 or more. CDs are liquid investment instruments with flexible maturities. Negotiable certificates of deposit are issued in denominations of $100,000 and are traded by securities dealers in secondary markets.

Commercial Paper

Commercial paper is an unsecured promissory note issued by industrial and financial firms. It matures anywhere from 30 to 270 days and is issued at a discount. There is no collateral and only the firm itself guarantees payment. Thus, the default risk of commercial paper is higher than that of many other securities. The secondary market for commercial paper is weak although it may be possible to sell the paper back to the issuer or to the dealer.

Banker's Acceptances

Banker's acceptances are short-term securities generated when a buyer agrees to pay for imported goods. When the buyer's bank promises to pay the seller for goods shipped, the acceptance is created. The buyer's bank may either keep the acceptance until maturity or sell it in the secondary market at a discount from face value. The risk of default is a function of the strength of the bank. Common maturities for these securities are 30 to 180 days.

Eurodollar Deposits

Eurodollar deposits are U.S. dollar denominated deposits in banks outside the U.S. A variety of maturities are available. The default risk is low and the secondary market is good. Eurodollar deposits usually pay higher rates than other short-term securities. Since the foreign banks are not as tightly regulated as U.S. banks Eurodollar deposits are seen to be riskier than other short-term securities.

Money Market Mutual Funds

Money market funds are offered by investment firms and banks as a way of pooling individual deposits and investing in larger blocks of short-term investments than would be possible for the individual investor. These funds usually offer check-writing privileges with daily competitive interest rates. They may be insured up to $100,000 by the organization sponsoring the fund or by the U.S. government in the case of banks and similar institutions.

Repurchase Agreements

Repurchase agreements can apply to a variety of securities. These arrangements occur where a seller agrees to repurchase the securities at a specified price on a stated date. The purchaser receives a rate of return somewhat below what would be available through outright purchase of the security.

As can be seen from the short description of some common marketable securities, there are many options available for investing excess cash. It is important for firms to develop good working relationships with bankers and other investment advisors. If they are aware of the firm's investment objectives and constraints, they can identify new opportunities and new investment vehicles as they become available. Such counselors can often help improve the short-term management of cash just by providing better record-keeping and more constant monitoring of actual and alternative yields for a modest cost.

Costs and Benefits of Marketable Securities Management

Since marketable securities are cash equivalents, many of the holding and shortage costs are the same as for cash. Although marketable securities earn a greater return on cash, the firm does incur an opportunity cost because alternative longer-term investments may provide higher returns. Additional holding costs for marketable securities are transaction costs such as sales commissions. Default, price and liquidity risk may also result in costs to the firm. For example, if a firm must sell some securities before they mature but after interest rates have changed, it may receive a lower return rate than planned. As always, the firm must balance the benefits holding marketable securities (not incurring shortage costs) with the opportunity and management costs for marketable securities.

Accounts Receivable Management _____

Accounts receivable arise when a health care firm extends credit to its customers. These customers receive goods and services but pay only part or none of the bill immediately. Accounts receivable are future cash inflows, or cash flows "waiting to happen."

The amount of accounts receivable and specific management issues are a function of the type of firm and the characteristics of its customers as well as its credit and collection policies. For example, an acute care hospital delivers goods and services to most of its patients before the patient's insurance company pays the bill. In addition, the patient pays any deductibles and coinsurance after receiving care. Further, the patient may be unable to pay immediately and may ask for credit from the hospital. Indeed, some of the hospital's clients may be indigent and unable to pay anything at all. Thus, the hospital usually has substantial accounts receivable from both patients and third party payers. In contrast, since a health maintenance organization's clients include employers and its product is the availability of health care services during a specific time period, it may collect its premiums in advance of the time period covered. The HMO would be less likely to provide its products to the indigent. As a result, the HMO would have a lower accounts receivable balance.

In general, firms face two primary activities in managing accounts receivable: (1) determining **credit policies** and (2) determining **collection policies** to minimize collection time. They are discussed next.

Credit Policies

Determination of an organization's credit policies must be made before the client appears. These policies include when and how much credit to approve (credit standards), the credit time period, and any discount policies.

Credit Standards. Credit standards are the minimum criteria for offering credit to clients. One area in which the economic criterion of marginality can be applied is the establishment of client categories based on the creditworthiness of each group. Based on the expected loss rates of each group, credit policies can be established that reflect loss expectations. Some categories may be such poor risks that credit is only granted in emergencies; otherwise, advance deposits or partial payments may be required.

Establishing the credit categories may rely on the *five C's* of credit: character, capacity, capital, collateral, and conditions. *Character* is an indicator of the probability that clients will try to pay their debts; it is a willingness-to-pay factor. *Capacity* refers to cash flows such as salary, dividends, and earnings that would indicate the client's ability to pay. *Capital* indicates the general financial status of the client's assets and liabilities. *Collateral* is a measure of the value of assets that may be pledged as security against the account. *Conditions* refer to general or specific economic circumstances that may affect either willingness or ability to pay. Information on all of these five factors is obtained from previous experience with the client's business or family, the shared knowledge of other health care firms, or credit bureaus. Knowledge of these factors, in advance, can be used to minimize the costs of credit and collection.

Some health care firms may be prohibited from setting credit standards. For example, emergency departments of acute care hospitals legally must treat certain patients. Since they are not allowed to turn these patients away, they are not permitted to evaluate their creditworthiness. In contrast, emergency departments can evaluate the creditworthiness of patients with non-urgent conditions.

Credit Period. The **credit time period** the firm offers is also important. For some services, the health care firm may set it at zero, as when deposits, advance payments or immediate copayments are required. Alternatively, as is true for many service providers, the credit period may be the time it takes to receive a third party payer's reimbursement. Then, the provider issues a bill for any deductibles and copayments. The firm may set a credit period for this portion of the bill, too, with terms (interest) for extending it.

The longer the credit time period, the higher the costs. These costs include the increasing risks of uncollectibility (bad debt), the costs of monitoring and "working" the account, and the opportunity costs of the funds. The opportunity costs of accounts receivable are analogous to the opportunity costs of cash in that a return on assets could be earned if the resources were invested elsewhere at a greater marginal return. For example, if the average size of accounts receivable doubles from $1 million to $2 million, and the lost earnings are 16% of the incremental balances, the opportunity cost of the decision to double the outstanding accounts is $160,000.

Discounts. The final aspect of credit policies concerns potential discounts for early payment. The goal of providing discounts is to attract customers and to speed payments of cash. Typically, the discount and payment period are expressed as the percent discount/period during which payment must be made to receive the discount. The "net" period is the number of days permitted for receiving the entire payment if the discount is not taken. Thus, 1/10 net 30 means a one percent discount for paying within 10 days. If the discount is not taken, the entire amount is due in 30 days. Economic theorists counsel that a firm should not grant any discounts in excess of its cost of capital. Since cost of capital is a weighted average across many different investment opportunities, a simplified approach is to look at the accumulated benefits that would be available under the discount or with various discount alternatives. Table 12-8 illustrates these computations, which show the benefits of investing the net proceeds for the difference between the full and net time periods. If the proceeds plus the interest earned exceed the amount that would be collected without a discount, the discount should be offered.

It should be obvious that the size of the discount and the length of the credit period are not as important as the alternative yields that could be earned on other investments. For instance, the conclusion drawn on 1/30 credit terms changes if the alternative short-term investment yield changes from 12% to 24%. Part B of Table 12-8 shows how changing this assumption changes the decision about whether to offer the discount.

The astute reader will note that the data in Table 12-8 assume zero bad debts. This assumption may be valid for a particular client with an excellent credit history of full payment. The model shown in Table 12-8 can be modified if offering discounts is expected to reduce bad debts. The second-to-last column can be reduced by the amount of expected bad debts. For example, if bad debts average 10% of receivables if no discount is offered, then the expected collections are reduced to $1,800. In such a situation, the discounted amount, to be paid within the specified period, should always be preferable. For example, the scenario in the first line of Table 12-8 would then compare $1,993 (with a discount) to $1,800 (no discount, but an average uncollectible ratio of 10%).

An alternative approach to the evaluation of accounts receivable discounts is shown in Table 12-9. This approach permits assumptions about the number of visits or the bad debt percentage to be changed. For the sample data shown in Table 12-9, the discount policy results in total collections of $22,551.78 whereas the no-discount policy provides only $22,500. Under these assumptions, a discount rate of 10% is estimated to provide slightly more revenue than the no discount policy of the past. Such apparently miraculous results can occur because the health care provider can minimize the number of defaulted accounts by encouraging early payment with an aggressive discount plan. The same kind of model should be useful for provider and payer firms when evaluating contracts with major purchasers, employers, or insurers.

Table 12-8   Evaluation of Discounts for Prompt Payment of Accounts Receivable.

A. Assume:
1. Credit and collection costs will not be significantly affected by a discount.
2. Alternative short-term investments yield 12% per year (1% per month).
3. $2,000 patient accounts normally due and paid in 30 days.

Payment Policy*	Discount	Net Proceeds ($2,000-discount)	Accumulation of proceeds and interest+	Expected collections if no discount and zero bad debts	Conclusions
1/10 1. Net 30	$20.00	$1,980	$1,993	$2,000	Reject discount
2/10 2. Net 30	$40.00	$1,960	$1,973	$2,000	Reject discount
2/20 3. Net 30	$40.00	$1,960	$1,967	$2,000	Reject discount

B. Change assumptions: Alternative short-term investment yields 24% (2 % per month).

Payment Policy*	Discount	Net Proceeds ($2,000-discount)	Accumulation of proceeds and interest+	Expected collections if no discount and zero bad debts	Conclusions
1/10 4. Net 30	$20.00	$1,980	$2,007	$2,000	Offer discount
2/10 5. Net 30	$40.00	$1,960	$1,987	$2,000	Reject discount
2/20 6. Net 30	$40.00	$1,960	$1,973	$2,000	Reject discount

*The numerator refers to the percent discount given, and the denominator refers to the number of days for this discount to be applicable. For instance, 2/10 net 30 means the creditor is offering a 2% discount if the bill is paid within 10 days and in any case the total (net) is due within 30 days.

+ Accumulation of proceeds and interest is the sum of the net proceeds and interest on net proceeds at the alternative short-term investment rate or, the rate x [(last day of net period – last day of discount period)/365 days].

Health care provider organizations have typically not considered variable pricing or discounting, perhaps because of fear of negative public relations. However, it is more equitable if credit users bear the costs of the credit. Non-credit users should not pay for those services that they are not utilizing.

Collection Policies

Collection policies refer the procedures the firm uses to minimize collection time for those accounts for which credit has been voluntarily or involuntarily granted. Speeding collection time decreases the opportunity cost of funds and the need to incur financing costs.

Table 12-9   A Model for Estimating Effects of Potential Credit and Collection Policies.

Givens

(A) Number of visits*	1,000	(H) Number taking discount (A)(B) — 600
(B) Percentage taking discount	60%	(I) Number of full-pay patients (A - H) — 400
(C) Average charge	$25.00	(J) Amount to be collected if no
(D) Bad debt percentage	10%	discount policy (A)(C)(100% - D) — $22,500
(E) Interest rate	7%	
(F) Discount percentages	10%	
(G) Days discount payment earns interest	20	

Derived figures	(K) Charge to full pay patients (C)(I)	(L) Expected bad debt (D)(K)	(M) Full-pay collections at end of month (K)(L)	(N) Charge to discount-pay patients (C)(H)	(O) Amount collected after discounted (10% discount)	(P) Interest earned on discounted collections [O(E/365)G]	(Q) Net collections & interest (O + P)	(R) Net collections with discount policy (M + Q)
1/10/30	$10,000	$1,000	$9,000	$15,000	$13,500	51.78	$13,551.78	$22,551.78

* The number of visits should be changed as credit policies change or prices increase or decrease, because these changes will increase or decrease the demand for the institution's services.

However, collection activities generate additional costs such as personnel expenses. In addition, overly aggressive collection policies may result in intangible costs from poor public relations. Therefore, the benefits of minimizing collection time must be balanced against the associated costs.

Some activities to speed the collection of receipts are discussed in the cash management section of this chapter. Additional activities to minimize collection time, which include (1) maintaining the accuracy and timeliness of billing, (2) collection and follow-up procedures, (3) monitoring performance ratios, and (4) selling accounts receivable, are discussed here.

Accuracy and Timeliness of Billing. If there is no bill, the firm cannot collect payment. If the bill that is generated is inaccurate or not timely, there are delays in receiving payment. Accuracy includes compiling the appropriate products and services on the bill and billing the appropriate client or payer. Timeliness involves getting the bill to the client as quickly as possible.

Although accuracy and timeliness of billing are important for all firms, they are especially important to providers paid on a fee-for-service basis. All goods and services provided must be identified and added into the bill. Sometimes, as in the case of an acute care hospital, it can take days for all items to be accumulated and charged to the patient.

A useful accounts receivable management technique for providers is to obtain prior authorization from the payer before services are delivered. Prior authorization includes confirmation of the patient's third party payer and approval of procedures and lengths of stay. Prior authorization eliminates the subsequent identification of ineligible parties and the rejection of their bills some 60 to 90 days later.

Electronic submission of bills is another means of increasing the accuracy and timeliness of billing. It is a frequent, and sometimes, required, method of billing for providers of health care services that deal with large third party payers.

Collection and Follow-Up Procedures. There are many collection and follow-up procedures available to the health care firm. They include demanding immediate payment, follow-up activities including letters, telephone calls, personal visits, using collection agencies, and legal action.

For providers, polite insistence on cash payment at the point of service delivery is the most effective way to minimize accounts receivable. The second best tactic is to accept payment by credit card. Each option can be prominently featured in printed materials and at "check-out" stations. Moving as many patients as possible toward a cash-on-delivery pattern will minimize accounts receivable. Payment in advance, or at the point of service, is most appropriate for outpatient units and elective procedures. Except for collecting any deductible or co-payment amounts, such tactics may be less crucial, or feasible, for inpatient care or for clients covered under managed care contracts,

A health care firm should evaluate the advantages of accepting credit cards. Although the firm will incur a cost for accepting credit cards, it will benefit from having cash sooner and from shifting the costs of credit investigation and collection efforts to the issuer of the charge card. The financial manager must identify the number and size of the accounts that would use credit cards, estimate the reduction in time lags due to credit card processing, and determine the marginal benefit of having cash resources earlier.

If the firm is unable to collect, it may use the services of a collection agency. Unfortunately, the fees charged by most agencies are high. Establishing an in-house collection agency can also be effective. This technique protects the provider's image and permits the institution to control and manage all collection procedures. Hourly pay rates, plus commissions, can be an effective motivator in such departments.

The firm may have to initiate legal action if the account is not paid. Some written contact with an attorney, with the correspondence handled by paralegal staff, can be a cost-effective mechanism.

Collection policies also include policies regarding when an account is to be written off or turned over to a collection agency. Size of accounts and the five C's have an obvious effect here. Finally, collection policies must take into account the internal control system regarding which personnel are responsible for recording and verifying patient payment data. Determining who can authorize writing off an account is important. If this authorization is not properly separated from payment processing and recording, a deterioration of internal control may occur.

Monitoring Accounts Receivable Performance Measures. By establishing and monitoring performance measures for accounts receivable management, the health care firm can determine if accounts are being collected in a timely manner. In this section, three performance measures are discussed.

The most common measure of accounts receivable management is the **days revenue outstanding** as accounts receivable also called days revenue in accounts receivable. This measure equates with the average collection period in Chapter 3. It is calculated as

$$\frac{\text{Accounts receivable}}{\text{Revenue / Days in period}} = \frac{\text{A / R}}{\text{Average daily revenue}}.$$

The denominator is the average daily revenue. For health care firms in which clients do not pay the full charge because of contractual arrangements, the net revenue should be used as should the accounts receivable less any expected deductions for uncollectible accounts. In Table 12-10, an example using quarterly ratios is shown for a health care provider. The quarterly data on days revenue shows an improvement in the second quarter (45.75) and deterioration in the last two quarters (51.0 and 58.50, respectively). Note that the fewer days revenue is in accounts receivable, the more positively the results are viewed.

A second means of evaluating accounts receivable performance is with an **aging schedule** that considers the amount of receivables outstanding at a particular time. As is shown in Table 12-11, the receivables are arranged by when the outstanding receivables were generated. Data are needed on both revenues and current account balances outstanding. Current unpaid accounts in accounts receivable are then arrayed in terms of date of service and are

Table 12-10 Days Revenue Outstanding.

Quarter	Net Patient Revenues	Net Accounts Receivable at End of Quarter	Days Revenues in Accounts Receivable	Calculation
1	$1,200,000	$750,000	56.25	$750,000/($1,200,000/90)
2	$1,200,000	$610,000	45.75	$610,000/($1,200,000/90)
3	$1,200,000	$680,000	51.00	$680,000/($1,200,000/90)
4	$1,200,000	$780,000	58.50	$780,000/($1,200,000/90)

classified into convenient groups (e.g., by months outstanding). In Table 12-11, as of the last day of the first quarter, 60% of the outstanding accounts receivable ($750,000) are from March ($450,000). Almost none (8%) of January's accounts are still outstanding at the end of the first quarter.

A third means of evaluating accounts receivable management is to incorporate an indicator of the percentage of revenues outstanding at any point in time. From Table 12-11, the percentage of the first month's revenues still outstanding at the end of the quarter is 20% ($60,000/$300,000). The percentage of revenues still outstanding from the second month is 60% ($240,000/$400,000). Finally, the percentage outstanding from the third month is 90% ($450,000/$500,000). In fact, this pattern (20%-60%-90%) is constant for all four quarters. In other words, accounts receivable managerial performance has not changed. The modest changes in aging and days revenue relationships are strictly due to changes in overall levels of activity. These changes are a function of patient services, level of demand, or admission policies. They are not the sole bailiwick of the business office manager.

Selling Accounts Receivable. The final means of speeding the collection of accounts receivable is to sell them. This can be done **with recourse** as in the case of pledging accounts receivable or **without recourse** when accounts receivable are factored or securitized.

One form of quickly turning accounts receivable into cash is to **pledge the accounts** or use them as collateral against a revolving credit bank loan. The lender evaluates the desirability of the accounts receivable and subtracts interest and other costs before advancing funds to the firm. In such cases, the clients continue to make payments to the provider in their normal manner. The sale is with recourse because the health care firm remains liable for paying the accounts receivable that turn out to be bad debts. Consequently, the transaction creates a secured loan that uses the accounts receivable as collateral. The accounts receivable remain on the health care firm's balance sheet and a loan liability is created.

Factoring is the second form of transforming accounts into cash. In this case, the accounts are literally sold to a lender (factor) at a discount. They are replaced by cash on the seller's balance sheet. The factor then performs all of the credit and collection activities and bears all of the risks. Since the selling firm is not liable for bad debts, the sale is without recourse. As with pledging accounts, the health care firm will receive the value of the accounts receivable less expected returns and program costs. Since the buying firm assumes the

Table 12-11   Aging of Accounts Receivable by Quarter.

Days	0-30	31-60	61-90
First Quarter			
Month	March	February	January
Net Revenues	$500,000	$400,000	$300,000
Accounts Receivable	$450,000	$240,000	$60,000
Percentage of Total Receivables at			
End of Quarter	60	32	8
Percent of Month's Revenues			
Outstanding at End of Quarter	90	60	20
Second Quarter			
Month	June	May	April
Net Revenues	$300,000	$400,000	$500,000
Accounts Receivable	$270,000	$240,000	$100,000
Percentage of Total Receivables at			
End of Quarter	44.4	39.3	16.3
Percent of Month's Revenues			
Outstanding at End of Quarter	90	60	20
Third Quarter			
Month	September	August	July
Net Revenues	$400,000	$400,000	$400,000
Accounts Receivable	$360,000	$240,000	$80,000
Percentage of Total Receivables at			
End of Quarter	52.9	35.3	11.8
Percent of Month's Revenues			
Outstanding at End of Quarter	90	60	20
Fourth Quarter			
Month	December	November	October
Net Revenues	$600,000	$300,000	$300,000
Accounts Receivable	$540,000	$180,000	$60,000
Percentage of Total Receivables at			
End of Quarter	69.2	23.1	7.7
Percent of Month's Revenues			
Outstanding at End of Quarter	90	60	20

For simplicity, in this example, all accounts are collected or written off by the end of the succeeding third month.

risk for bad debts, the cost is higher than for pledging accounts. Typically, the firm sells the receivables at a discount between 5% and 10% off the face value and pays a fee that is a percentage of the receivables sold. However, the selling firm also benefits by reducing its credit and collection personnel and stabilizing and enhancing its cash flow all without incurring any loans on its balance sheet.

The net effect of most factoring arrangements is that the institution sells its best accounts and keeps the less desirable ones. Generally, factoring is a long-term relationship, whereas pledging of accounts may be handled on a one-time basis.

The newest form of accounts receivable financing is based on an asset **securitization** program where an intermediary is used to manage the process. The intermediary sells A1-rated commercial paper and uses the proceeds to finance the provider's accounts receivable. In other words, the intermediary gets money by selling commercial paper to investors and sends that money to the provider, in exchange for the money from the provider's accounts receivable, which is then used to redeem the commercial paper.

Accounts receivable eligible for sale are usually those from third party payers but not from self-pay patients. The seller may receive up to 90 percent of the face value of the receivables. Although the selling firm is still responsible for collection and follow-up activities, an asset manager manages the cash for retiring the commercial paper and paying administrative costs.

Asset-based securitization is often more flexible and less costly than other forms of accounts receivable financing. Since collateral is supplied, it can provide a means of borrowing at a better rate than the firm can obtain on its own. As with factoring, securitization also provides off-balance-sheet financing that does not affect capital structure ratios.

Costs and Benefits of Accounts Receivable Management

Extending credit to its customers and accumulating accounts receivable can increase the firm's revenues by attracting customers who cannot pay immediately. Thus, an important shortage cost for accounts receivable is lost revenues.

The holding costs of accounts receivable include the opportunity cost of the delay in receiving cash payments, financing costs of securing funds to replace cash "tied up" in accounts receivable and the administrative costs of collecting the payments. The opportunity cost occurs because funds "tied up" in accounts receivable cannot be invested in financial or physical assets earning returns. Financing costs are incurred when the firm must borrow to meet its cash needs. Administrative costs such as salaries are required to collect accounts receivable. Not surprisingly, spending more on collection can reduce the opportunity and financing costs. However, the firm must determine the optimal amount of collection effort to minimize the opportunity and financing costs.

Summary

Managing current assets is one of the day-to-day functions of the health care organization. Managers must balance the costs of holding specific types of current assets against the costs of shortages of the current asset. Holding costs typically include both opportunity costs and the costs of managing the current asset. Shortage costs can include lost revenues, financing costs and poor vendor and community relations.

This chapter has concentrated on activities for the management of cash, marketable securities and accounts receivable. They are typically the most active current assets in a health care organization and affect the financial status of the service organization more significantly than other current assets such as inventories and prepaid items.

Bibliography

Ayers, D.H. and T.J. Kincaid. "Avoiding Potential Problems When Selling Accounts Receivable" *Healthcare Financial Management* (May): 50-55, 1996.

Ferconio, S. and M.R. Lane. "Financing Maneuvers" *Healthcare Financial Management* (October): 74-78, 1991.

Gallinger, G.W. and P.B. Healy. *Liquidity Analysis and Management*. Reading, Mass.: Addison-Wesley Publishing Co., 1987.

Kincaid, T.J. "Purchase of Receivables—Healthcare Providers" *Credit World* 82(4): 14-17, 1994.

Kolb, R.W. *Investments*. Miami: Kolb Publishing Co., 1992.

McCormack E.J. "The Hidden Costs of Accounts Receivable" *Healthcare Financial Management* (November): 80, 1993.

Ponton, K.T. "Medical Accounts Receivable—An Underused Asset for Hospitals" *Trustee* 46(6): 24-25, 1993.

Sen, S. and J.P. Lawler, "Securitizing Receivables Offers Low-Cost Financing Option" *Healthcare Financial Management* (May): 32-37, 1995.

Sutton, H.L. Jr. and A.J. Sorbo. *Actuarial Issues in the Fee-For-Service/Prepaid Medical Group*. Englewood, CO: Center for Research in Ambulatory Health Care Administration, 1993.

Terms and Concept

accounts receivable
aging schedule
banker's acceptance
buffer
cash budget
cash collection ratios
cash equivalents
cash flow synchronization
certificates of deposit
clearing float
collection float
collection policies
commercial paper

credit policies
credit time period
days revenue outstanding
default risk
disbursement control
Eurodollar deposits
factoring accounts receivable
disbursement float
factoring
Federal Agency issues
five C's
float
incurred but not reported expenses

lockbox
liquidity risk
mail float
money market funds
opportunity cost
overdraft account
pledging accounts receivable
price risk
primary market

processing float
recourse
repurchase agreements
secondary market
securitization
speculative motive
Treasury bills
with recourse
without recourse
zero-balance account

Questions and Problems

12-1 Define cash in terms of its placement in the current assets section on a balance sheet.

12-2 What are the three primary reasons for holding cash? Why is there a risk in holding cash?

12-3 Why is the cash budget so important in managing a health care institution?

12-4 Explain the costs of holding excess cash and cash shortage costs.

12-5 Identify ways to expedite check processing and the prompt deposit of cash.

12-6 Are there any health care organizations that would not require significant cash balances? Which ones? Why? Any that would not require any cash? Which ones? Why?

12-8 What does writing off accounts receivable mean? What kinds of write-off procedures would you recommend?

12-9 Why is it important to know how many accounts have been written off when interpreting the average collection period ratio (Chapter 3)?

12-10 Is there a particular group of customers to whom you would recommend offering liberal credit terms? Why? Under what circumstances would you restrict credit availability?

12-11 Could the five C's of credit management ever be in conflict? Why?

12-12 Do you think that health care providers should use the same criteria and screens for establishing credit limits that financial institutions (e.g., commercial banks, VISA) use? Why?

12-13 What are some examples of the costs of collection in health care firms? What are some examples of credit costs? Which do you expect are most significant? Why?

12-14 Change the data in the first row of Table 12-2 to better represent actual Medicare payment lags (e.g., 0, 25%, 50%, 25%). How does this change the data in Table 12-3, and how does it impact cash collection patterns? Why?

12-15 Why should you be suspicious of internal control problems if the cash surplus (deficit) line in a cash budget showed a negative figure for eleven months out of every twelve?

12-16 Given the following accounts receivable performance for Jackson Obstetrical and Gynecological Clinic, complete the following for each month and quarter.

   A. Aging schedule
   B. Days revenue in accounts receivable
   C. Percentage of billings outstanding
   D. Comparison of first and second quarter accounts receivable performance and reasons

Receivables
Outstanding at

	Month	Revenues	End of Qtr
	January	$150,500	$ 25,200
1st	February	112,800	73,900
Qtr	March	205,400	182,700
		$468,700	$281,800
	April	$182,300	$ 26,600
2nd	May	210,500	85,300
Qtr	June	194,600	185,500
		$587,400	$297,400

12-17 The laundry supplier for Fillmore Hospitals, Inc. (FHI), is considering offering the following discount scenarios. Evaluate whether or not the corporation should accept or reject the discount on a $4,500 account at an 8% annual cost of capital rate.

	Policy	Discount	Net Proceeds+ Proceeds	Interest	Collect if no Discount	Accept/ Reject
(1)	1/10 Net 30	[$45]	[$4,455]	[$4,475]	$4,500	
(2)	3/10 Net 30	[$135]	[$4,365]	[$4,385]	$4,500	
(3)	5/10 Net 30	[$225]	[$4,275]	[$4,295]	$4,500	

A. At which of the following cost of capital rates would a discount offer be profitable for FHI in Scenario 1?

5%	8%	16%	24%
4,467.50	4,475	4,495	4,515

B. Under what circumstances might a discount be offered even if the figures do not indicate profit from using the discount?

12-18 Recalculate lines 1 to 3 in Table 12-8, assuming that short-term investments yield 18% per year.

Appendix 12A

Evaluation of Cash Excess and Shortage Costs

The cash budget in Table 12-5 showed that each month the organization has a cash shortage and must borrow money to maintain the required minimum balance of $200,000. The example could also have been constructed to show a cash surplus each month. What difference does it make to the manager?

As with working capital in general, there are costs of having too much cash and costs of not having enough. The costs of excess cash are primarily the opportunity costs of investment yields that could have been earned by investing the funds elsewhere. This opportunity cost applies only to cash balances in excess of that necessary for transaction or buffer purposes. On the other hand, the costs of having insufficient cash pertain to purchase discounts that cannot be taken promptly, higher than normal interest rates on short-term loans, deterioration of credit ratings, and the worsening of relations with bankers and other suppliers. We refer to these two kinds of costs as cash excess and cash shortage costs, respectively. Both costs are important and must be considered by management.

Tables 12A-1, 12A-2, and 12A-3 illustrate the computation of cash excess and shortage costs in an environment where monthly, weekly, or daily cash flows have a degree of uncertainty associated with them. That is, an organization can only estimate the probability (not certainty) that any particular cash flow will occur during the time period in question. However, a probability distribution can be historically associated with the net cash flows in any time period. Once that probability distribution has been established, it can be used to calculate the **expected value** of each possible cash management strategy. Such a distribution is shown in Table 12A-1 where each of ten possible "actual net cash flows" are assumed to have an equal probability of occurring (10% each).

Table 12A-1 Probability of Estimated Cash Flows.

Estimated cash flows	Associated probability (%)	Estimated cash flows	Associated probability (%)
12,500	10	0	10
10,000	10	(2,500)	10
7,500	10	(5,000)	10
5,000	10	(7,500)	10
2,500	10	(10,000)	10

Table 12A-2 Shortage and Excess Costs Associated with Various Net Cash Flows and Cash Balances Held by a Provider.

Cash Balance Held Over Minimum*	Possible net cash flows ($)									
	12,500	10,000	7,500	5,000	2,500	0	(2,500)	(5,000)	(7,500)	(10,000)
0	2,000	1,600	1,200	800	400	0	700	900	1,100	1,300‡
2,000	2,320	1,920	1,520	1,120	720	320	540	740	940	1,140
4,000	2,640	2,240	1,840	1,440	1,040	640	240	580	780	980
6,000	2,960	2,560	2,160	1,760	1,360	960	560	160	620	820
8,000	3,280	2,880	2,480	2,080	1,680	1,280	880	480	80	660
10,000	3,600‡	3,200	2,800	2,400	2,000	1,600	1,200	800	400	0

* Over and above the minimum necessary for transactions and buffers.
† Cash shortages cost = $500 + ($10,000 x 8%) = $1,300
‡ Cash excess cost = $22,500 x 16% = $3,600

Table 12A-3 Expected Value of Cash Excess and Shortage Costs.

Cash Balance Held Over Minimum*	Possible net cash flows ($)									
	12,500	10,000	7,500	5,000	2,500	0	(2,500)	(5,000)	(7,500)	(10,000)
0	200	160	120	80	40	0	70	90	110	130†
2,000	232	192	152	112	72	32	54	74	94	114
4,000	264	224	184	144	104	64	24	58	78	98
6,000	296	256	216	176	136	96	56	16	62	82
8,000	328	288	248	208	168	128	88	48	8	66
10,000	360‡	320	280	240	200	160	120	80	40	0

* Beyond that needed for transactions and buffers.
† Expected value of shortage cost = $1,300 x 10% = $130
‡ Expected value of excess cost = $3,600 x 10% = $360

These ten possible net cash flows appear as headings in Table 12A-2. The cells in the figure represent either cash shortage or excess costs. They are computed first by adding the cash balance over the minimum to the "possible net cash flow." The cost of the excess or shortage is then computed according to cost assumptions shown in the footnotes. For example, if a health care organization adopted a strategy of holding $10,000 in cash beyond that needed for transactions and buffers, and a $12,500 cash inflow actually occurred in the next time period, the institution would incur an opportunity cost of $3,600 ($22,500 at 16%) as shown in the bottom left of Table 12A-2. As this $3,600 cash excess cost will probably occur only 10% of the time, its expected value is $360 (bottom row of the first column in Table 12A-3). Each cell in Table 12A-3 is calculated in the same way. The expected values of the costs for each strategy are then added (by rows) to obtain the total costs of holding excess cash balances for each strategy. For instance, given the assumptions in Table 12A-1, the cost of holding $10,000 in excess cash is $1,800 as shown in Table 12A-3.

The cash excess costs in this example are so much larger than the cash shortage costs that the minimum cost occurs for the strategy that would hold zero excess cash balances. This can be seen in the total column of Table 12A-3. This phenomenon will certainly not always be the case, as cash shortage costs may be underestimated. Some of the problems at the end of this chapter suggest that you look at alternative cost structures and the impact on recommended strategies. In addition, you should also feel comfortable knowing what happens as the probability distribution of actual net cash flow is weighted toward shortages or overages occurring more frequently.

Another way to use Table 12A-2 is to determine how often shortages will occur under any recommended strategy. For instance, there would be insufficient cash associated with a zero cash balance 40% of the time (the sum of the 10% probabilities on the four right-hand columns of Table 12A-1). Perhaps the board of trustees would not approve a strategy that would be short that often. Bankers on the board might require larger compensating balances if shortages were that prevalent. A compensating balance is a minimum amount required to be deposited and remain in an account in order to receive a certain benefit (i.e., a loan). If a compensating balance is required, we have underestimated the cost of shortages in Table 12A-2. In any event, the approach outlined in this section is useful to indicate the relative advantage of different cash-holding strategies. Can such costs be justified? Can they be passed on to patients or third parties? Can the CEO justify the additional expense in the face of competing demands for resources that may alleviate pain and suffering or save someone's life? Where large relative differences occur in the costs of alternative cash management strategies, the chief financial officer (CFO) must be able to explain the implications and possible effects of those costs to the institution's strategists. Perhaps, in this case, some shortages could be tolerated in exchange for higher yields that could be earned on cash balances invested elsewhere (16% is assumed in the analysis conducted).

To test your understanding:

I. Recalculate and estimate the lowest cost balance from Table 12A-3 assuming the following:

   a) Cash shortage cost = $1,000 + 12% of shortages;
   b) Cash excess cost = 10% of the excess;
   c) The probability distribution remains the same.

II. How would Table 12A-3 change with the skewed probability distribution (e.g., 1%, 1%, 1%, 2%, 5%, 10%, 10%, 20%, 25%, 25%)? What would be the lowest cash balance to hold?

13 The Capital Investment Decision

Most health care providers as well as payers must make sizable investments in long-lived assets such as buildings and equipment to provide effective, efficient, and proper health care to the community. Recommendations concerning what assets are needed are the outputs of the capital investment decision process. A poor capital investment decision can lead to overinvestment in the wrong kind of assets, a high fixed cost structure, and an inability to react to changes in the environment. For instance, it is difficult to convert excess intensive care facilities to outpatient clinics or ambulatory surgical centers once beds have been bought and construction has been completed. Similarly, third party payers cannot manage the care provided to their subscribers or negotiate contracts effectively with providers without the appropriate kinds of information systems.

From an accounting viewpoint, a **capital investment** is an expenditure that benefits more than one accounting period. Expenditures that benefit primarily one accounting period are usually considered operating expenses. Capital investment decisions should be a primary focus for top management because they are important in implementing the organization's strategic plan and they typically involve large sums of money for long periods of time.

The capital investment decision making process, sometimes called capital budgeting, with special emphasis on quantitative methods for analysis, is discussed in this chapter.

The Capital Investment Decision Making Process

An effective capital investment decision (capital budgeting) system should consist of three major phases:

- Identification of potential capital investments
- Evaluation of each potential investment
- Evaluation of the actual performance of the capital investments selected.

Capital investment requirements should flow primarily from the goals and objectives derived from the organization's strategic plan. The dissemination of these goals and objectives to the personnel in the organization is an important step in the capital budgeting process. Then, the managers who are in the best position to decide specifically how to accomplish these objectives can recommend appropriate capital investments for thorough evaluation.

Evaluation of each investment involves both quantitative and qualitative factors. The quantitative aspects can be more objective in nature than the qualitative factors. Thus, most formal evaluation techniques focus on quantitative analysis as does this chapter. However, qualitative issues are equally important and the organization's mission statement, strategic plan, and goals for its stakeholders should help guide investment analysis.

For each capital investment proposal, quantitative data are gathered and evaluated. Financial personnel can help prepare financial analyses of the proposed investments. Most organizations have a formal capital investment screening process to aid in determining the feasibility of a proposal. From a financial management perspective, the screening process usually involves establishing some minimum financial performance for the proposed investment. Typically, more potential investments pass the initial screening than the organization can undertake. Therefore, the organization often uses a ranking process to help prioritize the proposals. Top managers prioritize the proposals to best fit the overall needs of the organization.

Finally, once a decision to invest has been made, the decision must be implemented and the performance of the investment must be evaluated. During implementation, the costs and timetable for the investment must be controlled in order for the investment to perform as desired. For example, managers ensure that there are no cost overruns for renovation and installation of imaging equipment. After implementation, a review of the actual and planned performance, often called a postaudit, should be conducted. Planned costs and revenues should be compared with actual figures over the life of the investment. Such an evaluation is not only useful for managing the specific investment, it may provide useful information for the next round of decision-making. It may improve the forecasting ability of the organization or identify flaws in the decision-making process.

Note that the choice of financing is not considered to be part of the capital budgeting process. Financing decisions are made separately from capital investment decisions.

Methods for Analysis

Three types of evaluation methods are discussed in this chapter. Each has its own strengths and weaknesses, which should be thoroughly understood. The methods that are discussed are:

1. Accounting rate of return.
2. Payback method.
3. Time adjusted methods (Net Present Value and Internal Rate of Return).

Each method is described and examples are presented for illustration. First, however, the various data elements required for the analyses are discussed.

Financial Data for the Analyses

In this section, the projected financial data needed for the capital investment evaluation methods are described. The projected data all involve incremental income or cash flows for the organization. That is, only new revenues, expenses or cash flows that are attributable to the investment should be considered. Managers should also remember that the data needed for the analyses are largely projections, and, therefore, subject to forecasting error. Thus, alternative scenarios that lead to different quantitative projections of each variable in the analyses should always be evaluated. This type of analysis is called sensitivity analysis because the sensitivity of the decision to possible changes that may occur in any of the data elements should be ascertained.

The data shown in Table 13-1 for a capital equipment proposal for radiological equipment are used throughout this chapter to illustrate each evaluation method. These data come from equipment vendors, managerial estimates, marketing studies, and analytical calculations (*e.g.*, depreciation).

As can be seen from the table, the proposed investment is expected to cost $75,000, which includes the purchase cost, all installation costs, and any other out of pocket costs that are necessary to make the investment operational. The investment is expected to have an economic life of five years. Analyses should be conducted for the economic life of the investment. The **economic or technological life** of the proposal is defined as the period of time during which the health care provider is expected to receive benefits from the investment. It should not be confused with the physical life (although the physical life does set an upper limit on benefits) or the depreciation period established by the Internal Revenue Service or third party payers. Many types of health care equipment have very short economic lives because of rapid advancements in technology.

Opportunity costs are defined as the benefits that would be received from the next best alternative use of the investment funds. In this case, funds could earn 10% per year from the next best alternative use. This cost is discussed further later.

The table also presents information regarding the accrual accounting revenues and expenses expected from the investment. Revenues expected for the organization if the investment in the radiological equipment is made are $35,000 or $40,000 per year. All expenses related to the annual operation of the radiological equipment, which could include personnel, maintenance and other expenses, must also be determined. In the example, the incremental expenses are limited to depreciation and income taxes. The depreciation expense is determined with the straight line method for the economic life of the asset ($75,000/5). State and federal income taxes are 40% of the earnings before taxes. If the organization is tax-exempt, as are most not-for-profit health care providers, there would be no income taxes paid. As is customary, net income is determined by subtracting expenses from revenues.

Incremental, or additional, cash flows usually differ somewhat from the accrual accounting revenues and expenses. Cash flows reflect when cash is actually received and disbursed. Cash flows occur at the beginning, during each year and at the end of the investment project.

In the table, the incremental **cash inflows** consist of the revenues associated with the capital investment decision. They could also include any personnel or material savings and other cost savings that could be considered negative cash outflows. For example, a cash inflow results from a new piece of equipment that reduces the number of technicians required and thus reduces salary expense. In addition, salvage value can be treated as a cash inflow at the end of a piece of equipment's economic life.

Cash outflows for the project consist of the initial investment, which takes place at the beginning of the project, and any other actual outflows during the economic life of the project.

Table 13-1   Data for Radiological Equipment.

Asset and installation costs	$75,000
Estimated economic life of asset	5 years
Depreciation expense per year	$15,000
Opportunity cost of capital	10%
Combined state and federal marginal tax rate	40%

Projected Revenues and Expenses

Year	Revenue	Depreciation Expense	Income Taxes	Net Income
1	$35,000	$15,000	$8,000	$12,000
2	$40,000	$15,000	$10,000	$15,000
3	$40,000	$15,000	$10,000	$15,000
4	$35,000	$15,000	$8,000	$12,000
5	$35,000	$15,000	$8,000	$12,000

$$\text{Average Net Income} = \frac{\$12,000 + \$15,000 + \$15,000 + \$12,000 + \$12,000}{5} = \$13,200$$

Projected Cash Flows

Year	Cash Inflows	Cash Outflows	Net Cash Flows
0 (today)	$ 0	$75,000	($75,000)
1	$35,000	$8,000	$27,000
2	$40,000	$10,000	$30,000
3	$40,000	$10,000	$30,000
4	$35,000	$8,000	$27,000
5	$35,000	$8,000	$27,000

In the example shown in Table 13-1, cash outflows during the project are limited to income taxes since the depreciation expense is not a cash outflow. For a tax-exempt firm, there would be no taxes.

Accounting Rate of Return Method

In the past, analysts frequently used the accounting rate of return method to evaluate potential investments because it closely approximated the normal reporting of financial information. In this method, the increase in income as reported on the statement of revenue and expenses is divided by either the total or the average investment. The resulting rate of return is then considered in the decision to make the investment.

The **accounting rate of return** can be computed using the following formula:

$$\text{Accounting rate of return} = \frac{\text{Average annual increase in net income}}{\text{Initial investment}} \times 100\%$$

Using the data from Table 13-1, the accounting rate of return can be easily calculated as:

$$\frac{\$13,200}{\$75,000} \times 100\% = 17.6\%$$

The accounting rate of return is often calculated by using the average investment at the midpoint of the equipment's economic life. To determine the average investment, the initial investment is added to the value of the investment at the end of its life (usually $0) and divided by two. Therefore, the *adjusted* **accounting rate of return** is:

$$\text{Adjusted accounting rate of return} = \frac{\text{Average annual increase in net income}}{\text{Initial investment} / 2}.$$

Using the sample data from Table13-1, the adjusted accounting rate of return is:

$$\frac{\$13,200}{\$75,000 / 2} \times 100\% = \frac{13,200}{37,500} \times 100\% = 35.2\%$$

This adjusted rate of return remains constant throughout the economic life of the investment.

The accounting rate of return technique for evaluating capital investments is easy to understand and to compute. Unfortunately, it also has some serious weaknesses. First, it does not consider the time value of money. As will be demonstrated later in this chapter, a dollar received at some point in the future does not have the same value in terms of purchasing power as a dollar received today. Second, there is no clear guidance for determining how much rate of return is required for an investment to be acceptable to the organization. Clearly, if choices must be made among potential investments, the firm would choose the investments with the highest rates of return. However, the minimum required rate of return for the accounting rate of return method is often an arbitrary number.

Payback Method

The **payback period** is the amount of time it takes for cash inflows to recover the cash outflows of the investment. The payback period is expressed in units of time usually years. Using the data from Table 13-1, the payback period can be determined by showing when the net cash flows for the investment would be recovered. Year zero is the time at which the cash would be disbursed to purchase the equipment.

	Expected Net Cash Flows	
Year	Annual	Cumulative
0	($75,000)	($75,000)
1	$27,000	($48,000)
2	$30,000	($18,000)
3	$30,000	$12,000

This analysis shows that the project will payback the initial cost sometime during the third year. If one assumes that the net cash flows arrive steadily over the year, the fraction of the year can be calculated with the cash flows yet to be paid back divided by the total net cash flow generated during the year. For this example, it is $18,000 divided by $30,000 or 0.6 years. Thus, the payback period is 2.6 years.

The payback method is quite easy to compute and is easily understood, but it has several weaknesses. First, it disregards cash inflows after the payback period. In the example, the returns from years four and five are all "gravy." On the other hand, investments having negative net cash flows after the payback period may look acceptable. Second, the choice of a criterion for accepting an investment is arbitrary. Should it be three years, two years, four years, or some other length of time? Third, it creates a bias for projects that payback quickly. Many investments that require longer paybacks may be very valuable to the firm. Finally, the payback method ignores the time value of money.

Thus, both of the first two methods ignore the **time value of money**. That is, they treat dollars received at different points in time as having equal value. Dollars received at different points in time do not have equal value because (1) inflation erodes purchasing power and (2) people prefer to have access to funds today rather than tomorrow. To convince people to wait for the use of their funds, they must be compensated, such as a bank does when funds deposited in a savings account earn interest. Time adjusted methods correct the deficiency by using discounting techniques.

Time Adjusted Methods

There are two time adjusted methods most frequently used for evaluating capital investments, net present value and internal rate or return. Prior to discussing them, however, an introduction to discounting and compounding is presented.

Introduction to Discounting and Compounding. Discounting techniques used in evaluating capital investments can more easily be explained if we consider the **compounding** techniques with which most of us are familiar. Banks and other financial institutions use compounding to compute the **future value** of an investment. For example, if you set aside $10,000 today in a money market account at 10% interest, what will the account balance be at the end of one year? After earning interest at 10% for one year, the $10,000 deposit will have grown to $11,000, comprised of the original deposit of $10,000 plus $1,000 in interest. If the account continues earning interest at 10%, at the end of the second year an additional $1,100 of interest will accrue, resulting in an ending balance of $12,100. This process continues for as long as the funds are left on deposit. The process of earning interest on interest is known as compounding. The amount available at the end of the compounding process, the future value, can be computed by multiplying the initial or present value, by the compound interest factor

$$\text{Compound interest factor} = (1 + i)^n$$

where n equal the periods of time and i equals the interest rate paid during each time period on the account. For managers who do not want to calculate these amounts, present value tables, calculators and computer spreadsheet programs are available that solve the compounding equation with a minimum of difficulty.

Table 13-2 illustrates the compounding process for a period of four years. Assuming no withdrawals or additional deposits, interest continues to accrue at 10% each year. The basic compounding formula can be used to obtain any of these values. For example, for three years, $(1 + .10)^3$ can be computed as $(1.10)(1.10)(1.10)$, which is equal to 1.331. This factor can then be multiplied by the original deposit ($10,000) to determine the value in the account at the end of the third year ($13,310).

Table 13A-3 in the Appendix can also be used to determine the future value. It consists of compound interest factors. To use it, from the first column select the row with the appropriate number of periods. Then, find the column with the interest rate per period. Move to where the interest rate column intersects the time period row to find the future value factor. Multiply the initial amount by the future value interest factor (FVIF). Thus,

Future Value   =   Initial amount x Compound interest factor, or

FV   =   Present Value x FVIF.

Without referring to Table 13-2, determine the account value at the end of the fourth year. After computing your answer, refer to the last line in Table 13-2 to check your understanding.

Discounting is related inversely to compounding. Discounting is used in a situation where future cash flows are known, or can be estimated, but the value of these cash flows in today's terms must be computed. Rather than carrying values forward to some future date, the future values are known and are carried backward to the present. Thus, discounting is used to compare and evaluate cash flows occurring at different future dates, all on a consistent basis.

Table 13-2   Future Value of a Single Cash Deposit.

Year	Value at Beginning of Year	Interest	Value at End of Year
1	$10,000	$1,000	$11,000
2	$11,000	$1,100	$12,100
3	$12,100	$1,210	$13,310
4	$13,310	$1,331	$14,641

In discounting, we are interested in the present value of an amount to be received in the future. Since discounting is the inverse of compounding, its formula is also the inverse:

$$\text{Present Value} = \frac{\text{Future Value}}{(1+i)^n}$$

and the

$$\text{Present value interest factor} = \frac{1}{(1+i)^n} = \text{PVIF} .$$

Thus,

$$\text{Present Value (PV)} = \text{Future Value (FV) x PVIF.}$$

Many present value factors have been computed in Table 13A-1 in the Appendix. For example, the factor for present values for five years at 10% is computed as:

$$\frac{1}{(1+.10)^5} = \frac{1}{(1.1)(1.1)(1.1)(1.1)(1.1)} = .621$$

Assume a situation in which a health care provider estimates the cost of replacing a particular laboratory centrifuge at $16,104 five years from now. How much money must be deposited now to have sufficient funds in five years to replace the centrifuge? It is this type of question that discounting to today's value, or present value, is designed to answer. The cash flows pertaining to the centrifuge are

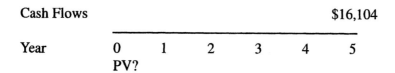

Cash Flows $16,104

Year   0   1   2   3   4   5
               PV?

Sketching time lines like the one above helps the analyst to make sure each cash flow is included appropriately in the analyses.

The **discount rate** for the analysis is chosen to reflect the firm's opportunity **cost of capital**. Here, we assume the appropriate discount rate for the provider is 10%. The present value of $10,000 is obtained by multiplying the present value factor (.621) by the future expected cost of the centrifuge ($16,104). The curious reader may verify this calculation by finding the future value of $10,000 in five years at 10%.

Present and future values merely represent different time perspectives. When present values are used, all cash flows are converted to equivalent values at the current time period. When future values are used, all cash flows are stated in terms of future time perspectives.

Since capital projects have differing time perspectives, it is rare that future values will all be stated in consistent terms. However, when present values are used, comparability is assured because all cash flows are translated or discounted to the current time perspective.

The relationship between compounding and discounting should now be clear. The same relationship exists when one considers a situation in which annual sums are to be invested or received. A stream of equal payments over time is termed an **annuity**. An **ordinary annuity** is one in which the equal cash flows arrive (or are paid) at the end of each period and the first cash payment occurs one period from today. For example, consider the situation below.

Cash Flows		2500	2500	2500	2500
Year	0	1	2	3	4
					FV?

Instead of a $10,000 initial investment, plan on investing $2,500 a year at the end of each year for four years. What will be the amount in the savings account after four years if 10% annual interest can be earned on the investment?

The calculations shown in Table 13-3 demonstrate how a stream of investments of $2,500 each year are integrated with the compound interest calculations. The savings account will grow to $11,602.50 at the end of the fourth year.

Table 13-3 is complicated, but simple annuity tables have been constructed to ease this burden. It is unnecessary to go into the more complicated mathematics necessary to calculate the future value annuity factors. The factors are presented in Table 13A-4 in the Appendix. These factors are used in the following expression:

Future value of an annuity = (Annuity amount during period) x
(Future value interest factor of annuity)

or   Future value of an annuity = (Annuity amount during period) x (FVIFA).

Table 13-3   Future Value of an Annuity.

Year	Principal at Beginning of Year	Interest Earned During Year	Deposit at End of Year	Total Principal at End of Year
1	$ 0	$ 0	$2,500	$2,500
2	$2,500	$250	$2,500	$5,250
3	$5,250	$525	$2,500	$8,275
4	$8,275	$827.50	$2,500	$11,602.50

Applying this expression to the data in Table 13-3 and using the four year factor for 10% from Table 13A-4, the equivalent future value of the annuity can be calculated as:

Future value of annuity = (Annual annuity amount) x FVIFA
$11,602.50 = $2,500 x 4.641.

This amount is identical to the future value laboriously calculated in Table 13-3. The factors in Table 13A-4 can be used for any ordinary annuity. That means that (1) the cash flow amounts must be equal each period, (2) the time periods must be equal (or the cash flows must be equally spaced), (3) the cash flows must arrive at the *end* of each time period, and (4) the first cash flow must occur one period from the present time.

A similar problem involves the concept of present value of an annuity: What would we pay today for the right to receive $2,500 a year for four years if the opportunity cost for the investment is 10%? The cash flow time line for this ordinary annuity is

Cash Flows		2500	2500	2500	2500
Year	0	1	2	3	4
					PV?

It is the same as the cash flow time line we used for determining the future value of an annuity. Now, however, the present rather than the future value is desired.

Table 13-4 indicates that the right to receive $2,500 at the end of each year for four years in the future is worth $7,922.50 now if our opportunity cost is 10%. The present value of each cash flow is determined and summed to find the total present value of the entire cash flow stream.

As before, tables are available to simplify the calculations. The following equation shows how to determine the present value of an annuity using the factors in Table 13A-2.

Present value of annuity = Annuity amount during period x Present value interest factor of annuity

or Present value of annuity = Annuity amount during period x PVIFA

where PVIFA is the present value annuity factor from Table 13A-2. This expression can be used for the data in Table 13-4:

Annual annuity amount x PVIFA = Present value of annuity
$2,500 x 3.17 = $7,925

which is only slightly different (because of rounding) from the result in Table 13-4.

Using these tables is much simpler than performing the calculations in Table 13-3 and 13-4. Nevertheless, it is always desirable and helpful in these analyses to sketch each cash flow on a timeline to make sure it is appropriately included in the analysis. Note that the tables in the appendix assume a one period (a year for our example) lag between the current time point (year 0) and the inception of any cash flows. Any cash flows that occur immediately can be added to the annuity once the value is calculated but they must be assigned a present value factor of 1.0.

Net Present Value Method. The net present value approach to evaluating capital investment decisions compares the discounted net cash flows of the investment over its economic life with the initial cash outflows required to purchase the investment. As is discussed in more detail below, since the funds used to make an investment could be used in alternative ways, the net cash flows that arrive over time are discounted by the opportunity cost of the firm's capital. The difference between the initial outflows and the discounted net cash flows is the **net present value (NPV)** of the investment. This amount can be either negative or positive.

An example of the determination of an investment's net present value using the data from Table 13-1 is shown in Table 13-5. As can be seen from that table, the net cash flows in each year are discounted by the PVIF for the year. For simplicity, the net cash flows are assumed to arrive at the end of the year with the exception of the initial investment, which is a cash outflow occurring immediately. This investment has a net present value of $32,061.

A positive net present value indicates that the investment returns a higher rate than the discount rate used for the analysis. A negative net present value indicates the opposite, that

Table 13-4   Present Value of an Annuity.

Year	Cash Flow Arriving at End of Year	PVIF	Present Value
1	$2,500	.909	$2,272.50
2	$2,500	.826	$2,065.00
3	$2,500	.751	$1,877.50
4	$2,500	.683	$1,707.50
		Total Present Value	$7,922.50

Table 13-5   Net Present Value (NPV) Example.

Year	Net Cash Flows*	PVIF	Present Value
0 (today)	($75,000)	1.0	($75,000)
1	$27,000	.909	$24,543
2	$30,000	.826	$24,780
3	$30,000	.751	$22,530
4	$27,000	.683	$18,441
5	$27,000	.621	$16,767
		Net Present Value	$32,061

* From Table 13-1.

the rate used in the computation is greater than the return received on the investment. A net present value of zero indicates that the investment return is equal to the discount rate used in the analysis. If the NPV of the investment equals or exceeds zero, the investment is desirable from a financial perspective.

The NPV method is conceptually the strongest method of all the methods presented in this chapter. It compares the cash flows generated by a project with the opportunity costs of the funds needed to fund it. A positive NPV shows that the project satisfies the opportunity costs of the firm's capital. In addition, a positive NPV adds value to the firm. All investments that add value to the firm should be adopted as long as they are consistent with the firm's mission and goals and the firm has sufficient capital. However, since it is difficult to find investments that do exceed their opportunity costs in well-functioning markets, the analyst must always be prepared to show *specifically* what allows the firm to add value from these investments.

The Opportunity Cost of Capital. The **weighted average cost of capital** is used as the discount rate in NPV analyses to reflect the opportunity cost of capital in NPV analyses. To determine the firm's weighted average cost of capital, several pieces of information are required. First, the sources of long-term capital, all of which have a cost, must be identified. Second, the cost, stated as a rate, of each source should be determined. Finally, the proportion of each source in the firm's target capital structure is required.

In Table 13-6, the sources of capital financing generally available to not-for-profit and for-profit firms are summarized. It is important to stress that every source of capital funds has some cost. Debt has a recognized cost in the form of interest payments. Other sources of capital such as common stock, retained earnings, donations, and grants have a cost because of the availability of alternative uses for the funds by investors, the community or the firm. Also, there are costs involved in applying for grants and holding fund drives. Several methods can

Table 13-6   Sources of Capital Available to Health Care Firms by Ownership Status.

Source of Capital	Not-for-Profit	For-Profit	Government
Debt			
Bank Loans	Yes	Yes	Yes
Taxable Bonds	Yes	Yes	No
Tax-Exempt Revenue Bonds	Yes	No	Yes
Tax-Exempt General Obligation Bonds	No	No	Yes
Equity			
Retained Earnings	Yes	Yes	Yes
Common Stock	No	Yes	No
Philanthropy	Yes	No	Yes
Grants	Yes	No	Yes

be used to measure capital costs. This chapter suggests some, but financial managers are encouraged to explore other alternatives.

First, a health care firm must estimate the current market interest rate for its debt. This rate can usually be determined from available information. Since the firm is interested in current opportunity costs, it should not use interest rates charged when any debt it has outstanding was issued. Rather, it should seek estimates of the market interest rate it would currently be charged on debt. If its bonds are publicly traded, current yields can be used to estimate the current opportunity cost of debt capital. Or, the cost can be estimated from current rates for bonds with the same Standard and Poors or Moodys rating as the firm's bonds. However, interest rates are sensitive to risk. One source of risk is the amount of debt the organization has. If the firm plans to increase its debt, thereby increasing the risk to its debt holders, expected interest rates should be adjusted upward.

The cost of debt for firms that are subject to income taxation is actually lower than the market interest rate. Because interest expenses are deducted before obtaining the income on which taxes are calculated, the firm's debt interest expenses lower taxes. Therefore, the cost of debt to the firm is lowered. The cost of debt to the taxable firm is determined with

$$i\,(1\text{-}T)$$

where i is the interest rate and T is the marginal combined state and federal income tax rate.

This adjustment is not made by tax-exempt firms. However, a tax-exempt firm will pay a lower interest rate on its debt than a comparably risky taxable firm because the interest income received by bondholders of tax-exempt firms is not taxable for investors. Further discussion of tax-exempt interest rates can be found in more advanced finance textbooks.

After estimating the cost of debt, a health care provider must estimate the opportunity cost of its equity. Since equity is a residual claim on the assets of the firm, after debt is paid, it is riskier than debt for suppliers of capital to the firm (investors). Thus, capital suppliers will require higher market return rates for equity than for debt.

For firms with publicly traded equity (stock), current return rates required by investors in equity markets are readily available. They are published in several sources and are available from financial analysts and brokers.

Determining the cost of equity for not-for-profit firms is more problematic since they are not publicly traded. The theory of business finance suggests that the institution must search out the "next best alternative" to determine the cost of capital for equity balances. One approach is to assign a cost to the net assets based on what could be earned through investing the funds in capital markets. One possible investment would be in risk free government bonds as an alternative investment for the firm's funds. This return would serve as the minimum return possible at the minimum level of risk. A better alternative would be to use the return available on a broad portfolio of stocks such as the return on the Standard and Poors 500. This is based upon the theory that the community invests in not-for-profit tax-exempt firms. The community's alternative investment would be in a well-diversified market portfolio of stocks. A second approach is to find a similar firm whose stock is publicly traded and to use its market return rate. The sensitivity of the decision to the estimate chosen should be evaluated by using different estimates to see if the decision would differ with a different estimate.

Next, weights are assigned to each type of capital based upon the proportion of each source of the firm's total capital. Unless any major changes in capital structure are anticipated, the firm's current capital structure is used. Financial analysts and scholars have developed and used the concept of optimal financial structure to indicate the capital structure where the cost of obtaining capital is minimized. Further discussion of this topic is beyond the scope of this text but can be found in more advanced finance texts. Unfortunately, not much practical guidance in how to determine the optimal capital structure for a firm is available. Therefore, the firm's current capital structure, or planned capital structure, is used most often in determining the weighted average cost of capital.

Use of the current capital structure of the firm as a whole also isolates financing decisions from the decision to undertake the individual capital project. For example, it might be possible to borrow 90% of the funds needed for a specific project. However, the ability of a health care firm to borrow such a high percentage is typically due to the earning power of the assets already owned by the institution. Finding a lender who will furnish a high percentage of funds for a specific investment without some commitment of resources from the borrower and a proper earning/repayment record in the past is very difficult.

Table 13-7 presents a worksheet that can be used to compute the cost of capital for a taxable and for a tax-exempt firm. The worksheet assumes a 50/50 split between long term debt and equity sources of capital.

For the taxable firm, the market interest rate on its debt is assumed to be 10%. As discussed previously, the cost of the debt to the firm, however, is reduced because the interest expense is deducted before taxes are calculated. Thus, the cost of debt for this firm is only 6%. The return on equity is the market return required on its stock. When weighted by the proportions of debt and equity, the firm's weighted average cost of capital is 10%.

For the tax-exempt firm, a lower market interest rate on its debt is assumed because bondholders do not have to pay income taxes on the interest earned. Its cost of equity is derived from that of a firm with similar riskiness, the taxable firm in Table 13-7. When weighted by the proportions of debt and equity, the firm's weighted average cost of capital is 9.5%.

Internal Rate of Return. Managers may prefer to have a rate of return on the investment. The **internal rate of return (IRR)**, illustrated in Table 13-8, is a time adjusted rate of return. It is the discount rate at which the net present value is equal to zero.

The internal rate of return is the percentage yield or rate that results in the present values of all cash inflows exactly equaling the present value of all outflows. It is a measure of the rate of return when all cash flows are taken into account. Using the approximation method, one selects a rate of return and calculates the NPV of the investment. If the NPV is positive, the rate chosen is too low. If the NPV is negative, the rate chosen is too high. Based upon the initial calculation, another rate is chosen and the NPV is calculated. This process is followed until the absolute value of the positive or negative NPV is nearly zero.

Table 13-7   Cost of Capital Worksheet.

Taxable Firm

Capital Source	Weight Based Upon Market Values	Cost	Weighted Cost
Debt	.50	10%(1−.40)	3.0%
Equity	.50	14%	7.0%
	Weighted Average Cost		10.0%

Tax-Exempt Firm

Capital Source	Weight Based Upon Book Values	Cost	Weighted Cost
Debt	.50	5%	2.5%
Net Assets (from Retained Earnings, Donations, Grants)	.50	14%	7.0%
	Weighted Average Cost		9.5%

The internal rate of return is obtained either by approximation or by using a financial calculator or a computer to calculate the return rate. Since the instructions for using calculators and computers vary, we discuss only the approximation method.

In Table 13-8, the net cash flows from the example in Table 13-1 are discounted by the PVIF for 24% and 28% from Table 13A-1. As can be seen from the results in Part a, 24% is too low but 28% is too high. In Part b, the factors for 25% and 26%, calculated using a spread sheet program, are used to determine the NPV. Since the NPV with a 25% discount rate is positive, 25% is too low. However, 26% is still too high. Finally, in Part c, the present value factors for 25.5% and 25.7% are used for the discount rate. The NPV when 25.7% is the discount rate is very close to zero. Indeed, the results from a computer calculation show the actual IRR is found to be 25.69%. (Rounding in Part c resulted in a small positive rather than negative value for the 25.7% discount rate.)

The firm would select projects with an IRR above a predetermined rate, which is often called a "**hurdle rate**." Ideally, this rate should be tied to a cost of capital. For competing projects, the one with the highest IRR should be selected.

Although the IRR is a method that recognizes the time value of money, it is inferior to NPV for several reasons. First, when using the IRR method, the analyst implicitly assumes that the dollars from the project can be reinvested at the project's IRR. (Remember that discounting is the opposite of compounding.) The IRR derived, however, is often not available from market investments. In contrast, the reinvestment rate assumption for the NPV method is that funds can be reinvested at the firm's cost of capital.

Second, for some projects, several different IRRs can be calculated or none at all. One example of a capital investment for which no IRR can be calculated is one that has no net cash inflows, such as an investment in heating and cooling equipment. Thus, it would be impos-

Table 13-8   Internal Rate of Return Example.

Part a

Year	Net Cash Flows	PVIF(24%)	Present Value (24%)	PVIF(28%)	Value(28%)
0 (today)	($75,000)	1.0	($75,000)	1.0	($75,000)
1	$27,000	.807	$21,789	.781	$21,087
2	$30,000	.650	$19,500	.610	$18,300
3	$30,000	.525	$15,750	.477	$14,310
4	$27,000	.423	$11,421	.373	$10,071
5	$27,000	.341	$9,207	.291	$7,857
		NPV =	$2,667	NPV =	($3,375)

Part b

Year	Net Cash Flows	PVIF(25%)	Present Value (25%)	PVIF(26%)	Value(26%)
0 (today)	($75,000)	1.0	($75,000)	1.0	($75,000)
1	$27,000	.800	$21,600	.794	$21,438
2	$30,000	.640	$19,200	.630	$18,900
3	$30,000	.512	$15,360	.500	$15,000
4	$27,000	.410	$11,070	.397	$10,719
5	$27,000	.328	$8,856	.315	$8,505
		NPV =	$1,086	NPV =	($438)

Part c

Year	Net Cash Flows	PVIF(25.5%)	Present Value (25.5%)	PVIF(25.7%)	Value(25.7%)
0 (today)	($75,000)	1.0	($75,000)	1.0	($75,000)
1	$27,000	.797	$21,519	.796	$21,492
2	$30,000	.635	$19,050	.633	$18,990
3	$30,000	.506	$15,180	.503	$15,090
4	$27,000	.403	$10,881	.401	$10,827
5	$27,000	.321	$8,667	.319	$8,613
		NPV =	$297	NPV =	$12

sible to select between two alternatives for this equipment using their IRRs. In contrast, investments in which the net cash flows switch from positive to negative during the life of the project may have more than one IRR. For example, consider the following.

Time	Net Cash Flows	NPV (25%)	NPV(400%)
0	($16,000)	($16,000)	($16,000)
1	$100,000	$80,000	$ 20,000
2	($100,000)	($64,000)	($ 4,000)
		0	0

For this project, the IRR is both 25% and 400%.

Finally, the IRR and NPV methods may lead to different projects being selected. Consider the following simple example.

Initial Investment (Time 0)	Net Cash Flow at End of Year 1	IRR	NPV
($10,000)	$15,000	50%	$3636
($20,000)	$29,000	45%	**$6364**

If only one of these investment projects could be accepted, based upon the IRR, the first project would be the one accepted. However, the NPV of the second project is higher.

Summary

The capital investment process is a vital management function for the health care provider. Only by properly evaluating proposals and selecting those that meet the qualitative and quantitative objectives of the organization will the quality of health care provided to the community be maximized.

The quantitative evaluation techniques suggested in this chapter are easy to apply. Each has its strengths and weaknesses. However, the net present value (NPV) method is the most conceptually sound. When using any of the methods, it must be recognized that the projections of future financial variables are uncertain. Since obtaining more accurate data may cost more than the benefits received, the sensitivity of the capital investment decision to slight inaccuracies or to changes in the environment should always be evaluated.

Appendix 13A: Present and Future Value Tables

Table 13A-1 Present Value of $1.

Period	1%	2%	4%	6%	8%	10%	12%	14%	15%	18%	20%	24%	28%	32%
1	.990	.980	.962	.943	.926	.909	.893	.877	.870	.847	.833	.806	.781	.758
2	.980	.961	.925	.890	.857	.826	.797	.770	.756	.718	.694	.650	.610	.574
3	.971	.942	.889	.840	.794	.751	.712	.675	.658	.609	.579	.525	.477	.435
4	.961	.924	.855	.792	.735	.683	.636	.592	.572	.516	.482	.423	.373	.329
5	.952	.906	.822	.747	.681	.621	.567	.519	.497	.437	.402	.341	.291	.250
6	.942	.888	.790	.705	.630	.565	.507	.456	.432	.370	.335	.275	.227	.189
7	.933	.871	.760	.665	.584	.513	.452	.400	.376	.314	.279	.222	.178	.143
8	.924	.854	.731	.627	.540	.467	.404	.351	.327	.266	.233	.179	.139	.109
9	.914	.837	.703	.592	.500	.424	.361	.308	.284	.226	.194	.144	.108	.082
10	.905	.820	.676	.558	.463	.386	.322	.270	.247	.191	.162	.116	.085	.062
11	.896	.804	.650	.527	.429	.351	.288	.237	.215	.162	.135	.094	.066	.047
12	.887	.789	.625	.497	.397	.319	.257	.208	.187	.137	.112	.076	.052	.036
13	.879	.773	.601	.469	.368	.290	.229	.182	.163	.116	.094	.061	.040	.027
14	.870	.758	.578	.442	.341	.263	.205	.160	.141	.099	.078	.049	.032	.021
15	.861	.743	.555	.417	.315	.239	.183	.140	.123	.084	.065	.040	.025	.016
16	.853	.728	.534	.394	.292	.218	.163	.123	.107	.071	.054	.032	.019	.012
17	.844	.714	.513	.371	.270	.198	.146	.108	.093	.060	.045	.026	.015	.009
18	.836	.700	.494	.350	.250	.180	.130	.095	.081	.051	.038	.021	.012	.007
19	.828	.686	.475	.331	.232	.164	.116	.083	.070	.043	.031	.017	.009	.005
20	.820	.673	.456	.312	.215	.149	.104	.073	.061	.037	.026	.014	.007	.004
25	.780	.610	.375	.233	.146	.092	.059	.038	.030	.016	.011	.005	.002	.001
30	.742	.552	.308	.174	.099	.057	.033	.020	.015	.007	.004	.002	.001	.000
40	.672	.453	.208	.097	.046	.022	.011	.005	.004	.001	.001	.000		
50	.608	.372	.141	.054	.021	.009	.004	.001	.001	.000	.000			
60	.550	.305	.095	.030	.010	.003	.001	.000	.000					

Table 13A-2   Present Value of An Annuity of $1 Per Period for n Periods.

Number of Payments	1%	2%	4%	6%	8%	10%	12%	14%	15%	18%	20%	24%	28%	32%
1	.990	.980	.962	.943	.926	.909	.893	.877	.870	.847	.833	.807	.781	.758
2	1.970	1.942	1.886	1.833	1.783	1.736	1.690	1.647	1.626	1.566	1.528	1.457	1.392	1.332
3	2.941	2.884	2.775	2.673	2.577	2.487	2.402	2.322	2.283	2.174	2.107	1.981	1.868	1.766
4	3.902	3.808	3.630	3.465	3.312	3.170	3.037	2.914	2.855	2.690	2.589	2.404	2.241	2.096
5	4.853	4.714	4.452	4.212	3.993	3.791	3.605	3.433	3.352	3.127	2.991	2.745	2.532	2.345
6	5.796	5.601	5.242	4.917	4.623	4.355	4.111	3.889	3.785	3.498	3.326	3.021	2.759	2.534
7	6.728	6.472	6.002	5.582	5.206	4.868	4.564	4.288	4.160	3.812	3.605	3.242	2.937	2.678
8	7.652	7.326	6.733	6.210	5.747	5.335	4.968	4.639	4.487	4.078	3.837	3.421	3.076	2.786
9	8.566	8.162	7.435	6.802	6.247	5.759	5.328	4.946	4.772	4.303	4.031	3.566	3.184	2.868
10	9.471	8.983	8.111	7.360	6.710	6.145	5.650	5.216	5.019	4.494	4.193	3.682	3.269	2.930
11	10.368	9.787	8.761	7.887	7.139	6.495	5.938	5.453	5.234	4.656	4.327	3.776	3.335	2.978
12	11.255	10.575	9.385	8.384	7.536	6.814	6.194	5.660	5.421	4.793	4.439	3.851	3.387	3.013
13	12.134	11.348	9.986	8.853	7.904	7.103	6.424	5.842	5.583	4.910	4.533	3.912	3.427	3.040
14	13.004	12.106	10.563	9.295	8.244	7.367	6.628	6.002	5.725	5.008	4.611	3.962	3.459	3.061
15	13.865	12.849	11.118	9.712	8.560	7.606	6.811	6.142	5.847	5.092	4.676	4.001	3.483	3.076
16	14.718	13.578	11.652	10.106	8.851	7.824	6.974	6.265	5.954	5.162	4.730	4.033	3.503	3.088
17	15.562	14.292	12.166	10.477	9.122	8.022	7.120	6.373	6.047	5.222	4.775	4.059	3.518	3.097
18	16.398	14.992	12.659	10.828	9.372	8.201	7.250	6.467	6.128	5.273	4.812	4.080	3.529	3.104
19	17.226	15.679	13.134	11.158	9.604	8.365	7.366	6.550	6.198	5.316	4.844	4.097	3.539	3.109
20	18.046	16.351	13.590	11.470	9.818	8.514	7.469	6.623	6.259	5.353	4.870	4.110	3.546	3.113
25	22.023	19.524	15.622	12.783	10.675	9.077	7.843	6.873	6.464	5.467	4.948	4.147	3.564	3.122
30	25.808	22.397	17.292	13.765	11.258	9.427	8.055	7.003	6.566	5.517	4.979	4.160	3.569	3.124
40	32.835	27.356	19.793	15.046	11.925	9.779	8.244	7.105	6.642	5.548	4.997	4.166	3.571	3.125
50	39.196	31.424	21.482	15.762	12.234	9.915	8.305	7.133	6.661	5.554	5.000	4.167	3.571	3.125

Table 13A-3   Future Value of $1 at the End of n Periods.

Period	1%	2%	4%	6%	8%	10%	12%	14%	15%	18%	20%	24%	28%	32%
1	1.010	1.020	1.040	1.060	1.080	1.100	1.120	1.140	1.150	1.180	1.200	1.240	1.280	1.320
2	1.020	1.040	1.082	1.124	1.167	1.210	1.254	1.300	1.323	1.392	1.440	1.538	1.638	1.742
3	1.030	1.061	1.125	1.191	1.260	1.331	1.405	1.482	1.521	1.643	1.728	1.907	2.097	2.300
4	1.041	1.082	1.170	1.263	1.361	1.464	1.574	1.689	1.749	1.939	2.074	2.364	2.684	3.036
5	1.051	1.104	1.217	1.338	1.469	1.611	1.762	1.925	2.011	2.288	2.488	2.932	3.436	4.008
6	1.062	1.126	1.265	1.419	1.587	1.772	1.974	2.195	2.313	2.700	2.986	3.635	4.398	5.290
7	1.072	1.149	1.316	1.504	1.714	1.949	2.211	2.502	2.660	3.186	3.583	4.508	5.630	6.983
8	1.083	1.172	1.369	1.594	1.851	2.144	2.476	2.853	3.059	3.759	4.300	5.590	7.206	9.217
9	1.094	1.195	1.423	1.690	1.999	2.358	2.773	3.252	3.518	4.436	5.160	6.931	9.223	12.166
10	1.105	1.219	1.480	1.791	2.159	2.594	3.106	3.707	4.046	5.234	6.192	8.594	11.805	16.059
11	1.116	1.243	1.540	1.898	2.332	2.853	3.479	4.226	4.652	6.176	7.430	10.657	15.111	21.198
12	1.127	1.268	1.601	2.012	2.518	3.138	3.896	4.818	5.350	7.288	8.916	13.214	19.342	27.982
13	1.138	1.294	1.665	2.133	2.720	3.452	4.364	5.492	6.153	8.599	10.699	16.386	24.758	36.937
14	1.150	1.320	1.732	2.261	2.937	3.798	4.887	6.261	7.076	10.147	12.839	20.319	31.691	48.756
15	1.161	1.346	1.801	2.397	3.172	4.177	5.474	7.138	8.137	11.973	15.407	25.195	40.564	64.358
16	1.173	1.373	1.873	2.540	3.426	4.595	6.130	8.137	9.358	14.129	18.488	31.242	51.923	84.953
17	1.184	1.400	1.948	2.693	3.700	5.055	6.866	9.277	10.761	16.672	22.186	38.740	66.461	112.13
18	1.196	1.428	2.026	2.854	3.996	5.560	7.690	10.575	12.375	19.673	26.623	48.038	85.070	148.02
19	1.208	1.457	2.107	3.026	4.316	6.116	8.613	12.055	14.231	23.214	31.948	59.567	108.89	195.39
20	1.220	1.486	2.191	3.207	4.661	6.728	9.646	13.743	16.366	27.393	38.337	73.864	139.37	257.91
25	1.282	1.641	2.666	4.292	6.849	10.834	17.000	26.461	32.918	62.668	95.396	216.54	478.90	1033.5
30	1.348	1.812	3.243	5.744	10.062	17.449	29.960	50.950	66.211	143.37	237.37	634.81	1645.5	4142.0
40	1.489	2.208	4.801	10.285	21.724	45.259	93.050	188.88	267.86	750.37	1469.7	5455.9	19426	66520
50	1.645	2.692	7.107	18.420	46.901	117.39	289.00	700.23	1083.6	3927.3	9100.4	46890		

Table 13A-4   Sum of the Future Value of An Annuity of $1 Per Period for n Periods.

Number of Payments	1%	2%	4%	6%	8%	10%	12%	14%	15%	18%	20%	24%	28%	32%
1	1.000	1.000	1.000	1.000	1.000	1.000	1.000	1.000	1.000	1.000	1.000	1.000	1.000	1.000
2	2.010	2.020	2.040	2.060	2.080	2.100	2.120	2.140	2.150	2.180	2.200	2.240	2.280	2.320
3	3.030	3.060	3.122	3.184	3.246	3.310	3.374	3.440	3.473	3.572	3.640	3.778	3.918	4.062
4	4.060	4.122	4.247	4.375	4.506	4.641	4.779	4.921	4.993	5.215	5.368	5.684	6.016	6.362
5	5.101	5.204	5.416	5.637	5.867	6.105	6.353	6.610	6.742	7.154	7.442	8.048	8.700	9.398
6	6.152	6.308	6.633	6.975	7.336	7.716	8.115	8.536	8.754	9.422	9.930	10.980	12.135	13.405
7	7.214	7.434	7.898	8.394	8.923	9.487	10.089	10.730	11.066	12.141	12.915	14.615	16.533	18.695
8	8.286	8.583	9.214	9.898	10.636	11.435	12.299	13.232	13.726	15.327	16.499	19.122	22.163	25.678
9	9.369	9.755	10.582	11.491	12.487	13.579	14.775	16.085	16.785	19.085	20.798	24.712	29.369	34.895
10	10.462	10.949	12.006	13.180	14.486	15.937	17.548	19.337	20.303	23.521	25.958	31.643	38.592	47.061
11	11.566	12.168	13.486	14.971	16.645	18.531	20.654	23.044	24.349	28.755	32.150	40.237	50.398	63.121
12	12.682	13.412	15.025	16.869	18.977	21.384	24.133	27.270	29.001	34.931	39.580	50.894	65.510	84.320
13	13.809	14.680	16.626	18.882	21.495	24.522	28.029	32.088	34.351	42.218	48.496	64.109	84.852	112.30
14	14.947	15.973	18.291	21.015	24.214	27.975	32.392	37.581	40.504	50.818	59.195	80.496	109.61	149.23
15	16.096	17.293	20.023	23.276	27.152	31.772	37.279	43.842	47.580	60.965	72.035	100.81	141.30	197.99
16	17.257	18.639	21.824	25.672	30.324	35.949	42.753	50.980	55.717	72.939	87.442	126.01	181.86	262.35
17	18.430	20.012	23.697	28.212	33.750	40.544	48.883	59.117	65.075	87.068	105.93	157.25	233.79	347.30
18	19.614	21.412	25.645	30.905	37.450	45.599	55.749	68.394	75.836	103.74	128.11	195.99	300.25	459.44
19	20.810	22.840	27.671	33.760	41.446	51.159	63.439	78.969	88.211	123.41	154.74	244.03	385.32	607.47
20	22.019	24.297	29.778	36.785	45.762	57.275	72.052	91.024	102.44	146.62	186.69	303.60	494.21	802.86

Bibliography

Cooley, P.L. and P.F. Roden. *Business Financial Management*. Chicago: The Dryden Press, 1988.

Gapenski, L.C. *Understanding Health Care Financial Management*. Ann Arbor, MI.: AUPHA Press/Health Administration Press, 1991.

Gapenski, L.C. "Using MVA and EVA to Measure Financial Performance" *Healthcare Financial Management* (March): 56-60, 1996.

Kamath, R.R. and J. Elmer. "Capital Investment De-cisions in Hospitals: Survey Results" *Health Care Management Review* 14(2): 45-56, 1989.

Smith, L.J., J. Frazier and W.S. Crone. "Strategic Considerations for Capital Formation and Development" *Healthcare Financial Management* (March): 30-36, 1994.

Trahan, E.A. and L.J. Gitman. "Bridging the Theory-Practice Gap in Corporate Finance: A Survey of Chief Financial Officers" *The Quarterly Review of Economics and Finance* 35: 73-87, 1995.

Terms and Concepts

accounting rate of return
adjusted accounting rate of return
annuity
capital budgeting
capital investment
cash inflow
cash outflow
compounding
cost of capital
discounting

discount rate
economic life
future value
hurdle rate
internal rate of return
net present value
opportunity cost of funds
ordinary annuity
payback period
present value

Questions and Problems

13-1 Why is the capital investment decision making process important to the long run financial viability of a health care provider or payer?

13-2 Describe the three major phases in a formal capital budgeting system.

13-3 Why are organizational objectives important in the capital investment decision process?

13-4 What are the five major inputs to the capital investment evaluation process?

13-5 Explain the following:
   A. Accounting rate of return
   B. Payback method
   C. Time adjusted methods

13-6 What is compounding? discounting?

13-7 What does a positive $310 net present value for an investment proposal indicate?

13-8 Explain the cost of capital concept.

13-9 For the examples below, compute the following. Assume a 12% discount rate.
       1. Accounting rate of return
       2. Payback period
       3. Net present value
       4. Internal rate of return

(A) Not-for-Profit Hospital

Initial investment	$100,000
Cash inflows	20,000
Economic life	10 years
Depreciation	10 years straight line
Disposal or salvage value	0

(B) Community Health Clinic

Initial investment	$50,000
Salary reduction per year	15,000
Economic life	5 years
Depreciation	None
Disposal or salvage value	0

(C) Mental Health Clinic

Initial cash outflow	$200,000
Net increase in revenues per year	45,000
Yearly cash outflows	16,000
Economic life	8 years
Depreciation	8 years straight line
Disposal value	20,000

(D) For-Profit (Taxable) Nursing Home

Initial cash outflow	200,000
Cash outflow 3rd year	10,000
Cash inflows per year	50,000
Economic life	6 years
Depreciation	6 years straight line
Tax rate	30%
Disposal value	0

13-10 The Mountain View Family Practice Clinic is considering the purchase of a new blood analyzer which will cost $150,000. The new equipment is expected to be in service for six years before it becomes technologically obsolete, although the major third party payers will allow a five year life for depreciation. Third party cost based payers currently represent 75% of the clients seen at the clinic. Net cash savings after cash expenses is anticipated to be $25,000 per year. The clinic's board of trustees would like each capital investment to meet a minimum return of 10%. No additional working capital will be required for the investment, and the analyzer is not expected to have any salvage value at the end of six years.
   A.   Would you recommend that Mountain View purchase the equipment?
   B.   What is the internal rate of return for the investment?

13-11 The Wanover County Board of Commissioners received a request from the County Health Director to invest in a new automated patient information system. The new system is anticipated to save $45,000 in personnel operating costs each year for the next three years and will cost $110,000 to install. Operating and maintenance costs for the three years are estimated to be $5,000 per year. The money to buy the equipment would come from a trust fund paying 8%. Should the new system be purchased? Why?

13-12 The Modern Health Investors Corporation (MHI) board of directors is considering the following alternative financial structures for the investor owned firm:
   A. 20% debt
       80% equity

   B. 40% debt
       60% equity

   C. 60% debt
       40% equity

MHI could issue new debt with a 10% rate of interest. Stocks similar to MHI have return rates of 18%. The return on high grade commercial paper is currently 12%, but is expected to decline over the next few years as economic conditions improve. The marginal tax rate for the firm is 34%.

   A. Compute the cost of capital for the three alternatives.
   B. Which structure would you recommend to the directors, and why?

14 Sources of Financing: Debt and Equity

Health care organizations have ongoing needs for financing. As discussed in Chapter 11, one financing need is for working capital. In addition, firms need funds to replace equipment with similar or technologically more sophisticated equipment, renovate, develop new services, form integrated delivery systems, and so on. Even though some types of health care firms, such as acute care hospitals, may downsize, decreasing some financing needs, other activities require considerable funds. For example, as integrated delivery systems form, their needs for funds to finance sophisticated information systems, the purchase of physician practices, off-campus facilities and the like may extend into the millions of dollars.

Health care organizations are very much like other economic organizations; they finance their assets from a variety of sources. Recall the simplified version of the accounting equation:

$$\text{Assets} = \text{Liabilities} + \text{Equities} \; .$$

This equation can be reformulated as:

$$\text{Assets Acquired} = \text{How Assets Financed} \; .$$

The right side of the accounting equation shows how assets are financed and indicates the relative amounts of different types of financing.

The sources of financing for health care firms have changed dramatically during recent history, requiring managers to acquire new knowledge and skills. In the early part of the twentieth century, much of the long-term financing for health care firms came from government, philanthropy or physicians. Government provided funds for public health activities while donations from individuals and localities financed the capital needs of not-for-profit hospitals. Individual physicians frequently financed for-profit hospitals. Government financing of hospitals grew during the years of the Great Depression and World War II with the funding of public hospital construction. Government financing expanded to not-for-profit hospital construction projects during the mid-1940s to the mid-1970s with the Hill-Burton program. Since that time, although government payment for services provided has grown, government no longer plays much role in supplying funds for financing. **Philanthropic financing** has diminished as well and is nearly non-existent. Hospitals and, increasingly, other types of health care firms have come to rely upon investors in capital markets who invest in the debt and equity of health care firms.

In this chapter, we discuss debt and equity financing. More specifically, we describe the major characteristics of debt and equity, investors' requirements for supplying funds, and the choice between debt and equity financing.

Debt Financing

Debt financing is characterized by an obligation to repay **principal**, the amount borrowed, and interest on the principal according to a prearranged schedule. The **maturity** date of the debt is the end of the obligation. Prior to the maturity date, the firm may choose to refinance its debt. **Refinancing** either involves extending the maturity date, as with bank financing, or retiring existing debt and issuing new debt, as with bond financing.

Debt may be secured or unsecured. **Secured debt** is guaranteed by the pledge of assets or **collateral**. If the debtor defaults, the security or collateral is sold by the lender to repay the debt. **Unsecured debt** is not guaranteed by collateral.

Debt claims usually take priority over equity claims in any bankruptcy proceedings. When economic organizations undergo any form of fiscal crisis, the holders of debt usually dictate changes in management, new forms of financing restrictions and new limitations on asset management. Creditors are extremely important in cases of fiscal crisis, but assume a lower profile when operations are flowing smoothly.

Next, we examine short-term debt and long-term debt in a systematic progression through the right-hand side of the balance sheet, moving from current liabilities to long term forms of financing. There are numerous types of debt financing and more are being developed all the time. In this chapter, to establish a foundation, we focus on the most common types of debt.

Short-Term Debt

Short-term debt matures within one year. Therefore, it is a current liability of the firm. In general, short-term debt can be obtained more quickly than long-term debt and has lower upfront and interest costs. It is more flexible with respect to early repayment and restrictions on obtaining additional debt than long-term debt arrangements. For the firm, an important disadvantage of short-term debt is that short-term interest rates usually change more rapidly than long-term interest rates. Therefore, if the firm continually relies on short-term debt, it may find that its interest rates are difficult to predict.

Although some short-term debt carries an explicit interest rate, other short-term debt does not. Both types are described here. Since sales of accounts receivable is described in Chapter 12, it is not discussed in this section.

Short-Term Non-Interest-Bearing Liabilities. Some forms of short-term debt do not bear an explicit interest rate. One of the most common forms of such debt is **trade credit**, commonly found in the form of accounts payable on purchases of supplies for operating purposes. Many managers do not view accounts payable as credit because these accounts do not carry an explicit interest rate. However, this view is erroneous because of the opportunity cost of funds. A positive return such as interest from investing the money elsewhere can generally be earned by postponing payment of trade accounts until they are due. Failing to consider this opportunity can lead to misguided decisions such as paying bills immediately upon receipt. The rule of thumb is: Pay all forms of short-term credit on the date due unless there is an incentive for paying earlier. Of course, some forms of short-term credit may be postponed beyond the due date, but the costs of doing so may include revocation of credit and a deterioration of credit ratings. These implicit costs are usually higher than realized, until experienced, and then it is too late. The costs of postponing payment of short-term liabilities to employees (wages) may include faster employee turnover. The costs of postponing payment of taxes payable may include high penalties, jail terms, and closure of the institution.

The typical incentive for early payment of accounts payable is a discount. As noted in Chapter 12, this discount is stated in terms of the number of days during which the discount may be taken and the length of time that may be taken to pay the account in the event that no discount is taken. A typical discount may be stated as 2/10 net 30. This formula means that a 2% discount may be taken on payments made within ten days; otherwise the net balance is due in 30 days. If the invoice amount is $1,000, a discount of $20 may be taken for payment within ten days. In other words, the organization is paying $20 for the privilege of postponing payment from day ten to day 30. This implicit credit decision translates into an interest rate that is often much higher than originally conceived. The way to calculate the approximate cost of trade credit is:

$$\textbf{Approximate interest rate } = \frac{\text{Discount amount}}{\text{Net amount due}} = \frac{\$20}{\$980} = 2.04\%$$

However, this interest rate is not stated on an annual basis. To do so, it must be multiplied by the number of times during the year such transactions could occur. This involves translating the credit period (20 days) into an annual number of such occurrences as in:

$$\text{Number of credit periods} = \frac{\text{Days in year}}{\text{Net days} - \text{Discount period}} = \frac{365}{20} = 18.25 \text{ times per year}$$

The approximate interest rate is then multiplied by the number of times per year that such borrowings could occur to arrive at an annual percentage rate (APR), also called the annual interest rate.

APR (Annual interest rate) = Approximate interest rate x Number of credit periods.

These relationships can simply be expressed as:

$$\text{APR} = \frac{20}{980} \text{ x } \frac{365}{20} = 2.04\% \text{ x } 18.25 \text{ times per year} = 37.23\%$$

This APR formula approximates the **effective (true) interest** cost as long as the time periods are short (30 days or less) and the discounts are low (3% or lower). Beyond these thresholds, some distortion is introduced by using the APR; however, the distortion will probably not be significant enough to change the decision to take the discount or not.

It is important to convert any interest rate to an APR to make it easier to comprehend and to compare to the cost of alternative financing sources. Figure 14-1 illustrates the use of the approximate APR method for a variety of short-term financing alternatives, including the factoring of accounts receivable, which is discussed in Chapter 12.

The first two examples in Figure 14-1 show the cost of two different accounts payable terms. The third example in Figure 14-1 illustrates the APR associated with an account receivable that is sold to a factor as described in Chapter 12. In this example, the factor is willing to purchase a $1,000 account for $930, which is a 7% discount. Therefore, the approximate rate is 7%, but since this is only a 30-day account, the number of periods in a year is 12, and the actual APR is more than 90%. Similarly, the fifth example illustrates the significant multiplier effects of selling an investment to obtain cash. Specifically, a Treasury bill with ten days remaining until maturity is sold at a 12% discount. In this example, the number of periods or times per year is 36.5, and this multiplier significantly increases the approximate rate of 13.6% to almost 500%.

Figure 14-1   Approximate APRs of Several Short-Term Financing Options.

1. $1,000 purchase at 1/10 net 30

$$\text{Approximate APR} = \frac{10}{990} \times \frac{365}{20} = (1.01\%) \times (18.25) = 18.43\%$$

2. $1,000 purchase at 2/10 net 60

$$\text{Approximate APR} = \frac{20}{980} \times \frac{365}{50} = (2.04\%) \times (7.3) = 14.9\%$$

3. Factor a $1,000 account receivable at 7%, assuming that payment would have been expected in 30 days.

$$\text{Approximate APR} = \frac{70}{930} \times \frac{365}{30} = (7.53\%) \times (12.17) = 91.6\%$$

4. Take out a bank loan of $1,000 for 30 days at 8% annual interest.

$$\text{Approximate APR} = \frac{6.67}{1000} \times \frac{365}{30} = (.667\%) \times (12.17) = 8.12\%$$

5. Sell a T-Bill with a face value of $1,000 maturing in 10 days for $880 immediately (a 12% discount).

$$\text{Approximate APR} = \frac{120}{880} \times \frac{365}{10} = (13.63\%) \times (36.5) = 497.73\%$$

These examples illustrate that non-interest-bearing short-term debt really has a cost; it just is not stated explicitly. This cost must be compared with the cost of alternative financing sources, some of which are illustrated in Figure 14-1.

Short-Term Interest-Bearing Liabilities. Among the types of short-term interest bearing liabilities are bank loans, lines of credit, revolving credit, and commercial paper, which was described in Chapter 12. The latter may only be available to large health care organizations. Local banks are the primary source of the other types of short-term credit for many health care organizations.

The specific characteristics and terms for each type of financing must be determined upon borrowing. The analytical procedures for evaluating short-term interest-bearing liabilities do not differ significantly from those for non-interest-bearing short-term loans. However, the rates are often obtained directly from debt service tables used by the bank or from present value calculations described elsewhere in this book. Therefore, we will not further describe the calculations necessary to establish an interest rate. These rates are often quoted on an annual basis as part of the loan proposal, and no separate calculations are needed.

Intermediate-Term Liabilities

Liabilities that mature within an interval of one to ten years are usually considered intermediate-term loans. However, the distinction between intermediate- and long-term debt is vague. Intermediate-term debt has historically been used for operating purposes or for other short-term projects. Generally, intermediate-term loans require systematic repayments. They are usually collateralized, although they may be unsecured. Bank loans usually have shorter maturities, and bankers may accept personal property (equipment, stocks, or other financial instruments) as collateral.

Insurance companies and pension funds provide much of the five to ten year debt financing; they usually require real property as collateral. Intermediate-term debt is often at variable interest rates pegged to the prime or the federal discount rate. Smaller loans usually carry proportionately higher rates to cover the fixed costs of evaluating the loan application and monitoring the loan repayment provisions. The terms associated with intermediate-term debt are often more flexible and more tailored to the debtor's needs than with long-term debt. They are also generally available more quickly, and the up-front costs associated with the loan application are lower. When intermediate-term loans are used to finance construction projects, closing costs and loan insurance costs are often similar to those for long-term debt.

Another major form of intermediate-term financing for equipment is the **capital lease**. Capital leases contain provisions that make them similar to debt financing. The firm that leases the equipment (the **lessee**) makes payment equal to the full price of the leased equipment plus a return on investment, has no service agreement and cannot cancel the lease. In essence, the lessee has all of the benefits and risks associated with owning the leased property. As a result, the leased property must be shown as an asset on the balance sheet and a corresponding liability must be recorded. A capital lease contrasts with an **operating lease** in which the contract length is for less than the life of the equipment, covers service and maintenance, and is cancelable.

Leasing is an expeditious way of obtaining the use of fixed assets. Leases can be negotiated quickly and there are almost no up-front costs. Leasing salespersons can often obtain almost instantaneous credit because the debt is secured by the equipment. However, leasing is a complex subject with important tax implications, most of which are beyond the scope of this text.

As for all long-term assets, evaluation of financing options occurs after the equipment acquisition has already been approved during the capital budgeting process. Only then can the lease financing option be compared to other financing alternatives with similar repayment terms. The incremental net cash flows must be determined for each financing option and compared on a present value basis. Such a comparison is illustrated in Table 14-1.

One option illustrated in Table 14-1 is buying the equipment for $100,000 and financing it with a loan having a 10% annual interest rate. For this loan, interest is paid annually and the principal is repaid at maturity. Alternatively, the firm could lease the equipment for $26,000 per year. In the example, a marginal combined federal and state tax rate of 40% is assumed. The net cash flows for debt financing include interest expenses and the tax savings generated by the tax deductibility of interest and depreciation. Naturally, a tax-exempt firm would not benefit from such tax savings. We assume no salvage value for this piece of equipment and that there are no reimbursement consequences for cash flows. At the end of the loan, the principal is repaid, generating a cash outflow. The cash flows for leasing include the additional expense for the lease payment and the tax savings resulting from its lowering of taxable income.

The net cash flows for both alternatives are discounted by the after tax cost of secured borrowing. In this case, the 10% rate on secured debt financing is decreased, as was explained in Chapter 12, to show the effect of the tax deductibility of the interest expense as follows

$$10\% \ (1 - \text{Marginal tax rate}) = 10\% \ (1 - .4) = 6\%.$$

After the present value of each financing option is determined, the two are compared to determine which is the least costly financing option for the firm. In the case illustrated in Table 14-1, the leasing option is more costly than financing with debt.

Long-Term Debt Financing

As with short-term debt, there are numerous specific types of long-term debt financing. A thorough discussion of the range of long-term debt financing options is beyond the scope of this text. Instead, in this section, we discuss the general characteristics of two common types of debt financing: mortgages and bonds.

A **mortgage** is a pledge or obligation with real property, usually real estate, as security. It is typically structured as an amortized loan in which the payment remains constant over the life of the loan. Part of the payment goes to pay principal and part pays interest on the outstanding principal. In the early part of the life of the loan, most of the payment is comprised of the interest portion. Over time, as the principal is reduced, more of the payment is comprised of the payment of principal and less of the interest expense.

Table 14-1   Evaluation of Borrowing Versus Lease Financing.

Cost of Buying and Borrowing

			Year			
	0	1	2	3	4	5
Purchase Price	($100,000)					
Loan Amount	$100,000					
Interest Expense (10% Interest Rate)		($10,000)	($10,000)	($10,000)	($10,000)	($10,000)
Interest Expense Tax Savings (40% Marginal Rate)		4,000	4,000	4,000	4,000	4,000
Depreciation Expense Tax Savings with Straight-Line Method (40% Marginal Rate)		8,000	8,000	8,000	8,000	8,000
Principal Repayment						(100,000)
Net Cash Flow		$2,000	$2,000	$2,000	$2,000	($98,000)
Present Value Interest Factors (1)		.9434	.8900	.8396	.7921	.7473
(Total) Present Value of Owning	($66,305)					

(1) The discount rate is the after-tax cost of borrowing with a secured loan. Thus, the discount rate in this case is 10% (1 − .4) = 6%.

Cost of Leasing

			Year			
	0	1	2	3	4	5
Lease Payment (1)	($26,000)	($26,000)	($26,000)	($26,000)	($26,000)	0
Lease Payment Tax Savings (40% Marginal Rate)	10,400	10,400	10,400	10,400	10,400	
Net Cash Flow	($15,600)	($15,600)	($15,600)	($15,600)	($15,600)	
Present Value Interest Factors (2)	1.0000	.9434	.8900	.8396	.7921	
(Total) Present Value of Leasing =	($69,656)					

(1) Lease payments are made at the beginning of the year, which is equivalent to being made at the end of the previous year.
(2) The discount rate is the after-tax cost of borrowing with a secured loan. Thus, the discount rate in this case is 10% (1 − .4) = 6%.

Cost Comparison

Net Advantage of Owning = ($66,305) − ($69,656) = $3,351

The discounted cash flow methods developed in Chapter 13 are used to determine the payment on such a loan. The payment for a $10,000 loan having a four year life with a 10% rate compounded annually is determined below. Since the amount is borrowed today, we equate the principal of $10,000 to the present value of the cash payments over four years with the following

Cash Flows $10,000 ? ? ? ?
Years 0 1 2 3 4

$$\$10,000 = PMT \times PVIFA_{10\%,4}$$

$$\$10,000 = PMT \times 3.170$$

$$PMT = \$3,154.57.$$

Table 14-2 also shows the amortization of the loan. Although the payments are equal each year, different amounts of interest and principal are paid with each.

The other major type of debt is bonds issued by the firm. A **bond** is a long-term promissory note issued by a firm. It obligates the firm, the borrower, to pay interest at specific times and to repay the principal at the maturity, or at the end of the life of the bond to investors who purchase the bonds. Thus, the purchasers of the bonds lend money to the firm in return for interest and principal payments. The firm divides the total amount of financing it needs into smaller parts, or individual bonds, with **face** or **par values** of $1,000, $10,000 or some other amount that is attractive to potential investors.

Table 14-2 Payment and Amortization Table for $10,000 Loan at 10% Annual Rate.

Annual Payment Calculation

$10,000 = PMT x PVIFA$_{10\%,4}$

$10,000 = PMT x 3.170

PMT = $3,154.57

Amortization Table

Year	Beginning Balance	Payment	Interest	Principal	Ending Balance
1	$10,000.00	$3,154.57	$1,000.00	$2,154.57	$7,845.43
2	7,845.43	$3,154.57	784.54	2,370.03	5,475.40
3	5,475.40	$3,154.57	547.54	2,607.03	2,868.37
4	2,868.37	$3,154.57	286.84	2,867.37 *	0.00

*Slight difference due to rounding.

A secured bond is backed by collateral. An unsecured bond, also called a **debenture**, is backed by the issuer but not by any specific collateral or pledge of assets. A **subordinated debenture** is a bond that is subordinated to bonds with a prior (senior) claim on assets. A subordinated debenture specifies the order of priority. It usually strengthens the claim and lessens the risks associated with senior debt and is issued when restrictive covenants prohibit issuance of additional debt with rights equal to those of debt instruments already issued. **Convertible bonds** allow the owner, the lender, to exchange them for other securities of the firm at some point in the future.

Bonds may also be **taxable** or **tax-exempt**. Investors in taxable bonds must pay income tax on the interest income from the bonds. Investors in tax-exempt bonds are exempt from federal income taxes on the interest income and may be exempt from state income taxes if they reside in the state in which the bonds were issued. Tax-exemption lowers the interest rate the firm must pay. This effect is discussed in greater detail later in this chapter. Only tax-exempt firms can issue tax-exempt bonds for a specific project and they must do so through an authority with the power to issue such bonds. Only projects with tax-exempt purposes can legally be financed with tax-exempt bonds. Because of the cost savings and lack of availability of many types of equity, tax-exempt debt is the largest source of capital for tax-exempt hospitals in the United States, comprising over 75% of the capital for new projects.

Unlike mortgages with their equal payments, bonds are not a form of amortized debt. Instead, interest payments are typically made every six months and the principal is repaid at maturity. Firms may issue **term bonds** or **serial bonds**. Term bonds have a single maturity date. Serial bonds mature at different times until the entire debt is paid off. Many not-for-profit hospitals issue serial rather than term bonds.

Interest rates on bonds may be **fixed** or **variable**. Fixed rates do not change with market conditions. Variable rates change as market interest rates change. For a fixed rate, the borrower's interest payment is based upon the **coupon rate**, which is the market rate of interest for the risk for the firm's bonds when they are issued. For a fixed rate bond, the interest expense for the six month period is calculated by dividing the annual interest rate by two and multiplying it by the face value of the bond. For example, the semi-annual interest expense for a $1,000 bond with a coupon rate of 8% is

$$\$1,000 \times (.08/2) = \$40.$$

The total interest expense for the borrowing firm is determined by applying this rate to the entire amount of principal outstanding. Unless the firm calls the bonds or refinances the bonds by paying them off and issuing new bonds, the interest expense remains the same over the life of the bond issue.

The interest rate and the timing of the payments are spelled out in the **indenture** agreement. The indenture is a legal document specifying the conditions of a bond issue. It is a contract between the seller, or issuer, and many buyers, or bondholders. The indenture also spells out the form of the bond, amount of the issue, restrictive covenants, and procedures that will be followed in case of default or early retirement.

Restrictive covenants are promises to perform certain acts and avoid others. Common restrictive covenants include maintaining a specified debt service coverage ratio, not issuing additional debt, maintaining property and equipment, and making payments to a sinking fund. A **sinking fund** is an accumulation of cash, usually held by a trustee, used to redeem bonds at their maturity. A **trustee** administers the indenture and enforces its various provisions. It is usually an entity such as the trust department of a major bank that acts as an agent for the holders (purchasers) of bonds. The trustee monitors the issuer to see that all of the indenture's provisions are followed and initiates default or redemption proceedings when appropriate.

Also included in the indenture are provisions outlining when and how the firm can call its bonds, which means the redemption of bonds before their maturity date. A **call provision** indicates when and for what price the bonds can be redeemed before maturity. Usually a premium over and above the bond's face (par) value is required for a firm to call its bonds. The call premium usually decreases over the life of the bond.

Even when the bonds are not called, long-term debt can be retired before maturity in order to issue a larger block of debt and simultaneously to eliminate certain restrictive covenants that limit the facility's flexibility. Debt refinancing may occur fairly regularly and routinely as part of the organization's changing response to competition, regulation, and managerial decision making.

The process of issuing bonds, whether it is an initial issue or a refinancing, is long and involves many participants. Prior to issuing bonds, the firm hires an investment banking firm. An investment banker has two functions. The first function is to act as an advisor to help structure the terms of the indenture and coordinate the efforts of the accountants, lawyers, rating agencies, and others involved in issuing long-term bonds.

The second function of an investment banker is to act as a sales broker. The sales function may be separated from the advising function in the interests of objectivity. Bonds can be sold to the public or privately placed. When bonds are **privately placed,** the terms of the bond are directly negotiated between the seller and a few buyers, who are usually large insurance companies, banks, and pension funds. When bonds are sold to the public, the investment banker either finds buyers for the bonds (**best efforts financing**) or buys them outright (**underwriting**) and resells them immediately to people who have already committed to their purchase. In some cases, a **syndicate**, which is a group of investment banks, jointly underwrites or brokers the bonds. Best-effort financings bear greater risks of low demand (unsold bonds) and higher interest rates than do bonds that are underwritten. In any event, the interest rate and the investment bankers' fees should be set as close to the issue date as possible.

The firm also typically contracts for a **feasibility study**, which is a long-range forecast of an issuer's ability to repay bonds. It is usually conducted by an accounting or other consulting firm that obtains estimates of the volume and scope of projected health care services, staffing plans, and relevant costs. All of these data are accumulated into a projection of cash flows that is then examined to determine the risks associated with principal and interest payments as stated in the indenture.

The investment banker works with the borrowing firm and other team members to compile an **official statement** or **prospectus,** the formal offering document. This statement discloses information that investors need to know to make an informed decision about whether to purchase the bonds. The **preliminary official statement** contains all of the information except the interest rate on the bonds. It is marked in red along the binding with a caution that the statement is preliminary and subject to revision. Because of the red lettering, it is often called a **red herring**.

The interest rate on the bonds is determined as close to the actual sale of the bonds as possible. A key participant in determining the interest rate is one of three large U.S. companies, Standard and Poor's, Moody's Investors Service, and Fitch's Investors Service, Inc., that examine the terms of a bond issue and the issuer's financial capabilities. They rate the bond issue on a graduated scale that represents an assessment of the quality of the issue and the risks of default. Note that the bond issue is rated and not the issuer. Rating agencies occasionally revise their ratings over the life of the bond as the issuer's financial status changes. Bonds with lower ratings have more risk, and consequently, the interest rate must be higher to compensate for the additional risk.

The interest rate that must be paid on the bonds, and, therefore, the firm's interest expense, is a direct function of the bond ratings when the bonds are issued. The higher the rating, the lower the cost. Bonds are rated according to risk groups as follows:

Description	S&P's	Moody's
Prime	AAA	Aaa
Excellent	AA & AA-	Aa
Good	A+, A, A-	A
Average	BBB+, BBB, BBB-	Baa
Non-investment grade	BB & below	Ba & below

After the bonds are rated, the current market interest rate associated with the rating is the interest rate that the firm pays. As we noted previously, a fixed interest rate determines the firm's interest expense for the life of the issue.

Frequently, a firm with a bond issue that is not expected to receive a favorable rating will choose not to be rated at all. In such cases, the market for bonds is restricted to private placement or to the general public as individual investors.

Health care firms can improve their bond ratings through **credit enhancement**. Credit enhancement is a means for transferring the risk of default to another firm. One means of transferring the default risk is with **bond insurance**. Firms can pay a premium upon issuance of bonds to an organization such as the American Municipal Bond Assurance Corporation (AMBAC) in return for a guarantee that the debt will be repaid. In essence, the default risk of the insurance firm and, therefore, its credit rating substitutes for the default risk of the issuing firm. However, insurers will not insure all bonds and the costs of the insurance must be weighed against the benefits. A second way to improve a credit rating is with a **letter of credit**, which is usually issued by a bank. It is a formal assurance that funds to repay the debt is provided by the bank. Again, the bank's credit rating substitutes for that of the issuing firm and a fee is required.

Cost of Debt

Since outside investors supply debt capital to the firm, any discussion of the **cost of debt** must start with investors' requirements for returns. The market interest rate is the rate of return earned by the investors for the loss of the use of their funds while the funds are invested in the debt of the firm.

There are three reasons why investors must be compensated for the loss of the use of their funds. First, since we assume individuals would prefer to consume goods and services today rather than in the future, interest rates reflect time preferences for consumption. Second, investors must be compensated for expected price inflation so that they do not lose purchasing power. Finally, because we assume that investors are risk averse, they must be compensated for bearing risk. Higher rates of return will be needed to convince them to invest in riskier investments. Adding the cost of these three factors results in a market interest rate for a particular debt arrangement.

A technical discussion of how market interest rates are determined is beyond the scope of this text. However, it is important to note that many factors enter into the market's assessment of the appropriate rate of compensation for a particular debt arrangement. The influence of the general economic climate, such as whether a recession is expected, and government policies, such as spending and taxation policies, on inflation and industry prospects are important to in setting interest rates in financial markets. Although health care financial managers need to be aware of such macroeconomic concerns, perhaps most important is the market's assessment of the default risk of her or his firm. Managers can do much to influence this assessment through sound management.

As discussed earlier in this chapter, bond ratings provide an important assessment of the default risk for a particular bond issue. Rating firms assess many factors in determining default risk. Among the factors are economic and demographic characteristics of a geographic service area, market and competition, and past and projected financial information. In addition, the assessment of management and governance are critical in determining bond ratings.

For a fixed interest rate bond issue, the initial rating determines the interest payment while the issue is outstanding even though rating firms may upgrade or downgrade the issue during its life. Although rating changes do not change the interest payments, for a fixed rate bond, such changes do signal the firm that its cost of debt in the future may be different than it was in the past.

Interest rates on a debt issue are also influenced by specific characteristics of the debt instrument. Characteristics such as conversion and call provisions can influence the interest rate. Of particular concern for many health care firms is whether the issue is taxable or tax-exempt. Interest rates on tax-exempt bonds are lower than on taxable bonds because investors are exempt from federal, and frequently, state and local, income taxes on the interest income. The interest rate on a tax-exempt bond that is equivalent to the interest rate on a taxable bond with the same risk can be determined with the following

$$\text{i (tax} - \text{exempt)} = \text{i (taxable)} \times (1 - T_p)$$

where i (tax-exempt) is the market interest rate for tax-exempt debt, i (taxable) is the market interest rate for taxable debt, and Tp is the marginal personal tax rate of investors. Thus, the equivalent tax-exempt rate for a 10% taxable rate where the marginal personal tax rate is 28% is

$$i \text{ (tax} - \text{exempt)} = 10\% \, (1 - .28) = 7.2\%.$$

As can be seen from the general equation and the example, tax-exempt bonds result in lower interest expenses for the firms that issue them. Thus, firms that qualify to issue tax-exempt debt can benefit from lower interest expenses.

However, tax-exempt firms are not the only firms than benefit from tax regulations. Taxable firms also receive a tax benefit that lowers the cost of their debt. Their benefit comes in the form of the tax deductibility of interest expenses. As is also demonstrated in Chapter 13, the cost of debt to the taxable firm is

$$i \text{ (taxable) } x \, (1 - \text{Tc)}$$

where i (taxable) is the market interest rate and Tc is the combined federal and state marginal corporate income tax rate of the firm. If the market interest rate on the firm's debt is 15% and it has a marginal tax rate of 40%, its cost of debt is only 9%.

Equity Financing

Like long-term debt, **equity** is a long term source of capital. It represents the residual ownership interest in the firm. As such, it appears as the last item on the right hand side of the balance sheet. Recall the simplified version of the accounting equation:

$$\text{Assets} = \text{Liabilities} + \text{Equities}$$

which is equivalent to

$$\text{Assets} - \text{Liabilities} = \text{Equities.}$$

Thus, if assets can be sold at book value, the equity value indicates the amount that owners would receive on liquidation of the assets. However, it is rare that all assets can be sold at book value and even rarer that equity ownership in a bankrupt organization yields anything to the equity owners.

In an investor owned organization, equity is derived from capital contributions, the sale of stock and retained earnings. Capital contributions from owners are a source of equity for many private for-profit firms such as partnerships.

Publicly traded firms may issue **preferred stock** or **common stock** along with other hybrid varieties that are not discussed here. Preferred stock is an equity instrument that usually has a senior claim to other equity securities. Preferred stock usually carries a fixed **dividend**, which is a distribution of earnings to shareholders, but no maturity date.

Common stock represents the residual ownership interest of an investor owned health care firm. When a firm first issues stock, it is called an **initial public offering (IPO)**. After the initial public offering, the firm may issue more stock periodically as needed. Each new issue of stock, whether an IPO or a later offering, is sold in the **primary market**. Proceeds from the sale of securities in the primary market go to the issuing firm. When shares of stock are resold, they are said to be sold in the **secondary market**. Proceeds of these sales accrue to the selling investors and dealers, not to the firm.

Common stock is purchased by many private investors, institutional funds, and other investors seeking a combination of annual dividends and an increase in the value of their stock. The appreciation in a stock's traded value is one of the prime differentiating factors, from the investors' viewpoint, between common stock and debt. High stock prices may also benefit managers who have been rewarded for past performance with stocks or stock options; their personal investment portfolio may then be more valuable.

Retained earnings refers to net income that is retained by the firm after distribution of dividends. On the balance sheet, the earnings retained each year are added to the accumulated retained earnings from all previous years. Thus,

Beginning Retained Earnings
+ Net Income
<u>−   Dividends</u>
Ending Retained Earnings

It is important to understand that the equity value recorded on the firm's financial statements may differ significantly from its market value under normal operating conditions. A simple presentation of owners' equity for a publicly traded firm on its balance sheet appears as follows:

Owners' Equity
Common Stock	$100
Retained Earnings	<u>$200</u>
Total	$300

The value of the common stock on the balance sheet is determined by multiplying the price per share of the stock when issued by the number of shares issued. That value does not change even as the market price per share changes. As more stock is issued, the proceeds at its initial sale are added to the previous balance. Similarly, the balance of retained earnings is the sum of the earnings retained annually by the firm. In contrast, the market value of the firm is the current price per share of stock multiplied by the number of shares outstanding. This market value is not shown on the firm's balance sheet.

There are three major types of equity capital available to not-for-profit health care organizations: philanthropic sources, government grants, and retained earnings. Both individuals and foundations can provide significant philanthropy for health care institutions. Although philanthropy was important in initiating many health care firms in the past, philanthropy is currently a minor source of equity capital for most health care firms. As with philanthropy, although government grants provided significant funding for health care firms in the past, they are now a much less important source of equity.

As a result, most not-for-profit health care firms rely primarily upon retained earnings for equity capital. As with for-profit firms, earnings retained by the firm are summed over its life and shown on the balance sheet. Unlike for-profit firms, since not-for-profit firms do not pay dividends, the income is retained in its entirety.

The discussion so far has assumed that the health care firm is either investor owned (for-profit) or not-for-profit. In reality, there are currently many interesting combinations of for-profit and not-for-profit health care firms. Some not-for-profits have for-profit subsidiaries. Others may joint venture or align with for-profit firms. Still other not-for-profit firms have recently converted to for-profit status. Consequently, a single health care firm may have a variety of types of equity financing.

Equity investments are also made in governmental health care firms; they are made through taxes paid by citizens of the governmental entity. This direct taxing power of the jurisdiction represents a significant source of capital. Capital formation in government hospitals does not necessarily rely on the same expectation of future cash flows and retained earnings that attends capital formation in other sectors. As long as it is politically feasible, the taxing power generates the cash flow.

Cost of Equity

As with debt, since outsiders provide equity capital to the firm, any discussion of the **cost of equity** must begin with a consideration of their requirements for returns on their invested funds. To simplify, we begin with the case of an investor owned firm that issues publicly traded stock.

The returns to an investor on the common stock of this type of firm are composed of dividends and changes in the price of the shares of stock owned. In order to attract equity financing, as with debt, the investor must be compensated for the loss of the use of the funds during the time of investment. He or she must be compensated for loss of consumption ability, expected inflation, and risk. Financial economists have developed models to show that investors require higher returns with higher levels of risk. More specifically, they are compensated for the risk of the stock measured by how its returns vary with the overall market's returns. For further description of these models, the reader is referred to the references listed at the end of the chapter.

It should be noted that the risk of equity capital is higher than that of debt capital to investors. Equity capital suppliers are residual claimants whose returns in the form of dividends and share price appreciation are uncertain. In contrast, debt capital suppliers are promised specific returns in the form of interest and the return of their original principal. Therefore, the cost of equity financing to the firm is higher than debt financing. However, as is described later in this chapter, this does not mean the firm should use all debt financing.

Some managers of not-for-profit health care firms act as if there is no required return on the equity capital investment in not-for-profit firms. This misconception fails to account for the opportunity costs to society of investing in health care organizations. The equity interests in a not-for-profit organization are held on behalf of the community. The board of trustees manages these equity interests on behalf of all constituencies that might be viewed as financial stakeholders in the equity including employees, patients, potential patients, donors, potential donors, governing boards, governmental units, regulators, and third-party payers.

Health care financial managers should be aware that communities could invest their funds in alternative investments. If these alternative uses have a positive return, then the cost of equity capital is also positive. Therefore, as is discussed in Chapter 13, the manager can quantify the return required on the equity of not-for-profit firms with alternative investments in a broad portfolio of stocks or in a stock of a similar firm whose stock is publicly traded.

Capital Structure Decisions

Armed with an understanding of the basic characteristics and requirements of debt and equity capital suppliers, the manager is ready to tackle the difficult question of the appropriate amounts of each to use in financing the firm. **Financial leverage** refers to the proportion of long-term debt to equity for an organization. An organization is considered highly leveraged when it has a high proportion of long-term debt relative to equity sources of capital.

The **optimal capital structure** is the mix of long-term debt and equity that minimizes the firm's overall cost of capital, which is discussed in Chapter 13. Unfortunately, there is no simple formula to determine the optimal capital structure of a firm. Therefore, the advantages and disadvantages of debt financing must be carefully weighed.

One advantage of debt is that it is less costly than equity. Since debt has a higher claim on the firm's assets than equity and the interest and principal payments are spelled out in the indenture, it is less risky for the investor than equity. In contrast, equity holders are residual claimants. Dividend payments, share price appreciation, and even the return of the original investment are not promised. Recall, too, that for taxable firms, the tax deductibility of the interest expense further lowers the cost of debt to the firm.

Another advantage of debt financing is that the tax deductibility of interest expenses prior to determining taxable income increases the total cash available to debt and equity investors. This can be seen with a comparison of the total dollar returns to investors from the same firm when it uses little debt and when it uses more debt[1]. In Table 14-3, the returns generated from a capital structure debt/total assets of 10% is compared to those from a capital structure of 70% debt/total assets. The total cash available to debt and equity investors is the sum of the net income and interest expense. Because taxes require less cash when the interest expense is high, more is available for investors. The example in the table also demonstrates that the return on equity (net income/equity) is higher when more debt is in the firm's capital structure. Firms in higher marginal tax brackets benefit the most from this tax policy.

Table 14-3   The Effect of Capital Structure on Returns and Variability of Return on Equity.

Financing Mix

	Debt to Total Assets = 10%	Debt to Total Assets = 70%
Current Liabilities	$ 20,000	$ 20,000
Long-Term Debt	10,000	70,000
Equity	70,000	10,000
Total Liabilities and Equities	$100,000	$100,000

Income Statements for Three States of the Economy

State of the Economy	Debt to Total Assets = 10%			Debt to Total Assets = 70%		
	Good	Fair	Poor	Good	Fair	Poor
Revenues	$60,000	$50,000	$30,000	$60,000	$50,000	$30,000
Expenses Other than Interest	20,000	20,000	20,000	20,000	20,000	20,000
Interest Expense (@10%)	1,000	1,000	1,000	7,000	7,000	7,000
Earnings Before Taxes	39,000	29,000	9,000	33,000	23,000	3,000
Income Taxes (@34%)	13,260	9,860	3,060	11,220	7,820	1,020
Net Income	$25,740	$19,140	$5,940	$21,780	$15,180	$1,980

Returns to Investors

State of the Economy	Debt to Total Assets = 10%			Debt to Total Assets = 70%		
	Good	Fair	Poor	Good	Fair	Poor
Total Cash Available to Debt and Equity Investors	$26,740	$20,140	$6,940	$28,780	$22,180	$8,980
Return on Equity (ROE)	36.77%	27.34%	8.49%	217.80%	151.80%	19.80%
Standard Deviation of ROE		24.20%			129.80%	

Unfortunately, the increased return on equity with higher financial leverage is achieved at the cost of higher risk. The standard deviation of return on equity, a measure of variability, is higher when there is more debt. Eventually, as debt becomes a greater portion of the capital structure, debt capital suppliers require a higher interest rate in compensation for the higher risk they bear, driving the cost of debt up. Similarly, because it is a residual claim, the risk and cost of equity increase in this situation as well. One strategy managers can use to counteract the increase in risk associated with an increase in debt financing is to use assets as security.

As can be seen from this brief discussion, the firm should use a mix of debt and equity financing. As the firm moves from no debt to some debt, the overall cost of capital decreases. However, beyond some point, a higher debt/total assets ratio increases both the cost of debt and of equity. The manager's task in determining the firm's optimal capital structure is to determine the point at which the cost of capital is minimized. It is not a simple decision, but it is one that merits careful consideration.

Summary

Many health care firms have come to rely upon investors in capital markets who invest in the debt and equity of health care firms. In this chapter, we described the major characteristics of debt and equity, investors' requirements for supplying funds, and the choice between debt and equity financing.

Notes

1. Gapenski, L.C. *Healthcare Finance for the Non-Financial Manager.* Chicago: Probus Publishing Co., 1994.

Bibliography

Barkley, R. *Capital Survey of Emerging Organizations.* Englewood, CO: Medical Group Management Association, 1995.

Blake, J.W. "Financing Medical Office Buildings" *Journal of Health Care Finance* 22 (1): 43-48, 1995.

Brigham, E.F. and L.C. Gapenski. *Financial Management.* Chicago: The Dryden Press, 1991.

Brown, J.B. *Health Capital Financing.* Ann Arbor, MI: Health Administration Press, 1988.

Cerne, F. "Capital Decisions—Where is the Smart Money Being Invested?" *Hospitals & Health Networks* (June 5): 33-42, 1995.

Gapenski, L.C. *Healthcare Finance for the Non-Financial Manager.* Chicago: Probus Publishing Co., 1994.

Kelly, V.K. "Banks as a Source of Capital" *Topics in Health Care Financing* 19 (4): 21-34, 1993.

Lutz, S. "Doc Companies Dominate Top IPOs" *Modern Healthcare* (January 22): 42-44, 1996.

Mieling, T.M. and J.O. Keshner. "Accessing Capital for Integrated Delivery Systems" *Healthcare Financial Management* (January): 32-35, 1996.

Pierce, E. "Financing of Integrated Delivery Systems" *Topics in Health Care Financing* 20 (3): 28-36, 1994.

Smith, S.D. "The Use of Interest Rate Swaps in Hospital Capital Finance" *Journal of Health Care Finance* (Winter): 35-44, 1994.

Sterns, J.B., and T. K. Majidzadeh "A Framework for Evaluating Capital Structure" *Journal of Health Care Finance* (Winter): 80-85,1995.

Varwig, D. and R. Barkley. "Capital Financing Along the Integration Highway" *Journal of Health Care Finance* (Summer): 60-75, 1995.

Terms and Concepts

approximate (annual) interest rate
best efforts financing
bond
bond insurance
call provisions
capital lease
capital structure
collateral
common stock
convertible bonds
cost of debt
cost of equity
coupon rate
credit enhancement
debenture
debt
dividend
effective interest cost
equity
face value
feasibility study
financial leverage
fixed interest rate
indenture
initial public offering
lessee
letter or credit
maturity
mortgage

official statement
operating lease
optimal capital structure
par value
philanthropic financing
preferred stock
preliminary official statement
primary market
principal
private placement
prospectus
red herring
refinancing
restrictive covenants
retained earnings
secondary market
secured bond
serial debt
sinking fund
subordinated debenture
syndicate
taxable bonds
tax-exempt bonds
term bonds
trade credit
trustee
underwriting
unsecured debt
variable interest rate

Questions and Problems

14-1   What are equity claims? If a hospital went bankrupt and sold its assets for $10 million to retire bonds of $10 million, how much could equity owners claim?

14-2   Restate in your own terms the concept of equity in a not-for-profit organization.

14-3   What is trade credit and why is it considered a form of short-term debt?

14-4   What does 3/10 net 30 mean? How much of a discount would be granted on $10,000 under these terms? What would the approximate annual interest rate be?

14-5   What financial institutions are the primary source of short-term credit?

14-6   Calculate the effective interest rate of a $5,000 bank loan assumed at 15% and paid back in quarterly payments over a year. How does the effective interest rate change when only one payment is made at the end of a year?

14-7   What are restrictive covenants?

14-8   What is credit enhancement? What are two common forms?

14-9   Why is bond insurance helpful in reducing financing costs?

14-10 What is meant by financial leverage? If a health care firm is highly leveraged, how have its assets been financed?

14-11 Why is the cost of equity for not-for-profit firms not zero?

14-12 Explain the differences between preferred and common stock.

14-13 How does stock differ from debt in terms of the investor's return on investment?

14-14 What would happen to a bankrupt organization that sold its assets for $12 million but had bonds of $18 million?

14-15 Calculate the approximate APR of the following short-term financing options:
   A. $5,000 purchase at 1/10 net 30
   B. Sell a U.S. Treasury bill now for $8,200; it will mature in 6 months and be worth $10,000
   C. Take out a loan of $8,000 for 60 days at 16% annual interest
   D. Purchase $15,000 in supplies on account at 2/10 net 20.

14-16 What would the APR be in 6-15D if the $15,000 in supplies could be turned over only twice a year?

14-17 Calculate the effective interest rate on a $1,500 loan at 10% paid in six equal installments over one year.

14-18 A. Carfield Ambulatory Group is using short-term financing in several aspects of its operations. Determine the approximate APR actually involved in each situation.

1. Purchase of $50,000 value of equipment; total payments over one year total $62,000.
2. Short-term loan to meet payroll of $23,000, to be repaid in six months at 8% interest for the period.
3. Accounts receivable incur 2% per month interest starting 60 days after billing.
4. Sell a $15,000 T-bill maturing in 60 days for $12,500 at an 8% discount rate.
5. When would such approximate interest rates be adequate measures of annual interest?

B. What other considerations could affect the choice of options?

14-19 In these days of high competition in the automobile market, other industries are catching "low-interest-itis." Harrison Hospital is considering three bids for financing its purchase of the latest ultrasound equipment. Assume the equipment to be bought is the same for each bid.

A. $10,000/month for 16 months, no interest
B. $12,500/month for 12 months + 10% annual interest
C. $7,200/month for 18 months + 5% annual interest.

Which payment plan is preferable? Why?

Glossary of Financial Management Terms

The definitions used in this Glossary reflect current usage at the time of preparation of the text. They are intended to serve as a general guide only. Users should check with appropriate professionals when clarification is needed.

Absorption Costing. Absorption or full costing assigns costs, both fixed and variable, to units or services produced..

Accelerated Cost Recovery System (ACRS). Depreciation schedules that permit recovery of an asset's original cost over a period less than the asset's useful life.

Accelerated Depreciation. Any method of calculating depreciation expense which results in progressively smaller periodic charges. Examples are double-declining-balance and sum-of-the-years'-digits methods.

Account. Used for accumulating information regarding a single asset, liability, owners' equity item, revenue or expense.

Accounting. An information system conveying financial information about a specific entity. Or the process of identifying, measuring and communicating information to permit informed judgments and decisions by users of the information.

Accounting Conventions. Methods or procedures used in accounting.

Accounting Cycle. The sequence of accounting procedures starting with journal entries for various transactions and events and ending with the post-closing trial balance. Its output is the financial statements.

Accounting Equation. Assets = Equities. Assets = Liabilities plus Owners' Equity.

Accounting Errors. Unintentional arithmetic errors and mis-applications of accounting principles in previously published financial statements which are corrected directly to retained earnings.

Accounting Event. Any occurrence that is recorded in the accounting records. It must be a) objectively measurable, and b) affect the financial position of the company.

Accounting Methods. Accounting principles or procedures for carrying out accounting principles.

Accounting Rate of Return. Average net income divided by investment.

Accounts Payable Payment Period. A turnover ratio indicating the length of the payment period which can identify potential problems before they become serious and result in poor vendor relationships. Calculated by dividing the number of days in the year (365) by the **accounts payable turnover** ratio.

Accounts Payable Turnover. A turnover ratio indicating the number of days' of supplies usage (or other category of costs) which can identify potential problems before they become serious and result in poor vendor relationships. Calculated by dividing the cost of supplies by the balance in accounts payable.

Accounting Period. The period of time covered by financial statements which measure cash flows, such as the income statement and the statements of changes in financial position.

Accounting Principles. A common set of concepts, standards and procedures used as a general guide for recording transactions or events reported in the financial statements. The term "Generally Accepted Accounting Principles", often called GAAP, tends to be used when the method or procedure has been given official authoritative sanction by a group such as the APB, FASB, or SEC.

Accounting Rate of Return. Income for a period divided by average investment during the period. Based on accounting income, rather than discounted cash flows. A useful measure of managerial efficiency, as a control device (minimum rate to establish segmental efficiency), and a planning device (evaluating proposed purchases).

Accounts Payable. A liability representing an amount owed to a creditor, usually arising from purchase of medical supplies.

Accounts Receivable. A claim against a debtor usually arising from patient services rendered or products provided.

Accounts Receivable Turnover. Net sales on account for a period divided by the average balance of net accounts receivable. Useful in studying credit and collection policies.

Accrual. An expense or revenue that increases over time and which must be given recognition when financial statements are prepared. For example, the recognition of wages payable or interest receivable at the end of a period even though no actual cash transaction is made at that time.

Accrual Basis of Accounting. The method of recognizing revenues as services are delivered and as services are rendered, not when cash is received. Expenses are recognized in the period when the related revenue is recognized independent of the time when cash is paid out. Contrast with the cash basis of accounting.

Accrued. A revenue (expense) that has been earned (recognized) even though the related payment has not yet been received. This adjective should not be used as part of an account title. For example, Interest Receivable or Payable, not Accrued Interest Receivable/Payable, is the preferred account title.

Accrued Payable/Accrued Receivable. A payable or receivable resulting from the passage of time that has not been entered in the accounting records. For example, salaries and interest accrue as time passes. They are typically recognized in the accounting records when the books are closed.

Accumulated Depreciation. A preferred title for the contra-asset account that shows the amount of depreciation that has been expensed on an asset since it was acquired.

Acid Test Ratio. Sum of cash, marketable securities, and receivables divided by current liabilities. Some non-liquid receivables may be excluded from the numerator. Sometimes called the quick ratio.

Acquisition Cost. The net invoice price of an asset plus all expenditures to put the asset in place for its intended use. Other expenditures might include legal fees, transportation charges, and installation costs. Often called historical cost.

Activity-Based Depreciation. Production method of depreciation which focuses on units of output produced.

Activity-Based Costs (Activity Bases). New variation of a cost-based approach to pricing called "activity-based" costs, sometimes called ABC costing. Under ABC, cost "drivers" are identified, and then overhead costs are assigned based on many different cost drivers. ABC uses an expanded set of cost drivers, rather than the more typical limited set of activities on which to allocate overhead costs. ABC is more accurate because the overhead costs are traced more finely to the services that are provided to each patient.

Activity Ratios. Also called turnover ratios; designed to identify relationships between the income statement and balance sheet.

Actual Costs. Costs recognized under accrual accounting by a firm during a period.

Acute Care. The highest level of nursing care available to the patient in a hospital.

Additional Paid-In Capital. An alternative title for capital contributed in excess of par or stated value.

Adequate Disclosure. Fair presentation of financial statements requires disclosure of material items.

Adjunct Account. An account that accumulates additions to another account. For example, premium on bonds payable is an adjunct to the liability bonds payable. The actual liability is the sum of the two account balances at a given date.

Adjusted Acquisition (Historical) Cost. Cost adjusted for general or specific price level changes.

Adjusted Basis. The basis used to compute gain or loss on disposition of an asset for tax purposes.

Adjusted Cash Balance. The balance shown in the firm's account for cash in the bank plus or minus appropriate adjustments, such as for notes collected by the bank or bank service charges. The account balance is reconciled with the adjusted bank balance. The balance shown on the statement from the bank plus or minus appropriate adjustments, such as for outstanding checks or unrecorded deposits is the adjusted cash balance.

Adjusted Trial Balance. Trial balance taken after adjusting entries and before closing entries.

Adjusting Entry. An entry made at the end of an accounting period to record a transaction or other accounting event which for some reason has not been recorded or has been improperly recorded during the accounting period. Sometimes the term is used to refer to the process of restating financial statements for general price level changes.

Administrative Expense. An expense related to the enterprise as a whole, as contrasted to expenses related to more specific functions such as manufacturing or selling.

ADR. Asset Depreciation Range, a term used by the IRS to set the length of time eligible to depreciate an asset.

Advances from (by) Customers. A preferred term for the liability account representing receipts of cash in advance of delivering the goods or rendering the service. Sometimes called deferred revenue or deferred income.

Advances to Suppliers. A preferred term for disbursements of cash in advance of receiving assets or services.

Agent. One authorized to transact business for another.

Aging Schedule. A report showing the length of time that accounts receivable have been outstanding.

Aging Accounts Receivable. The process of classifying accounts receivable by the time elapsed since the claim came into existence for the purpose of estimating the amount of uncollectible accounts receivable as of a given date.

AICPA. American Institute of Certified Public Accounts, the national organization that represents CPAs. It sets accounting standards and oversees the writing and grading of the Uniform CPA Examination. Each state, however, sets its own requirements for becoming a CPA in that state. See **certified public accountant**.

All-Inclusive Concept. No distinction is drawn between operating and non-operating revenues and expenses and the only entries to retained earnings are for net income and dividends. Under this concept all income, gains, and losses are reported in the income statement. Events that could be reported as prior-period adjustments and/or corrections of errors are included in net income.

Allocate. To spread a cost from one account to several accounts, products, activities, or to several periods.

Allocation Basis or Allocation Base. Basis on which costs are allocated. Usually some measure of services or other resources; may use AHA recommended allocation bases. Whenever a cost allocation basis that will more realistically reflect costs or result in a more accurate cost allocation can be identified, then the new allocation base may be used to allocate costs.

Allocation Sequence. The allocation sequence determines which cost center costs are allocated first. Most standardized reporting forms suggest an order of allocation beginning with depreciation. This sequence is only a recommended one, based on the rule-of-thumb that the cost center that serves the most other cost centers should be allocated first. Other sequences may be more advantageous.

Allocation Statistics. Proportions indicating the services provided by one cost center to another. Used in conjunction with **allocation basis** in order to allocate costs from one cost center to another.

Allocation Strategies. Under cost-based reimbursement, managers must consider how their choices may significantly affect the results of any cost allocation. Also related to **Revenue Maximization.**

Allowable Costs. Those costs which are allowable under the principles of reimbursement in the Medicare and Medicaid Acts or contractual agreements with other payers, such as Blue Cross, Blue Shield, CHAMPUS, Workman's Compensation.

Allowance. The difference between gross revenue charges at established rates for services rendered and amounts received (or to be received) from patients or third-party payers. Allowances should be distinguished from uncollectible losses (bad debts). Types of allowances are: 1) Charity Allowances as the difference between charges and amounts received from indigent patients, voluntary agencies, or governmental units on behalf of specific indigent patients, 2) Courtesy Allowances or Policy Discounts as the difference between charges and amounts received form doctors, clergymen, employees, and employees' dependents and 3) Contractual Adjustments as the difference between charges and amounts received from third-party payers under contractual agreements.

Allowance for Doubtful Accounts. See Allowance for Uncollectible Accounts.

Allowance for Uncollectible Accounts. The estimated amount of accounts receivable that will not be collected. The actual write-off of specific accounts receivable does not affect revenue or expense in the period of the write-off. The revenue reduction is recognized at the time the allowance account is credited. The amount of this credit to the allowance account may be based on a percentage of sales on account, or

determined from an aging accounts receivable. This method enables an estimate to be shown of the amount of receivables that will be collected without identifying the specific uncollectible accounts.

Allowances Ratio. The **allowances ratio** is used to determine the effects of allowances deducted from gross patient revenue for charity care, courtesy allowances, and contractual discounts. This ratio is less important now that allowances and discounts are not shown on the income statement. Calculated by dividing the appropriate allowances by gross patient revenues.

Ambulatory. Able to walk and not confined to bed.

Ambulatory Care. Any type of medical care provided to a patient who is not hospitalized.

American Accounting Association (AAA). An organization primarily for academic accountants, but open to all interested in accounting. It seeks to influence the development of accounting theory by encouraging and sponsoring accounting research.

Amortization. The general process of allocating acquisition cost of assets to the periods of benefit as expenses. It is called depreciation for plant assets, depletion for wasting assets (natural resources), and amortization for intangibles.

Analysis of Changes In Cash. A part of the **cash flow statement** that explains the causes of the changes in cash during a period.

Ancillary Services. Services provided to patients by the various specialty departments of the hospital, such as radiology, laboratory, pharmacy, therapy, etc., as distinguished from routine inpatient services.

Anesthesiologist. A medical doctor with specialized training in the administration of anesthetics.

Annual Report. A report for stockholders and other interested parties prepared once a year. It includes a balance sheet, an income statement, a cash flow statement, a reconciliation of changes in owners' equity accounts, a summary of significant accounting principles used, other explanatory notes, the auditor's report, and comments from management about the year's events.

Annuity. A series of payments made at specified intervals.

Annuity Due. An annuity where the first payment is made at the start of period one (or at the end of period zero).

Annuity in Arrears. An ordinary annuity where the first payment occurs at the end of the first period.

Annuity Method of Depreciation. A compound interest method of computing depreciation.

APB. Accounting Principles Board of the AICPA that established accounting principles from 1959 through 1973, through the issuance of 31 APB Opinions. It was superseded by the **FASB**.

APB Opinion. The name given to pronouncements of the APB that make up much of generally accepted accounting principles.

Application of Funds. Transaction that reduces cash or working capital. Also called Use of Funds.

Applied Cost. A predetermined average cost that has been allocated to a service or activity. Can be based on actual costs or standard costs.

Applied Overhead. Overhead costs charged to services or departments at an appropriate rate.

Appraisal. The process of obtaining an amount for an asset or liability that involves expert opinion. It is not usually used under accrual accounting.

Appreciation. An increase in economic worth caused by rising market prices for an asset.

Appropriation. In governmental accounting, an expenditure authorized for a specific amount, purpose, and time.

Appropriation Account. In governmental accounting, an account set up to record specific authorizations to expend funds. It is credited and appropriated amounts at the start of the budget cycle, and debited with expenditures during the period and encumbrances outstanding at the end of the period.

ARB. Accounting Research Bulletins issued by the former Committee on Accounting Procedure of the AICPA between 1939 and 1959.

Arbitrage. The simultaneous purchase in one market and sale in another of a security or commodity in hope of making a profit on price differences in the different markets.

Arm's Length. A transaction negotiated by unrelated parties, each acting in his or her own self interest which forms the basis for fair market value determination.

Assess. To value property for the purpose of property taxation. The amount of the assessment is determined by the taxing authority.

Asset. A future benefit or service potential that is recognized in accounting only after a transaction has occurred. It may be tangible or intangible, short term (current) or long-term (noncurrent).

Asset Depreciation Range. (ADR). The range of depreciable lives allowed by the Internal Revenue Service for a specific depreciable asset.

Asset Turnover. Ratio of net sales to average assets. A measure of the effectiveness of the utilization of assets.

Asset Valuation. Under generally accepted accounting principles (GAAP) fixed assets are valued at their **historical cost**: the actual purchase price plus related costs necessary to put the assets into service. Accountants are very concerned about asset valuation because assets are transformed into expenses, which are a form of expired costs. Costs are recognized as assets are used. There is a causal link between assets, their valuation, and the costs and expenses that appear in income statements. Value can mean: (1) how much something means to us; (2) how much we could sell an item for; (3) the benefit we think we will receive as a result of owning an item; and (4) how much we paid for it. This ambiguity must be confronted whenever assets are valued on the balance sheet.

Attachment. Laying claim to the assets of a borrower or debtor by a lender or creditor when the borrower has failed to meet repayment obligations on time.

Attest. Rendering of an opinion by an auditor that the financial statements are fair.

Audit. Systematic inspection of accounting records involving analyses, tests, and confirmations. Accomplished in accordance with auditing standards.

Audit Committee. A committee of the board of directors of a corporation usually consisting of outside directors who nominate the independent auditors and discuss the auditors' work with them.

Auditing Standards. A set of ten standards promulgated by the AICPA for auditors including three general standards, three standards of field work, and four standards of reporting. These standards deal with the measures of the quality of the performance and the objectives to be attained, rather than with specific auditing procedures.

Auditor. One who checks the accuracy, fairness, and general acceptability of accounting records and statements.

Audit Program. The procedures followed by the auditor in carrying out the audit.

Auditor's Report. The auditor's statement of the work done and an opinion of the financial statements. Opinions are usually unqualified, but may be qualified, or the auditor may disclaim an opinion in the report. Often called the accountant's report or the auditors opinion.

Audit Trail. A reference accompanying an entry or posting to an underlying source record or document. An audit trail is essential for efficiently checking the accuracy of accounting entries.

Authoritarian Approach. Also called **top-down approach.** Method of budgeting in which there is little participation by most of the organization's staff.

Authorized Capital Stock. The number of shares of stock that can be issued by a corporation.

Average. The arithmetic mean of a set of numbers obtained by summing the items and dividing by the number of items. Could also be the weighted average or the geometric or harmonic mean.

Average Collection Period. A turnover ratio indicating the average time necessary to collect accounts receivable. Calculated by dividing the number of days in the period (365) by the accounts receivable turnover ratio.

Average Cost Flow Assumption. An inventory flow assumption where the cost of units is the weighted average cost of the beginning inventory and purchases.

Average Daily Operating Revenue. A turnover ratio indicating the amount of revenue earned on a daily basis. Calculated by dividing operating revenues by the number of days in the period (365).

Average Daily Patient Revenue. A turnover ratio indicating the amount of revenue earned on a daily basis. Calculated by dividing patient revenues by the number of days in the period (365).

Average Costs (or Average Service Costs). Most cost-based approaches are based on average costs where the full costs of the service are divided by the number of units of service provided. Any average cost is the result of dividing costs by a quantity of output or services.

Avoidable Cost. An incremental or variable cost. Sometimes called an out-of-pocket cost.

Bad Debt. An account which is written off when it is unpaid, although the patient may have the ability to pay. See also **uncollectible accounts.**

Bad Debt Ratio. A profitability ratio measuring the amount of patient service revenues that are lost to uncollected accounts receivable. Calculated by dividing bad debt expenses by net patient service revenue. Sometimes calculated by dividing bad debt expenses by either inpatient or outpatient revenues.

Bad Debt Recovery. Collection, perhaps partial, of a specific account receivable previously written off as uncollectible.

Bailout Period. The total time that must elapse before net accumulated cash inflows from a project, including potential salvage value of assets at various times, equal or exceed the accumulated cash outflows.

Balance. The difference between the sum of debit entries minus the sum of credit entries in an account. If positive, the difference is called a debit balance; if negative, a credit balance.

Balance Sheet. Statement of financial position which shows the assets, liabilities, and owner's equity of a firm.

Balance Sheet Account. An account that can appear on a balance sheet. Balance Sheet accounts are usually considered permanent accounts.

Balloon Payment. When a debt is not fully amortized, the balloon payment is the final payment and is larger than the preceding payments.

Bank Balance. The amount of the balance in a checking account shown on the bank statement.

Bank Reconciliation Schedule. A schedule that shows how the difference between the book balance of the cash in bank account and the bank statement can be explained.

Banker's Acceptance. Short-term security created when a buyer agrees to pay for imported goods. They buyer's banker promises to pay the seller for the goods, creating the acceptance.

Bankrupt. Said of a company whose liabilities exceed its assets where a legal petition has been filed and accepted under the bankruptcy law. A bankrupt firm is typically insolvent but does not have to be.

Bank Statement. A statement sent by the bank to a checking account customer showing deposits, checks cleared, and service charges for a period of time, usually at monthly intervals.

Basis. Acquisition cost, or some substitute thereof, of an asset used in computing gain or loss on disposition or retirement.

Bear. One who believes that security prices will fall. Contrast with **bull.**

Bearer Bond. The possessor of the bond is entitled to interest and principal.

Bed. A hospital bed is one regularly maintained in a hospital for the use of patients. The term "hospital bed" includes all bed facilities maintained for use of both inpatients and outpatients, excluding labor room and recovery room beds. Typical bed categories are:

An **outpatient** bed is one regularly maintained for use by outpatients in a patient center. An **inpatient** bed is one regularly maintained for use by inpatients who are lodged in the nursing service areas of the hospital. Inpatient beds are generally divided into categories which reflect the type of inpatient using the bed. **Adult beds** are those assigned for regular use by inpatients who are 14 years of age or over, and which are maintained in areas for adult or adolescent lodging. **Pediatric beds** are those assigned for regular use by patients other than newborns who have not reached the age of 14 years. **Newborn beds** are those assigned for regular use by infants newly born in the hospital. Bassinets maintained for the use of newborn infants should comprise the greatest number of these beds.

Beginning Inventory. Valuation of inventory on hand at the beginning of the accounting period.

Best Efforts Financing. Occurs when the investment banker finds purchasers for the firm's newly issued securities instead of buying the securities and then selling them.

Betterment. An improvement to a fixed asset.

Big Six. Denotes the six largest public accounting (CPA) firms in alphabetical order: Arthur Andersen & Co.; Coopers & Lybrand; Ernst & Young; Deloitte & Touche; Peat, Marwick, KPMG; and Price Waterhouse & Co.

Bill of Materials. A specification of the quantities of direct materials expected to be used to produce a given job or quantity of output.

Board-Designated Funds. Unrestricted funds set aside by the Governing Board for specific purposes or projects.

Board Designated Investment Funds. Unrestricted funds which, at the discretion of the Governing Board, have been designated for investment to produce income as if they were endowment funds.

Board of Directors. The governing body of a corporation elected by the stockholders.

Bond. A certificate to show evidence of debt. The par value is the principal or face amount of the bond payable at maturity. The coupon rate is the amount of interest payable in one year divided by the principal amount. Coupon bonds have coupons attached to them which can be redeemed at stated dates for interest payments. Normally bonds are issued in $1,000 units and carry semiannual coupons.

Bond Conversion. The act of exchanging convertible bonds for preferred or common stock. Also called bond refinancing or refunding.

Bond Discount. From the standpoint of the issuer of a bond at the issue date, the excess of the par value of a bond over its initial sales price. As a bond holder, the difference between par value and selling price when the bond sells below par.

Bond Indenture. The contract between an issuer of bonds and the bondholders.

Bond Insurance. Insurance purchased by firm's issuing bonds that guarantees debt payments will be made if the firm is unable to pay. In essence, the firm "purchases" the bond insurance firm's creditworthiness.

Bond Premium. Similar to bond discount except that the issue price is higher than par value.

Bond Redemption. Retirement of bonds.

Bond Refunding. The issue of new bonds and using the proceeds to retire an outstanding bond issue.

Bond Table. A table showing current price of a bond as a function of the coupon rate, years to maturity, and effective yield to maturity (or effective rate).

Bonus. An amount over the normal wage or salary, usually paid for meritorious performance.

Book. As a verb, to record a transaction. As a noun, usually plural, the journals and ledgers. As an adjective, see book value.

Book Inventory. An inventory amount that is determined from the amount of initial inventory plus invoice amounts of purchases less invoice amounts of requisitions or withdrawals. Implies a perpetual inventory method.

Bookkeeping. The process of analyzing and recording transactions in the accounting records.

Book of Original Entry. A journal.

Book Value. The amount shown in the books or in the accounts for any asset, liability, or owners' equity item.

Book Value per Common Share. Common stockholders' equity divided by the number of shares of common stock outstanding.

Breakeven Point. The volume of sales required so that total revenues and total costs are equal. It may be expressed in units (fixed costs/contribution per unit) or in sales dollars (selling price per unit x fixed costs/contribution per unit).

Breakeven Quantity. The number of unit sales or services needed to break even (or meet a desired profit objective). Calculated by dividing the fixed costs plus desired profit by the contribution margin per unit.

$$\text{Break-even Quantity} = \frac{\text{Fixed Costs} + \text{Desired Profit}}{\text{Contribution Margin per Unit}}$$

Break Even Analysis. Techniques that are used to calculate the break even quantity or break even revenue dollars. Also known as **cost-volume-profit analysis**.

Budget. A financial plan that is used to plan for future operations. It is frequently used to help control and evaluate operating results.

Budget Variance. A variance between actual costs and the amount budgeted. With regard to fixed costs, refers to the variance between actual costs and the budgeted amount of fixed costs. May also be called a **Spending Variance**.

Budgetary Accounts. The accounts that reflect estimated operations and financial condition in government accounting, as affected by estimated revenues, appropriations, and encumbrances. Proprietary accounts record the transactions.

Budgetary Control. The management of governmental or nongovernmental unit in accordance with an official (approved) budget in order to keep total expenditures within authorized (planned) limits.

Budgeted Costs. Costs recorded under the budget or financial plan used to plan the results of future operations. Budgeted costs are often compared with actual costs to determine variances.

Budgeted Statements. Pro forma statements prepared before the event or period occurs.

Buffer. Use of cash for unexpected needs.

Bull. One who expects security prices to increase. Contrast with **bear.**

Burden. Indirect overhead expenses.

Business Combination. As defined by the APB in Opinion No. 16, bringing together of two or more incorporated or unincorporated businesses into a single accounting entity. The merger will be accounted for either with the purchase method or the pooling of interests method.

Business Risk. The risk that the firm will be unable to cover operating costs.

Bylaws. The rules adopted by the stockholders of a corporation which specify the general methods for carrying out the functions of the corporation.

Byproduct. A joint product whose value is so small relative to the value of the other joint products. The costs assigned to byproducts reduce the costs of the main products. Byproducts are shown in the accounts at net realizable value.

CA. Chartered Accountant in Canada or the United Kingdom.

Call Provisions. Provisions that indicate when and for what price bonds can be redeemed by the issuing firm before maturity.

Callable Bond. A bond for which the issuer reserves the right to pay a specific amount, the call price, to retire the obligation before maturity date. The amount of the call price over the face amount of the bond is the call premium.

Canadian Institute of Chartered Accountants. The national organization that represents chartered accountants in Canada.

Capacity. The amount stated in units of service, which can be produced per unit of time. If stated in units of input, such as direct labor hours, capacity is the amount of input that can be used in production per unit of time.

Capacity Costs. Fixed costs in patient care context.

Capacity Variance (Volume Variance). Standard fixed overhead rate per unit of output or input activity times units of output budgeted for a period, minus actual units of output completed during the period.

Capital. Owners' equity in a business.

Capital Account. An account used to record some element of a firm's capital. May refer to the owner's account in a sole proprietorship.

Capital Asset. A designation for income tax purposes which describes most property held by a taxpayer. Assets, goods held primarily for sale, most depreciable property, real estate, receivables, certain intangibles, and a few other items are not included.

Capital Budget. A plan of proposed outlays for acquiring long-term assets and the sources of capital to finance this.

Capital Budgeting. The process of choosing investment projects for an enterprise.

Capital Contributed in excess of Par (or Stated) Value. The amount received by the issuer for capital stock in excess of par (or stated) value.

Cash Equivalents. Short-term interest bearing securities easily converted to cash.

Cash Flow Synchronization. Synchronizing cash inflows and outflows.

Capital Expenditure. An expenditure to acquire long-term assets.

Capital Gain. The excess of proceeds over cost from the sale of a capital asset as defined by the Internal Revenue Code.

Capital Investment. Outlay of money to acquire long-lived assets.

Capital Lease. Lease containing provisions that transfers the benefits and risks to the lessee.

Capital Loss. Occurs when the cost of a capital asset exceeds its sale price. A negative capital gain.

Capital Rationing. The imposing of constraints on the amounts of total capital expenditures in each period.

Capital Stock. The ownership shares of a corporation. It consists of all classes of common and preferred stock.

Capital Structure. The relative proportions of long-term debt and owners' equity in a corporate structure.

Capitalization of a Corporation. The total of stockholders' equity plus bonds outstanding.

Capitalization of Earnings. A technique used to estimate the economic worth of a firm by computing the net present value of the predicted net income of the firm in the future.

Capitalization Rate. An interest rate used to convert a series of payments into a present value amount.

Capitalization Ratio. Ratios used to analyze long-run liquidity and capital structure. Capitalization ratios help evaluate the firm's financial flexibility and the amount of potential risk in the financing assets. Another commonly used term for this group of ratios is **leverage ratios.** Both ratios refer to the substitution of debt for equity financing with the goal of increasing return on equity.

Capitalize. To record an expenditure that may benefit a future period as an asset rather than to treat the expenditure as an expense of the period of occurrence.

Capitation Rate. Average cost of providing health care services per member per month to an enrolled population.

Carryback, Carryforward, Carryover. The use of losses or tax credits from one period to reduce income taxes payable in other periods. There are three common kinds of carrybacks; for net operating losses, for capital losses, and for the investment tax credit. The first two are applied against taxable income and the third against the actual tax. In general, carrybacks are for three years with the earliest year used first. Operating losses, the investment tax credit, and the capital loss for corporations can generally be carried forward for five years.

CASB. Cost Accounting Standards Board.

Case Mix. An output measure expressed in terms of case mix based on the different mix of services provided or populations served. One of the most common case mix measures is based on the intensity or acuity of care. Further differentiation can be achieved by adding case severity measures to the unit of service measure.

Cash. Currency and coins, negotiable checks, and balances in bank accounts.

Cash Basis of Accounting. In contrast to the accrual basis of accounting, a system of accounting in which revenues are recognized when cash is received and expenses are recognized as expenditures are made. No attempt is made to match revenues and expenses in determining income.

Cash Budget. A schedule of expected cash receipts and disbursements.

Cash Collection Basis. The installment method for recognizing revenue. This is not to be confused with the cash basis of accounting.

Cash Cycle. The period of time that elapses during which cash is converted into inventories, inventories are converted into accounts receivable, and receivables are converted back into cash.

Cash Discount. A reduction in sales or purchase price which is allowed for prompt payment.

Cash Equivalent Value. A term used to describe the amount for which an asset could be sold. This is usually based on market values.

Cash Flow. Cash receipts minus disbursements for a given period.

Cash Flow Statement. A statement similar to the typical statement of changes in financial position where the flows of cash rather than of working capital are explained. This is required by FASB 95.

Cashier's Check. A bank's own check drawn on itself and signed by the cashier or other authorized official. It is a direct obligation of the bank.

Cash Receipts Journal. A special journal used to record all receipts of cash.

Cash (Surrender) Value of Life Insurance. An amount that could be realized if the policy were immediately canceled and traded with the insurance company for cash.

Cash Turnover. A turnover ratio used to compare patient revenues to cash. Calculated by dividing patient revenues, or operating revenues, by cash balances shown on the balance sheet.

Census. The count of patients in the hospital at any one point in time (usually midnight).

Census, Average Daily. The average number of inpatients in the hospital each day for a given period of time.

Central Corporate Expenses. General overhead expenses incurred in running the corporate headquarters and related supporting activities of a corporation.

Central Processing Unit (CPU). That portion of a computer containing the arithmetic, logic, control units, and in some cases, main storage devices.

Certificate. The document that is the physical embodiment of a bond or a share of stock.

Certificate of Deposit. Banks typically pay a higher rate if the depositor promises to leave funds on deposit for several months or more. The amount of the funds is reflected in a certificate of deposit. Usually the depositor can withdraw the funds before maturity if a penalty is paid.

Certificate of Need (CON). A formal confirmation by an approved government agency that a program or construction proposal submitted by a facility meets an unmet need in a defined service area.

Certified Check. The check of a depositor drawn on a bank on the face of which the bank has written the words accepted or certified with the date and signature of a bank official. The check then becomes an obligation of the bank.

Certified Financial Statement. A financial statement attested to by an independent auditor who is a CPA.

Certified Public Accountant. An accountant who has satisfied the statutory and administrative requirements of his or her jurisdiction to be registered or licensed as a public accountant. In addition to passing the Uniform CPA Examination administered by the AICPA, the CPA must meet certain educational and moral requirements which differ from jurisdiction to jurisdiction. The jurisdictions are the fifty states, the District of Columbia, Guam, Puerto Rico, and the Virgin Islands.

CHAMPUS. An insurance program sponsored by the Department of Defense to cover military dependents and retirees at nonmilitary or VA hospitals. agencies. Now known as **OCHAMPUS**, but most operations have been transferred to the private sector.

Charge. As a noun, a debit to an account; as a verb, to debit.

Charge Off. To treat an amount originally recorded as an asset as a loss or expense. Usually the term is used when the amount is not in accord with original expectations.

Charges or Revenues, Gross. The total charges at established rates for services rendered to a patient.

Charges or Revenues, Net. The charges covered by a third-party payer and the net amount billed to the patient as deductible and coinsurance amounts.

Charity Deduction. Deduction from gross revenues (stated at full charge) for free or discounted care provided to the medically indigent.

Charter. A document issued by a state government authorizing the creation of a corporation.

Chart of Accounts. A systematically organized list of names and numbers of accounts.

Check. The Federal Reserve Board defines a check as a draft or order upon a bank or banking house purporting to be drawn upon "a deposit of funds for the payment at all events of a certain sum of money to a certain person therein named or to him or his order or to bearer and payable instantly on demand."

Check Register. A journal to record checks issued.

CICA. Canadian Institute of Chartered Accountants.

Clean Surplus Concept. The notion that the only entries to the retained earnings account are to record net earnings and dividends. This concept, with minor exceptions, is now controlling in GAAP.

Clearing Account. An account containing amounts to be transferred to another account before the end of the accounting period. Examples are the income summary account, whose balance is transferred to retained earnings, and the purchases account, whose balance is transferred to inventory or to cost of goods sold.

Clearing Float. The time it takes for a check to clear the banking system after it is received.

Close. To transfer the balance of a temporary or contra account to the main account to which it relates. For example, to transfer revenue and expense accounts directly, or through the income summary account to an owners' equity account.

Closing a Cost Center. Used under most cost allocation processes to indicate when costs are no longer allocated from one cost center to another. When a cost center is "closed", then no more costs can be allocated to it.

Closing Entries. The entries that accomplish the transfer of balances in temporary accounts to the related balance sheet accounts.

CMA. Certified Management Accountant. Awarded by the Institute of Management Accounting of the National Association of Accountants to those who pass a set of examinations and meet certain experience and continuing education requirements.

Coding of Accounts. The numbering of accounts, as for a chart of accounts, which is particularly necessary for computerized accounting.

Coefficients. The "a" and "b" terms in the Total Cost Equation, $y = a + b(x)$ are known as coefficients or cost factors. Also related to regression coefficients where statistical techniques are used to determine the coefficients. Also known as **cost factors.**

Coinsurance. Insurance policies that protect against hazards such as fire or water damage often specify that the owner of the property may not collect the full amount of insurance for a loss unless the insurance policy covers at least some specified percentage, usually about 80 percent, of the replacement cost of the property. Coinsurance clauses induce the owner to carry full, or nearly-full, coverage.

Collateral. Assets pledged by a borrower.

Collectible. Capable of being converted into cash; now if due or later if otherwise.

Collection Float. Float associated with collections of accounts.

Commercial Paper. Short-term notes issued by corporate borrowers.

Commission. Remuneration to employees based upon an agreed activity rate, such as sales.

Committed costs. Usually refers to fixed costs or fixed expenses during the next budget period. For example, amounts obligated to pay for leases, loans, and insurance, etc. They reflect commitments that management really cannot reallocate to other purposes or purchases. On the other hand, if management has complete discretion over how the money is spent, the cost is considered to be **non-committed**.

Common Cost. Cost resulting from use of a facility, (i.e., plant or equipment), or a service, (i.e., fire insurance), that benefits several services or departments. It must be allocated to those patient care services or departments to obtain the full cost of the patient care services.

Common-Size Statement. A percentage statement comparing the individual accounts on the financial statement.

Common Stock. Stock representing the class of owners who have residual claims on the assets and earnings of a corporation.

Common Stock Equivalent. A security whose primary value arises from its ability to be exchanged for common shares. It includes stock options, warrants, and sometimes convertible bonds or convertible preferred stock who meet certain yield requirements.

Comparative Statements. Financial statements showing information for the same company over time.

Compensating Balance. When a bank lends funds to a customer it often requires that the customer keep on deposit in a checking account an amount equal to a percentage of the loan. The amount required to be left on deposit is the compensating balance and effectively increases the interest rate on the loan.

Completed Contract Method. Recognizing revenues and expenses for a job or order only when it is finished. However, when a loss on the contract is expected, revenues and expenses are recognized in the period where the loss is first forecast.

Composite Depreciation. Group depreciation of dissimilar items.

Composite Life Method. Group depreciation for items of unlike kind. For example, when a single item, such as a crane, which consists of separate units with differing service lives, such as the chassis, the motor, the lifting mechanism, and so on, is depreciated as a whole rather than treating each of the components separately.

Compound Entry. A journal entry with more than one debit or more than one credit, or both.

Compounding Period. The time period for which interest is calculated.

Compound Interest. Interest calculated on principal plus previously undistributed interest.

Compound Interest Depreciation. A method designed to hold the rate of return on an asset constant. The periodic depreciation charge is the cash flow for the period less the internal rate of return multiplied by the asset's book value at the beginning of the period. When the cash flows which form the asset are constant over time, the method is sometimes called the annuity method of depreciation.

Comptroller. Controller.

Computer. A data processor that can accept data, perform prescribed operations on that data, and furnish results with little or no human intervention.

Confirmation. A formal memorandum delivered by the customers or suppliers of a company to its independent auditor verifying the amounts shown as receivable or payable. If the auditor asks that the document be returned whether the balance is correct or incorrect, then it is called a "positive confirmation." If the auditor asks that the document be returned only if there is an error, it is called a "negative confirmation."

Conglomerate. This term is used when the owned companies of a holding company are in dissimilar lines of business.

Conservatism. A reporting objective that calls for anticipation of all losses and expenses but defers recognition of gains or profits.

Consignee. See consignment.

Consignment. Goods delivered by the owner (the consignor) to another (the consignee) to be sold by a third party. The owner is entitled to the return of the property or payment of an amount agreed upon in advance.

Consignor. See consignment.

Consistency. Like accounting transactions are treated in the same way over different periods. The reporting policy implies that procedures, once adopted, should be followed from period to period by a reporting entity.

Consolidated Financial Statements. Statements issued by legally separate companies that show financial position and income as they would appear if the companies were one legal entity. Such statements reflect an economic, rather than a legal, concept of the entity.

Consumer Price Index (CPI). A price index computed and issued monthly by the Bureau of Labor Statistics of the U.S. Department of Labor. The index attempts to track the price level of a group of goods and services purchased by the average consumer.

Constructive Receipt. An item is included in taxable income when the taxpayer can control funds whether or not cash has been received. For example, interest added to principal in a savings account is deemed to be constructively received.

Contingent Annuity. An annuity whose number of payments depends upon the outcome of an event whose timing is uncertain at the time the annuity is established.

Contingent Issue (Securities). Securities issuable to specific individuals upon the occurrence of an agreed upon event.

Contingent Liability. A potential liability, such as losing a lawsuit. Until the outcome is known, the contingency is merely disclosed in notes rather than shown in the balance sheet accounts.

Continuing Appropriation. A governmental appropriation automatically renewed without further legislative action until it is altered, revoked, or expended.

Continuity of Operations (Going Concern). The assumption in accounting that the business entity will continue to operate long enough for current plans to be carried out.

Continuous Compounding. Compound interest where the compounding period is every instant of time.

Contra Account. An account that accumulates deductions from another account. For example, accumulated depreciation is the contra account for machinery.

Contra Asset. See contra account. Refers to a deduction from an asset account. For example, allowance for uncollectible accounts is a contra-asset account associated with accounts receivable.

Contractual Allowance. The difference between gross revenues and what a third party payer contracts to pay for its clients or beneficiaries.

Contractual Replacement Funds. Funds set aside by agreement with third-party payers for renewal and replacement of property, plant, and equipment.

Contributed Capital. The sum of the balances in capital stock accounts plus capital contributed in excess of par (or stated) value accounts. This is typically owners' equity less retained earnings.

Contribution Margin. Revenue from sales less variable expenses.

Contribution Margin Ratio (Percentage).
The percentage of each revenue dollar that is available to meet fixed costs and profit. How much of each revenue dollar is left-over after covering variable costs? This percentage is called the **contribution margin ratio (CMR)**. It is stated in percentage terms and is equal to the contribution margin per unit divided by revenue per unit:

$$\text{Contribution Margin Ratio} = \frac{\text{Contribution Margin per Unit}}{\text{Revenue per Unit}}$$

$$= \frac{CMU}{RU}$$

The contribution margin ratio can also be obtained from an entirely different, but related, calculation. This alternative calculation does not require per unit data. Instead, it divides the contribution margin (in dollars) by the total revenue (in dollars):

Contribution Margin = Contribution Margin (dollars)
Ration   Total Revenue (dollars)

$$= \frac{CM}{TR}$$

The contribution margin ratio is used to calculate break-even in terms of revenue dollars.

Contribution Margin Per Unit. Selling price less variable costs per unit.

Contributory. A pension plan where employees, as well as employers, make payments to a pension fund.

Control (Controlling) Account. A summary account that shows totals of entries and balances that appear in individual accounts in a subsidiary ledger. Accounts Receivable is a control account backed up with accounts for each customer. The balance in a control account should not be changed unless a corresponding change is made in the subsidiary accounts.

Controllable Cost. A cost whose amount can be influenced by the way in which operations are carried out or by particular managerial decisions. Contrast with **noncontrollable costs.**

Controlled Company. A company, a majority of whose voting stock is held by an individual or corporation.

Controller. The title often used for the chief accountant of an organization. Often spelled comptroller.

Controlling. Management's activities to ensure that the firm's procedures and outcomes are in line with its service and financial goals and objectives.

Conversion. The act of exchanging a convertible security for another security.

Conversion Cost. Direct labor costs plus factory overhead costs incurred in producing a product.

Convertible Bond. A bond that may be converted into a specified number of shares of capital stock.

Convertible Preferred Stock. Preferred stock that may be converted into a specified number of shares of common stock.

Copyright. Exclusive right granted by the government to an author, composer, playwright, etc. (and their heirs) for the life of the creator plus 50 years to enjoy the benefit of a piece of written work. The economic life of a copyright may be considerably less than the legal life.

Corporate Strategy. The hospital's formalized mission or purpose, and the program directives that result from and are held together by the mission statement.

Corporation. A legal entity authorized by a state to operate under the rules of the entity's charter.

Cost. The sacrifice, measured by the price paid or required to be paid, to acquire goods or services. The term "cost" is often used when referring to the valuation of a good or service acquired. For example, the cost would be the book value of machinery and the expense would be depreciation expense. The terms cost and expense are sometimes used incorrectly as synonyms.

Cost Accounting. The process of classifying, summarizing, recording, reporting, and allocating.

Cost Accounting Standards Board. A board of five members previously authorized by the U.S. Congress to promulgate cost-accounting standards designed to achieve uniformity and consistency in the cost-accounting principles followed by defense contractors and subcontractors under federal contracts. The board is now defunct, but CASB standards are still in effect and are supervised by the General Accounting Office (GAO).

Cost Allocation. The process of apportioning or allocating the costs of nonrevenue-producing cost centers to each other and to the revenue-producing centers on the basis of statistical data that measures the amount of service rendered by each cost center to other centers. Also called cost determination or cost finding.

Cost-Based Reimbursement Payers. Under this approach, the third party pays the hospital for the cost of care received by covered patients, with the expense elements to be included and excluded from cost determined by the third party.

Cost Categories. Any classification of costs into categories. Usually refers to fixed and variable costs summing to total costs.

Cost Center. A center of activity for which expenditures and expenses are accumulated.

Cost Driver. Cost drivers are activities in an organization that cause costs to increase or decrease. Volume can be said to be an important, and often critical, cost driver.

Cost Factors. The "a" and "b" terms in the Total Cost Equation, $y = a + b(x)$ are known as coefficients or cost factors. Also related to regression coefficients where statistical techniques are used to determine the coefficients. Also known as **coefficients.**

Cost Finding. Obsolete term for the process of apportioning or allocating the costs of nonrevenue-producing cost centers to each other and to the revenue-producing centers on the basis of statistical data that measures the amount of services rendered by each center to other centers. Also called cost determination or cost allocation.

Cost Flows. Costs passing through various classifications within an entity.

Cost Method (For Investments). Accounting for an investment in the capital stock of another company where the investment is shown at acquisition cost, and only dividends declared are treated as revenue. It is generally used if less than twenty percent of the voting stock is held by the investor.

Cost Method (For Treasury Stock). The method of showing treasury stock as a contra account to all other items of stockholders' equity in an amount equal to that paid to reacquire the stock.

Cost Models (or Cost Modeling). See **Financial Modeling.**

Cost of Capital. The weighted average return market's require of the firm's debt and equity adjusted for tax savings for debt and issuance costs for debt and equity.

Cost of Debt. The market required return rate on the firm's debt less any tax benefits of debt.

Cost of Equity. For for-profit firms, the market required return rate on the firm's stock plus adjustments for flotation costs if new stock would have to be issued to finance a project. For not-for-profit firms, the opportunity cost of funds, which is often quantified as a required return rate on a similar firm's stock.

Cost of Goods Purchased. Net purchase price of goods acquired plus costs of storage and delivery to the place where the items can be productively used.

Cost of Goods Sold. Inventoriable costs that are expensed because the units are sold. It can be computed be taking beginning inventory plus cost of goods purchased or manufactured minus ending inventory.

Cost Principle. The principle that requires reporting assets at historical or acquisition cost, less accumulated depreciation.

Cost-Recovery Method. A method of revenue recognition that credits cost as collections are received until all costs are recovered. Only after costs are completely recovered is profit recognized. To be used only when the total amount of collections is highly uncertain.

Cost Sheet. Statement that shows all the elements comprising the total cost of an item.

Cost Shifting. Recall that many major purchasers of health insurance predominantly pay full charges. **Cost shifting** represents costs not reimbursed or paid by some (usually cost-based) payers, such that the difference (unpaid balance) is shifted to the charge-based payers. As health care costs have escalated, many private insurance carriers and self-insured employer groups have been forced to reconsider their passive acceptance of cost shifting.

Cost-to-Cost Ratio. The percentage of completion method where the estimate of completion is the ratio of costs incurred to date divided by total costs expected to be incurred for the entire project.

Cost-Volume-Profit Analysis. Techniques that are used to calculate the breakeven quantity or breakeven revenue dollars. Also known as **breakeven analysis**.

Cost-Volume-Profit Graph (Chart). A graph that shows the relation between fixed costs, contribution per unit, breakeven point, and sales.

Costing. The process of determining the cost of activities, products, or services.

Coupon. The portion of a bond redeemable at a specified date for interest payments. Its physical form is much like a ticket. Each coupon is dated and is deposited at a bank just like a check for collection or is mailed to the issuer's agent for collection.

Coupon Rate. For a bond, the amount of annual coupons divided by par value.

Covenant. A promise with legal validity.

Covered Charges. The charges incurred by a patient which are covered under the contractual agreements with third-party payers.

CPA. Certified public accountant.

CPI. Consumer price index.

CPM. Critical Path Method. An operations research technique for solving management control problems.

Cr. Abbreviation for credit entry in a journal or ledger.

Credit. An entry on the right-hand side of an account. Used to make an entry on the right-hand side of an account. Records increases in liabilities, owners' equity, and revenues; records decreases in assets and expenses.

Credit Enhancement. Methods of improving the creditworthiness of a firm such as bond insurance or obtaining a letter of credit from a bank.

Credit Loss. The amount of accounts receivables that is or is expected to become uncollectible.

Credit Memorandum. A document used by a seller to inform a buyer that the buyer's account receivable is being credited (reduced) because of errors, returns, or allowances.

Credit Time Period. Length of time a client is allowed to pay a bill.

Creditor. A lender.

Cross-Reference (Index). A number placed by each account in a journal entry indicating the ledger account to which the entry is posted and placing in the ledger the page number of the journal from which the entry was made. It is used to link the debit and credit parts of an entry in the ledger accounts back to the original entry in the journal.

Cross Section Analysis. Analysis of financial statements of various firms for a single period of time, as opposed to time series analysis where statements of a given firm are analyzed over several periods of time.

Cumulative Dividend. Preferred stock dividends in areas that must be paid before dividends to common stockholders can be declared.

Current Asset. Cash and other assets that are expected to be turned into cash, sold, or exchanged within the normal operating cycle of the firm, usually one year. Current assets include cash, marketable securities, receivables, inventory, and current prepayments.

Current Asset Turnover. A turnover ratio used to compare patient revenues to current assets. Calculated by dividing patient revenues, or operating revenues, by current assets shown on the balance sheet.

Current Cost. Cost stated in terms of current market prices rather than in terms of acquisition cost. Contrast to historical costs.

Current Fund. In governmental accounting, a synonym for general fund.

Current Funds. Cash and other assets readily convertible into cash. In governmental accounting, funds spent for operating purposes during the current period. Includes general, special revenue, debt service, and enterprise funds.

Current Liability. A debt or other obligation that must be discharged within a short time, usually one year.

Current Operating Performance Concept. The notion that reported income for a period ought to reflect only ordinary, normal, and recurring operations of that period. A consequence is that extraordinary and non-recurring items are entered directly in the retained earnings account. This concept does not reflect generally accepted accounting principles.

Current Ratio. Sum of current assets divided by sum of current liabilities. Used as an indicator of solvency.

Current Replacement Cost. The amount currently required to acquire an identical asset (in the same condition and with the same service potential).

Current Selling Price. The amount for which an asset could be sold as of a given time in an arm's length transaction rather than in a forced sale.

Current Value Accounting. The form of accounting where all assets are shown at current replacement cost (entry value) or current selling price or net realizable value (exit value) and all liabilities are shown at present value. It does not represent GAAP.

Current Yield. The annual interest received as a percent of the price of the bond.

Cushion Ratio. A liquidity ratio often used by lenders and rating agencies to evaluate the firm's ability to pay its annual debt service (principal and interest). Calculated by dividing cash and other short-term investments (marketable securities and other cash equivalents) by the annual debt service requirements. It includes cash in restricted accounts (which may have otherwise been ignored in a liquidity analysis), and it ties the balance sheet and income statement together. The numerator emphasizes "substance over form"; it should include all forms of liquid, spendable cash or cash equivalents.

Customers' Ledger. The ledger that shows accounts receivable of individual customers. It is the subsidiary ledger for accounts receivable, the controlling account.

Data. Basic elements of information, (i.e., facts, numbers, letters, symbols), that can be processed by a computer.

Debenture Bond. A bond not secured with collateral.

Debt. Financing characterized by an obligation to repay principal and interest on the principal according to a prearranged schedule.

Debit. An entry on the left-hand side of an account. If used as a verb, to make an entry on the left-hand side of an account. Debits record increases in assets and expenses and record decreases in liabilities, owners' equity, and revenues.

Debit and Credit Conventions. The equality of the two sides of the accounting equation is maintained by recording equal amounts of debits and credits for each transaction. The conventional use of the T-account form and the rules for debit and credit in balance sheet accounts are summarized on the following page.

Debit Memorandum. A document used by a seller to inform a buyer that the seller is debiting (increasing) the amount of the buyer's account receivable because of a service charge or any other type of charge other than a payment for a check. An accounting error.

Debt. The general name for notes, bonds, mortgages, and similar instruments where the evidence of amounts owed is known.

Debt Capacity. A concept related to capitalization and leverage based on a target debt-to-assets ratio. Debt capacity is often subjectively determined. It is often a normative target set by lenders or rating agencies.

Debt-Equity Ratio. Total liabilities divided by total equities. The denominator can be total stockholders' equity and the numerator can be restricted to long-term debt only.

Debt Financing. Raising funds by issuing bonds or notes.

Debtor. One who borrows from a creditor or lender.

Debt Ratio. Debt-to-assets ratio.

Debt Service Coverage. A capitalization ratio used to evaluate the firm's ability to meet all of its debt service (interest and principal) obligations. Unlike the cushion ratio, the debt service ratio is based on accrual accounting (income statement) results and not on cash flows.

Debt Service Fund. In governmental accounting, a fund established to account for payment of interest and principal on all general obligation debt other than that payable from special assessments.

Debt Service Requirement. The amount of cash required for payments of interest, current maturities of principal on outstanding debt, and payments to sinking funds (corporations), or to the debt service fund (governmental).

Debt-to-assets Ratio. A capitalization ratio used to indicate the proportion of assets financed by debt. Related to **leverage**. May also be calculated as **Long-term debt-to-assets.**

Decision Making. Managerial processes involved in choosing one alternative over another. Usually involves incremental costs and incremental benefits.

Declaration Date. Time when a dividend is declared by the board of directors.

Declining-Balance Depreciation. The method of calculating the periodic depreciation charge by multiplying the book value at the start of the period by a constant percentage.

Deductible and Coinsurance Amounts. The portion of charges which are to be borne by the patient and not paid by a third party.

Deep Discount Bonds. Bonds selling a significant amount below par value. Also called zero coupon bonds.

Defalcation. Embezzlement.

Default. Failure to pay interest or principal on a debt when due.

Default Risk. Risk that the issuer of a debt security will not be able to make interest or principal payments as promised.

Deferred Asset. Deferred charge.

Deferred Charge. An expenditure not recognized as an expense of the period when made but carried forward as an asset to be written off in future periods. Typical examples include insurance premiums and/or prepaid rent.

Deferred Credit. Sometimes used to indicate advances from customers or deferred income tax liabilities.

Deferred Expense. Deferred charge.

Deferred Income or Revenue. Advances from customers.

Deferred Income Tax (Liability). An balance sheet liability account that occurs when the pre-tax income shown on the tax return is less than what it would have been had the same accounting principles been used in tax returns as used for financial reporting.

Deferred Revenue (Unearned Revenue). Sometimes used to indicate advances from customers.

Deficit. A debit balance in the Retained Earnings account.

Defined Benefit Plan. A pension plan where the employer promises specific benefits to each employee. The employer's cash contributions and pension expense are adjusted in relation to investment performance of the pension fund.

Deflation. A period of generally declining prices.

Demand Deposit. Funds in a checking account at a bank.

Denominator Volume. Capacity measured in expected number of units to be produced this period, divided into budgeted fixed costs to obtain fixed costs applied per unit of product.

Departmental RCC (Ratio of Charges to Charges). An allowable method of reimbursement under which the hospital reports costs on a department-by-department basis and is reimbursed at the ratio of payer charges to total charges for each department. This method is also referred to as RCCAC (ratio of charges to charges applied to cost).

Deposits in Transit. Deposits made by a firm but not yet reflected on the bank statement.

Depreciable Cost. That part of the cost of an asset, usually acquisition cost less salvage value, that is to be charged off as an expense over the life of the asset through the process of depreciation.

Depreciable Life. The time period over which depreciable cost is to be expensed.

Depreciation. The process of allocating the cost of an asset to the periods of benefit. Depreciation methods typically used the annuity method, composite method, compound interest method, declining-balance method, double-declining-balance method, replacement method, retirement method, straight-line method, sinking-fund method and sum-of-the-years'-digits method.

Depreciation Funds. The segregation of periodic transfers of cash, equivalent to depreciation charges, for the purpose of plant improvement, replacement, or expansion.

Diagnostic Related Groups (DRG). A patient classification system based on 23 major diagnostic categories (MDC) according to the body organ affected. The 23 MDCs were then divided into 467 DRGs based on whether or not an operating room procedure was performed. This resulted in a medical and surgical partition for each MDC. Further differentiation was accomplished by utilizing data on specific operating room procedure, primary diagnosis, age, and presence of substantial complications and/or comorbidities. Note that in 1995, there were 490 different DRGs.

Differential Analysis. Analysis of incremental costs and revenues.

Differential Cost. Incremental cost; cost that changes with respect to a specific decision.

Dilution. A potential reduction in earnings per share or book value per share by the potential conversion of securities or by the potential exercise of warrants or opinions.

Dilutive. Said of a security that would reduce earnings per share if it were exchanged for common stock.

Direct Cost. Cost that can be traced to a specific cost object.

Direct Costing. The method of allocating costs that assigns only variable costs to products and treats fixed costs as period expenses.

Direct Distribution. See direct method.

Direct Labor (material) Cost. Cost of labor (material) applied and assigned directly to a service.

Direct Method. A cost allocation technique involving the distribution of costs of nonrevenue producing cost centers directly to revenue centers without recognizing any services that may be provided from one cost center to another.

Disbursement. Payment of cash or by a check.

Disbursement Control. Methods to slow the availability of funds to suppliers and others so the firm has the use of the cash for a longer period.

Discharges. An inpatient discharge is the termination of lodging and the formal release of an inpatient by the hospital. Since deaths are a termination of lodging, they are also inpatient discharges, although recorded as a specific kind of discharge.

Disclosure. The showing of facts in financial statements, or the auditor's report.

Discount. The difference between face or future value and present value of a payment. It can also mean a reduction in price granted for prompt payment within a specified time period.

Discounted Bailout Period. The total time that must elapse before discounted value of net accumulated cash flows from a project equal or exceed the present value of net accumulated cash outflows.

Discounted Payback Period. Amount of time over which the discounted present value of cash inflows from a project equal the discounted present value of the cash outflows.

Discount Rate. Rate used to convert future payments to present values.

Discounts (Lost). The sum of discounts offered for prompt payment that were not taken because of expiration of the discount period.

Discussion Memorandum. A neutral discussion of all the issues concerning an accounting problem of current concern to the FASB.

Dishonored Note. A promissory note whose maker does not repay the loan at maturity for a term loan, or on demand for a demand loan.

Distribution Expense. Expense of selling, advertising, and delivery activities.

Dividend. A distribution of earnings to owners of a corporation. It may be paid in cash (cash dividend), with stock (stock dividend), with property, or with other securities. Dividends, except stock dividends, become a legal liability of the corporation when they are declared.

Dividends in Arrears. Dividends on cumulative preferred stock that have not been declared in accordance with the preferred stock contract. Such arrearages must usually be cleared before dividends on common stock can be declared.

Dividend Yield. Dividends declared for the year divided by market price of the stock as of a given time of the year.

Divisional Reporting. Line of business reporting.

Dollar Value LIFO method. A form of LIFO inventory accounting with inventory quantities (layers) measured in dollar, rather than physical, terms.

Donated Capital. A stockholders' equity account credited when contributions, such as land or buildings, are freely given to the company.

Donated Services. The estimated monetary value of services of personnel who receive no monetary compensation or partial compensation for their services.

Double-Declining-Balance Depreciation (DDB). Declining-balance depreciation, where the constant percentage is 2/n and n is the depreciable life in periods.

Double Entry. The system of recording transactions that maintains the equality of the accounting equation. Each entry results in recording equal amounts of debits and credits.

Double Taxation. Corporate income is subject to the corporate income tax and the after-tax income, when distributed to owners, is subject to the personal income tax.

Doubtful Accounts. Accounts receivable estimated to be uncollectible.

Dr. The abbreviation for a debit entry in a journal or ledger.

Draft. A written order by the first party, called the drawer, instructing a second party, called the drawee (such as a bank), to pay a third party, called the payee.

DRG. See **Diagnostic Related Groups**.

Earnings. Income or profit.

Earnings Cycle. The series of transactions during which cash is converted into goods and services, goods and services are sold to customers, and customers pay for their purchases with cash.

Earnings per Share (of Common Stock). Net income to common stockholders (Net income minus preferred dividends) divided by the average number of common shares outstanding. Frequently the item of greatest interest contained in corporate annual reports. See also primary earnings per share and full diluted earnings per share.

Economic Cost. The entire cost of all operations or activities, including both tangible and intangible costs, accounting costs, and opportunity costs.

Economic Life. The time span over which the benefits of an asset are expected to be received. The economic life of a patent, copyright, or franchise may be less than the legal life and/or the physical life.

Economic Order Quantity. In mathematical inventory analysis, the optimal amount of stock to order when inventory is reduced to a level called the re-order point.

Effective Interest Method. A systematic method for amortizing bond discount or premium that makes the interest expense for each period divided by the amount of the net liability at the beginning of the period equal to the yield rate on the bond at the time of issue.

Effective (Interest) Rate. The internal rate of return or yield to maturity at the time of issue. If the bond is issued for a price below par, the effective rate is higher than the coupon rate. If it is issued for a price greater than par, then the effective rate is lower than the coupon rate.

Efficiency Variance. A term used for the quantity variance for labor or variable overhead in a standard cost system.

Electronic Spreadsheet. Budgeting or financial planning program used on micro-computers.

Emergency Room Admissions. A patient receiving service in the emergency room who is sufficiently ill or injured to require admission to a hospital bed.

Emergency Services. Services provided by a hospital for critically injured or ill persons who arrive on an unscheduled basis without referral by a physician.

Encumbrance. Funds restricted for an anticipated expenditure, such as for outstanding purchase orders. Appropriations less expenditures less outstanding encumbrances yields unencumbered balance.

Ending Inventory. The cost of inventory on hand at the end of the accounting period, often called closing inventory. The cost of inventory becomes the beginning inventory for the next period.

Endorser. The payee of a note or draft who signs it, after writing "Pay to the order of X," transferring the note to person X, and presumably receiving some benefit in return.

Endowment Funds. Funds in which a donor has stipulated, as a condition of his gift, that the principal of the fund is to be maintained inviolate and in perpetuity and that only income from investments of the fund may be expended.

Enterprise. Any business organization.

Enterprise Fund. A fund established by a governmental unit to account for acquisition, operation, and maintenance of governmental services that are supposed to be self-supporting from user charges, such as for water or airports.

Entity. A person, partnership, corporation, or other organization. The accounting entity for which accounting statements are prepared may not be the same as the entity defined by law. For example, a sole proprietorship is an accounting entity but the individual's combined business and personal assets are the legal entity in most jurisdictions.

Entity Theory. The view of the corporation that emphasizes the form of the accounting equation that says assets=equities. The entity theory is less concerned with a distinct line between liabilities and stockholders' equity than is the proprietorship theory.

Entry Value. The current cost of acquiring an asset or service at a fair-market price.

EOQ. Economic order quantity.

EPS. Earnings per share.

Equities. Liabilities plus owners' equity.

Equity. A residual claim on assets.

Equity Financing. Funds secured by a firm issuing capital stock.

Equity Method. A method of accounting for an investment in the stock of another company in which the proportionate share of the earnings of the other company is debited to the investment account and credited to a revenue account as earned. It is used in reporting when the investor owns twenty percent or more of the stock of an unconsolidated company.

Equity Ratio. Stockholders' equity divided by total assets.

Equivalent Production. Equivalent units of output produced.

Equivalent Units (of Work). The number of units of finished goods that would require the same costs as were actually incurred for production during a period.

ERISA. Employee Retirement Security Income Act of 1974. The federal law that sets pension plan requirements.

Estimated Liabilities. Estimated cost to be incurred for such uncertain events as repairs under warranty. Estimated liability is shown in the balance sheet.

Estimated Revenue. A term used in governmental accounting to designate revenue expected to accrue during a period whether or not it will be collected during the period.

Estimated Salvage Value. Synonymous with salvage value or residual value of an asset at its retirement date.

Eurobond. An international bond sold primarily in countries other than the country of the currency in which the issue is denominated.

Eurodollar Deposits. U.S. dollar denominated deposits in banks outside of the U.S.

Excess of Revenues over Expenses. Net income. Often used as a euphemism for net income in a not-for-profit organization.

Excess present value. Present value of anticipated net cash inflows minus cash outflows for a project.

Excess Present Value Index. Excess present value divided by initial cash outlay.

Except For. Qualification in auditor's report.

Exchange. The generic term for a transaction (or more technically, a reciprocal transfer) between one entity or another.

Exchange Rate. The price of one country's currency in terms of another country's currency.

Ex-Dividend. Said of a stock at the time when the declared dividend becomes the property of the person who owned the stock on the record date.

Exemption. A tax term used for various amounts subtracted from gross income to determine taxable income.

Exercise. When the owner of an option or warrant purchases the security that the option entitles him or her to purchase, he or she has exercised the option or warrant.

Expected Return. The rate of return an investor expects from an investment.

Expected Value. The mean of arithmetic average of a statistical distribution or series of numbers.

Expendable Fund. In governmental accounting, a fund whose resources, principal, and earnings may be expended.

Expenditure. Payment of cash to obtain goods or services.

Expense. The cost of resources and other assets used in producing revenue.

Expense Account. An account to accumulate expenses, that is closed at the end of the accounting period.

Expense Budget. A dollar estimate of the resources needed to provide products or services during the coming period.

Expenditure Budget. Planned cash expenditures.

Expired Cost. An expense or loss.

Exploded Costs. Used as part of the reciprocal cost allocation method to refer to the costs associated with nonrevenue producing cost centers *before* their costs are allocated to other centers. Exploded costs only occur at an intermediate step under a reciprocal allocation process and are *not* actual costs.

Exposure Draft. A preliminary statement of the FASB (or APB between 1962 and 1973) which shows the contents of a pronouncement the Board is considering making effective.

External Reporting. Reporting to stockholders and the public as opposed to internal reporting for management's benefit.

Extraordinary Item. A material expense or revenue item characterized both by its unusual nature and infrequency of occurrence that is shown separately from ordinary income and from income from discontinued operations on the income statement to demonstrate its income tax effects.

Face Amount (Value). The amount due at maturity from a bond or note.

Factoring. The process of buying notes or accounts receivable at a discount from the holder to whom the debt is owed.

Fair Market Price (Value). Price (value) determined at arm's length between a willing buyer and a willing seller, each acting rationally in their own self interest.

Fair Presentation (Fairness). When the auditor's report says that the financial statements "present fairly. . .," the auditor means that the accounting alternatives used by the entity are all in accordance with GAAP.

FASB. Financial Accounting Standards Board. An independent board responsible, since 1973, for establishing generally accepted accounting principles. Its official pronouncements are called "Statements of Financial Accounting Standards" and "Interpretations of Financial Accounting Standards."

FASB Interpretation. An official statement of the FASB interpreting the meaning of Accounting Research Bulletins, APB Opinions, and Statements of Financial Accounting Standards.

Favorable Variance. An excess of standard cost over actual cost.

Feasibility Study. A long-range forecast of a bond issuer's ability to repay the bonds.

Federal Agency Issue. Security issued by a federal agency that is not backed by the U.S. Treasury.

Federal Income Tax. Income tax levied by the U.S. government on individuals and corporations.

Fee-For-Service (FFS). Method of payment for health care products or services in which the health care organization is paid for each product or services. Payment may be on a full or discounted charge basis.

FICA. Federal Insurance Contributions Act. The law that sets "Social Security" taxes and benefits.

Fiduciary. The responsible person for the custody or administration of property belonging to another, such as an executor (of an estate), agent, receiver (in bankruptcy), or trustee (of a trust).

FIFO. First-in, first-out; an inventory flow assumption by which ending inventory cost is determined from most recent purchases and cost of goods sold is determined from oldest purchases including beginning inventory.

Final Settlement. The amount due to the hospital from the payer, as a result of determining the final total allowable cost for the reporting period and comparing that number with the amount that has been received from the payer for the reporting period.

Finance. To supply the organization with funds through the issue of stocks, bonds, notes, or mortgages, or through the retention of earnings.

Financial Accounting. The accounting of assets, equities, revenues, and expenses of a business. Primarily concerned with the historical reporting of the financial position and operations of an entity to external users.

Financial Leverage. The proportion of long-term debt to equity.

Financial Management. Management of the firm's assets, liabilities and equities.

Financial Executives Institute (FEI). An organization of financial executives, such as chief accountants, controllers, and treasurers, of large businesses.

Financial Modeling. Financial modeling is used to obtain estimates of prices or cost structures under varying scenarios determined. Uses microcomputers and spreadsheet software packages to more quickly build and test alternative financial models. One basic financial model can be expressed as a cost-volume-profit model:

Revenues = Fixed Costs + Variable Costs

or alternatively;

Price x Quantity = Fixed Costs + (Variable Cost per Unit x Quantity)

Financial Plan. A plan based on cash-flow projections that specifies inflows and outflows of cash required to meet operating expenses. The plan also outlines capital-budgeting decisions that result in implementing the firm's objectives over a certain period of time.

Financial Position. Statement of the assets and equities of a firm displayed on the balance sheet statements.

Financial Risk. The risk that a borrower will default on interest payments when they are due.

Financial Statements. The balance sheet, income statement, statement of retained earnings, statement of changes in financial position, and any additional notes related to the statements.

Financial Structure. Capital structure as the amount of debt and equity in the corporation.

Financing Lease. A lease treated by the lessee as both the borrowing of funds and the acquisition of an asset to be depreciated. Both the liability and the asset are recognized on the balance sheet.

Finished Goods. Manufactured products ready for sale which are maintained in inventory.

Fiscal Intermediary. An organization which acts as intermediary between the provider and third-party payer. It receives billings from the provider and makes payments for covered charges.

Fiscal Year. A period of twelve consecutive months chosen by a business as the accounting period for annual reports. It can be either a natural business year or calendar year.

Fixed Assets. Assets of a relatively permanent nature held for long-term use in hospital operations and not intended to be converted into cash in the immediate future.

Fixed-Benefit Plan. A defined benefit (pension) plan.

Fixed Budget. A plan that provides for specified amounts of expenditures and receipts that do not vary with activity levels. Sometimes called a "static budget."

Fixed Charge Coverage. A capitalization ratio used to evaluate the firm's ability to meet all of its fixed charges(interest and leases). Unlike the cushion ratio, the fixed charge ratio is based on accrual accounting (income statement) results and not on cash flows.

Fixed Cost (Expense). An expenditure or expense that does not vary with the volume of activity within a specified range.

Fixed Cost Variance. A variance between actual fixed costs and budgeted fixed costs. May refer to the **budget variance** or the **volume variance** or to both variances.

Fixed Interest Rate. Interest rate that is constant over the life of the debt. Does not vary with market rates.

Fixed Liability. Long-term liability.

Flexible Budget. Budget that adjusts budgetary accounts as a function of activity levels.

Float. Checks that have been credited to the depositor's bank account, but not yet debited to the drawer's bank account.

Flow of Costs. Costs passing through various classifications within an entity.

Flow-Through Method. Accounting for the investment tax credit to show all income statement benefits of the credit in the year of acquisition, rather than spreading them over the life of the asset acquired (deferral method).

Footing. Adding a column of figures.

Footnotes. Also called **Notes.** More detailed information than that provided in the income statement, balance sheet, statement of retained earnings, and cash flow statement. These are considered an integral part of the statements and are covered by the auditor's report.

For-Profit Firm. Firm that is owned by investors and whose goal is to maximize the wealth of the owners.

Forecast. An estimate or projection of costs or revenues or both.

Franchise. A privilege granted or sold, to use a name or to sell products and services.

Freight-In. The cost of freight or shipping in acquiring inventory, preferably treated as a part of the cost of inventory.

Freight-out. The cost of freight or shipping in selling inventory, treated as a selling expense in the period of sale.

Full costs. Costs comprising both direct and indirect costs for each cost object. Full costs are the sum of direct costs plus a share of indirect costs that have been allocated to a cost object. Cost allocation is used to calculate full costs.

Full Disclosure. The reporting policy requiring that all significant or material information is to be presented in the financial statements.

Full-Time Equivalent (FTE). The equivalent of one employee working full time, (i.e., 2,080 hours per year). For example, two employees working half-time are one full-time equivalent.

Fully Diluted Earnings per Share. Smallest earnings per share figure on common stock that can be obtained by computing an earnings per share for all possible combinations of assumed exercise or conversion of potentially dilutive securities.

Fully Vested. Said of a pension plan when an employee (or his or her estate) has rights to all the benefits purchased with the employer's contributions to the plan even if the employee is not employed by this employer at the time of retirement.

Functional Classification. The grouping of expenses according to the operating purposes (e.g., patient care, education) for which costs are incurred. Income statement reporting form in which expenses are reported by functions, that is, cost of goods sold, administrative expenses, selling expenses.

Fund. An asset or group of assets set aside for a specific purpose.

Fund Balance. In governmental accounting context, the excess of assets of a fund over its liabilities and reserves. The not-for-profit equivalent of stockholders' equity.

Funded. Said of a pension plan or other obligation when funds have been set aside for meeting the obligation when it becomes due. The federal law for pension plans requires that all normal costs be funded as recognized. In addition, past and prior service costs of pension plans must be funded over 30 or over 40 years, depending upon the circumstances.

Funding. Replacing short-term liabilities with long-term debt.

Funds. Generally working capital. Current assets less current liabilities.

Funds Provided by Operations. An important subtotal in the statement of changes in financial position. This amount is the total of revenues producing funds less expenses requiring cash disbursement.

Funds Statement. An informal name often used for the statement of changes in financial position.

Funny Money. Said of securities such as convertible preferred stock, convertible bonds, options, and warrants which have aspects of common stock equity but which did not reduce reported earning per share.

FUTA. Federal Unemployment Tax Act which provides for taxes to be collected at the federal level, to help subsidize the individual states' administration of their unemployment compensation programs.

GAAP. Generally accepted accounting principles. A plural noun.

Gain. Excess of revenues over expenses from a specific transaction.

General Debt. Debt of a governmental unit legally payable from general revenues and backed by the full faith and credit of the governmental unit.

General Expenses. Operating expenses other than those specifically assigned to cost of goods sold, selling, and administration.

General Fixed Asset (Group of Accounts). Accounts showing those long-term assets of a governmental unit not accounted for in enterprise, trust, or intragovernmental service funds.

General Fund. Assets and liabilities of a nonprofit entity not specifically earmarked for other purposes. The primary operating fund of a governmental unit.

General Journal. The formal record where transactions or summaries of similar transactions are recorded in journal entry form as they occur.

General Ledger. The name for the formal ledger containing all of the financial statement accounts. It has equal debits and credits as evidenced by the trial balance.

Generally Accepted Accounting Principles (GAAP). As previously defined by the APB and now by the FASB, the conventions, rules, and procedures necessary to define accepted accounting practice at a particular time. It includes both broad guidelines and relatively detailed practices and procedures.

Generally Accepted Auditing Standards (GAAS). The standards, as opposed to particular procedures, promulgated by the AICPA (in Statement on Auditing Standards No. 1) which concern "the auditor's professional qualities" and "the judgment exercised by him in the performance of his examination and in his report." Currently, there are ten such standards; three general ones (concerned with proficiency, independence, and degree of care to be exercised), three standards of field work, and four standards of reporting. The first standard of reporting requires that the auditor's report state whether or not the financial statements are prepared in accordance with generally accepted accounting principles.

General Partner. Member of partnership personally liable for all debts of the partnership.

General Price Index. A measure of the aggregate prices of a wide range of goods and services in the

economy at one time relative to the prices during a base period.

General Price Level Changes. Changes in the aggregate prices of a wide range of goods and services in the economy. These price changes are measured using a general price index.

General Purchasing Power of the Dollar. The command of the dollar over a wide range of goods and services in the economy. The general purchasing power of the dollar is inversely related to changes in a general price index.

Global Pricing. Global pricing represents an approach to risk sharing between the physician and the organizational unit providing care. Global pricing requires that a price be set for a particular service that includes both the physician component and the institutional (hospital, home care, clinic, etc.) component. Under global pricing, three categories of payments could be established in order to compensate providers for various services and risks:

> a risk pool to be used for outliers,
> a physician compensation pool, and an
> institutional payment rate.

Payments to the risk pool are usually taken "off the top" and paid first.

GDP Implicit Price Deflator (Index). A price index issued quarterly by the Office of Business Economics of the U.S. Department of Commerce. This index attempts to trace the price level of all goods and services comprising the gross national product.

Goal Congruence. The goals and objectives of employees are closely aligned with organization goals and objectives. Actions taken by employees that are in their best interests are also in the firm's best interests.

Going-Concern Assumption. For accounting purposes a business is assumed to remain in operation long enough for all its current plans to be carried out. This assumption is part of the justification for the acquisition cost basis, rather than a liquidation or exit value basis, of accounting.

Going Public. Issuing shares to the general investing public. The selling of stock shares to the general investing public.

Goodwill. The excess of cost of an acquired firm or operating unit over the current or fair market value of net assets of the acquired unit.

Goodwill Method. A method of accounting for the admission of a new partner to a partnership when the new partner is to be credited with an amount of capital greater than the value of the tangible assets contributed.

Graphical Analysis. Used in conjunction with **breakeven analysis** or with the **high-low method.** Any managerial performance report shown as a graph.

Gross. Not adjusted or reduced by deductions or subtractions. Contrast with **net,** where such deductions have been included.

Gross National Product (GNP). The market value of all goods and services produced within a nation for a year as measured by final sales of goods and services to individuals, corporations, and governments plus the excess of exports over imports.

Gross Patient Revenue. All patient services at charges not reduced by discounts, allowances, or other adjustments.

Gross Depreciation. A method of calculating depreciation charges where similar assets are combined rather than depreciated separately. No gain or loss is recognized on retirement of items from the group until the last item in the group is sold or retired.

Ground-up Approach to Standard Costing. Technique for setting standards for each procedure within a cost center. Used with procedure-based standard costing where fixed and variable costs are used to determine the standard costs for each procedure.

Health Maintenance Organization (HMO). A prepaid type of health care program with the objective of preventing rather than treating serious illness by primary patient care and control of utilization of medical services.

Historical Cost. Acquisition cost, original cost, sometimes referred to as sunk cost.

Historical Summary. A part of the annual report to stockholders that shows important items, such as net income, revenues, expenses, asset and equity totals, earnings per share, etc., for past periods of time.

Holding Company. A company that confines its activities to owning stock in, and supervising management of, other companies. A holding company usually owns a controlling interest, that is, more than 50 percent of the voting stock in the companies whose stock it holds.

Holding Gain or Loss. Difference between end-of-period price and beginning-of-period price of an asset held during the period. Ordinarily, realized holding gains and losses are not separately reported in financial statements.

Home Care. This level of care involves visits by nurses to the home of the patient.

Horizontal Analysis. Time series analysis of financial statement data showing percentage change from one year to the next.

Horizontal Integration. Combination of many similar units into one firm. Examples include multihospital systems and physician group practices.

Hospital-Based Physician (HBP). Physicians performing services for patients in the hospital where the hospital pays the physician for his or her services. Payment may be in the form of salary, percentage of billings, rate per unit of service or treatment, or other. Hospital-based physicians are most commonly found in the radiology, laboratory, EKG, EEG, and emergency departments.

Human Resource Accounting. A term used to describe a variety of proposals that seek to report and emphasize the importance of human resources, knowledgeable, trained, and loyal employees in a that is, company's earning process and total assets.

Hurdle Rate. Minimum internal rate of return the firm requires to accept a capital investment project.

Hypothecation. The pledging of property, without transfer of title or possession, to secure a loan.

ICU. Denotes the **intensive care unit** of the hospital.

Ideal Standard Costs. Standard costs set equal to those that would be incurred under the best possible conditions.

Identity Matrix. A square matrix with ones on the main diagonal and zeros elsewhere. A matrix such that for any other matrix, A, IA = AI = A. The matrix equivalent to the number one.

IIA. Institute of Internal Auditors.

Imprest Fund. Petty cash fund.

Improvement. An expenditure to extend the useful life of an asset or to improve its performance (rate of output, cost) over that of the original asset. Such expenditures are capitalized as part of the asset's cost.

Imputed Cost. A cost that does not appear in accounting records, such as the interest that could be earned on cash spent to acquire inventories or the rent that would be paid if the building was owned by the company.

Inclusive Pricing. An all-inclusive approach to billing and reimbursement. Payers or patients are not given itemized bills.

Income. Excess of revenues over expenses for a period.

Income Accounts. Revenue and expense accounts.

Income from Discontinued Operations. Income, net of tax effects, from parts of the business that have been discontinued during the period or are to be discontinued in the near future.

Income Statement. The statement of revenues, expenses, gains, and losses for the period ending with net income for the period. The earnings per share amount is usually shown on the income statement. The reconciliation of beginning and ending balances of retained earnings may also be shown in a combined statement of income and retained earnings.

Income Summary. An account used in problem solving that serves as a surrogate for the income statement. All revenues are closed to the income summary as credits and all expenses as debits. The balance in the account, after all other closing entries are made, is then closed to the retained earnings or other owners' equity account and represents net income for the period.

Income Tax. An annual tax levied by the federal and other governments on the income of an entity or an individual.

Incremental Analysis. Incremental effects of one alternative versus another are used to choose the preferred alternative. Contrast with **total cost approach**.

Incremental Cost. Costs that will be incurred if an activity is undertaken.

Incurred But Not Reported (IBNR) Expenses. Expenses that a health maintenance organization estimates to have been incurred by enrollees but have not yet been reported to the HMO.

Indenture. A formal agreement between the issuer of a bond and a purchaser of the bonds.

Independence. The mental attitude required of the CPA in performing the attest function. It implies impartiality and that the members of the auditing CPA firm own no stock in the corporation being audited.

Independent Accountant. The CPA who performs the attest function for a firm.

Indexation. An attempt by lawmakers or parties to a contract to cope with the effects of inflation. Amounts fixed in law or contracts are "indexed" when these amounts change as a given measure of price changes.

Indirect Costs. Costs of service not easily associated with the providing of specific services such as overhead costs.

Indirect Labor (material) Costs. An indirect cost for labor (material).

Individualized Pricing. Contrast with **inclusive pricing**. Payers or patients are given itemized bills.

Inflation. A time of generally rising prices.

Information. The collection of facts and intelligence which result from accountants' activities and work.

Information System. The system, both formal and informal, for collecting, processing, and communicating data that are useful for the managerial functions of decision making, planning, control, and for financial reporting.

Initial Public Offering (IPO). Term describing the first issue of stock by a firm.

Inpatient. A patient admitted to a hospital and occupying a hospital bed overnight or longer.

Inpatient Admission Classifications. An inpatient admission is the formal acceptance by a hospital of a patient who is to receive physician, dentist, or allied services while lodged in the hospital. Only one hospital admission may be counted for an inpatient during the period of his continuing as an inpatient. Admissions could be classified along the following lines:

> Classification by age, by adult inpatient admissions, pediatric inpatient admissions, newborn inpatient admissions, by financial relationship with the hospital such as payment status or by type of hospital accommodation such as private, semi-private or ward. Classification by types of medical care provided is now more common using diagnostic codes and acuity levels.

Insolvent. Unable to pay debts when due.

Installment. Partial payment of a debt or in accordance with the terms of the debt instrument.

Insurance. A contract for reimbursement of specific losses. Self insurance is not insurance but merely the willingness to assume risk of incurring losses while saving the premium.

Intangible Asset. A nonphysical, noncurrent asset such as copyright, patent, trademark, goodwill, and capitalized advertising cost. It is amortized over a period not to exceed 40 years.

Interest. The charge or cost for using money, frequently expressed as a rate per period, usually one year, called the interest rate.

Interest Imputed. The difference between the face amount and the present value of a debt is called imputed interest.

Inter-fund Accounts. In governmental accounting, the accounts that show transactions between funds, especially inter-fund receivables and payables.

Internal Audit. An audit conducted by employees to ascertain whether or not internal control procedures are working as opposed to an external audit conducted by a CPA.

Internal Control. The procedures used by a business in attempting to insure that operations are carried out or recorded as planned.

Internal Rate of Return. The discount rate that equates the net present value of a stream of cash flows, including the initial cash outflow, to zero.

Internal Reporting. Reporting for management's use in planning and control.

Internal Storage. Memory devices, such as magnetic cores, forming an integral physical part of a computer and directly controlled by the computer.

International Classification of Disease Adapted (ICDA). A coding structure used to code diseases for statistical analysis and billing purposes. Also known as **ICD-9-CM.**

Inventory. The balance in an asset account such as raw materials, supplies, work in process, and finished goods.

Inventory Equation. Beginning inventory + net additions - withdrawals = ending inventory.

Inventory Turnover. Number of times the average inventory has been sold during a period. Cost of goods sold for a period divided by average inventory for the period. Used to determine the effectiveness of inventory management.

Invested Capital. Contributed capital.

Investment. An expenditure to acquire property or other assets in order to produce revenue.

Investment Tax Credit. A reduction in income tax liability granted by the federal government to firms that buy new equipment.

Invoice. A document showing the details of a sale or purchase transaction.

Issue. When a corporation exchanges its stock for cash or other assets, the corporation is said to issue, not sell that stock.

Issued Shares. Those shares of authorized capital stock of a corporation that have been distributed to the stockholders. Shares of treasure stock are legally issued but are not considered to be outstanding for the purpose of voting, dividend declarations, and earnings per share calculations.

Job Cost Sheet. A schedule showing actual or budgeted inputs for a special service.

Job-order Costing. Accumulation of costs for a particular identifiable batch of services.

Joint Cost. Cost of simultaneously producing or otherwise acquiring two or more products, called joint products, that must by the nature of the process be produced or acquired together.

Joint Venture. A partnership or other agreement under which the participants have contractually agreed to provide specified money or services or expertise in exchange for a designated share of ownership and profits.

Journal. The place where transactions are recorded as they occur.

Journal Entry. A recording in a journal of equal debits and credits with an explanation of the transaction.

Journalize. To make an entry in a journal.

Journal Voucher. A voucher documenting a transaction leading to an entry in the journal.

Kiting. It refers to the practice of taking advantage of the float, the time that elapses between the deposit of a check in one bank and its collection at another.

Labor Variances. The price (or rate) and quantity (or usage) variance for direct labor inputs in a standard cost system.

Land. An asset shown at acquisition cost plus the cost of any nondepreciable improvements. Use as a plant or office site is implied in accounting rather than as a natural resource, such as timberland.

Lapping (Accounts Receivable). The theft, by an employee, of cash sent in by a customer to discharge the latter's payable. The theft from one customer is concealed by using cash received from another customer.

Lead Time. The time that elapses between order-placing and receipt of the ordered goods or services.

Lease. A contract calling for the lessee (user) to pay the lessor (owner) for the use of an asset.

Leasehold. The asset representing the right of the lessee to use leased property.

Leasehold Improvement. An improvement to leased property which is amortized over the economic life of the asset or the life of the lease. Should be amortized over service life or the life of the lease, whichever is shorter.

Ledger. A book of accounts.

Legal Capital. Par or stated value of issued capital stock. The amount of contributed capital that, according to state law, remains permanently in the firm as protection for creditors.

Length of Stay (Average). A statistical measure of patient turnover determined by dividing the total number of patient days of care in a given period of time by the total number of inpatients who were discharged during that period.

Lessee. The receiver of user of the services of leased assets under a lease contract.

Lessor. The owner of assets which are being used.

Letter of Credit. Formal assurance by a bank that it will repay the firm's debt if the firm is unable to pay.

Leverage. The use of long-term debt securities for raising funds to be used in the company. Usually based on the debt-to-assets ratio. See also **Capitalization Ratio.**

Liability. A legal obligation to pay a definite or reasonably certain amount at a definite or reasonably certain time in return for a current benefit.

Lien. The right of person A to satisfy a claim against person B by holding B's property as security or by seizing B's property.

Life Annuity. A contingent annuity in which payments cease at death of specified persons(s).

LIFO, Last-in First-out. An inventory flow assumption where the cost of goods sold is the cost of the most recently acquired units and the ending inventory cost is determined from costs of the oldest units.

Limited Liability. Stockholders of corporations are not personally liable for debt of the company.

Limited Partner. Member of a partnership not personally liable for debt of the partnership. Every partnership must have at least one general partner who is fully liable.

Line of Credit. An agreement with a bank or set of banks for short-term borrowings on demand.

Liquid. A business with a substantial amount of working capital, especially quick assets.

Liquid Assets. Cash, marketable securities, and current receivables.

Liquidating Dividend. Dividend declared in the winding up of a business to distribute the assets of the company to the stockholders. It should be treated as a return of investment, not as revenue.

Liquidation Value Per Share. The amount each share of stock will receive if the corporation is dissolved.

Liquidity. A firm's ability to meet obligations as they mature. Based on current assets and current liabilities and cash flows. Many different ratios can be used to evaluate liquidity.

Liquidity Risk. Risk that a security can not easily be resold.

List-Price Method. See trade-in transaction.

Loan. An arrangement where the owner of property, allows the borrower the use of the property for a period of time that is usually specified in the agreement setting up the loan.

Lockbox. A post office box emptied by the organization's bank to which clients mail payments.

Logs (Third-Party). Records maintained by the hospital for each third-party payer listing for each patient, days in the hospital and charges segregated by routine services, ancillary services, non-covered services, deductibles and coinsurance, etc.

Long-Term Care. Custodial care. Typically provided in a nursing home.

Long-Term (Construction) Contract Accounting. The percentage of completion method of revenue recognition.

Long-term Debt-to-Asset Ratio. A capitalization ratio used to indicate the proportion of assets financed by long-term debt. Related to **leverage.** May also be calculated as **Debt-to-assets.**

Loss. Excess of cost over net proceeds for a single transaction or negative income for a period.

Mail Float. The delay during which checks are in the mail.

Make-or-Buy Decision. A managerial decision about whether the firm should produce a product internally or purchase it from others.

Malpractice Insurance. Insurance for medical or professional malfeasance. One type is based on incidents or occurrences where the insurer is liable for all cases which result from an action which occurred in the policy year. The other is based on "Claims made" where the insurer is only liable for claims asserted in the policy year, regardless of when the action or incident occurred on which the claim is based.

Managed Care. The coordination of a patient's medical care by payers and providers.

Management. Executive authority that operates a business.

Management (Managerial) Accounting. Reporting designed to enhance the ability of management to do its job of decision making, planning, and control.

Managerial Control. Relates to planning and control decisions made by managers in an organization.

Margin. Revenue less specified expenses. Also known as **operating margin.** See also: **contribution margin.**

Marginal Cost. Incremental cost per unit.

Marginal Revenue. Incremental revenue associated with sale of one extra unit of product or service.

Margin of Safety. Excess of actual, or budgeted, sales over break even sales. Usually expressed in dollars; though it may be expressed in units of product.

Marginal Tax Rates. The rate at which additional income is taxed.

Markdown. The reduction below an originally established retail price.

Marketable Securities. Holdings in stocks and bonds of other companies that can be readily sold on stock exchanges or over-the-counter markets and that the company plans to sell as cash is needed. Classified as current assets and as part of working capital.

Market. Any organized system for exchanging economic resources.

Market Rate. The rate of interest a company must pay to borrow funds currently.

Mark-on. An amount added to cost to obtain price and typically expressed as a percentage of cost.

Markup. An amount added to cost. That is typically expressed as a percentage of selling price.

Markup Percentage. Markup divided by selling price.

Matching Convention. The concept of recognizing cost expirations (expenses) in the same accounting period that the related revenues are recognized.

Materiality. The concept that accounting should disclose separately only those events that are relatively important for the business or for understanding its statements.

Material Variances. Price and quantity variances for direct materials or supplies in standard cost systems.

Maturity. The end of the debt obligation. Principal must be repaid on many forms of debt at maturity.

Maturity Matching. Matching of an asset's life with the maturity of its financing source.

Matrix. In computers, a logic network of circuits capable of performing a specific function. In mathematics, numbers arranged in rows and columns.

Maturity. The date at which an obligation, such as the principal of a bond or a note, becomes due.

Maturity Value. The amount expected to be collected when a loan reaches maturity. Depending upon the context, the amount may be principal and interest.

Medical Staff Classifications. Appointments to the medical staff fall into several classes, the most common of which are:

- **Attending.** Full admitting privileges in accordance with their abilities and qualifications, and also participate as members of the medical staff committees, serve as officers of the medical staff and serve as directors or chiefs of departments. They are required to attend meetings of the general staff and departmental staffs, and may be required to devote time to the education programs and supervise residents in outpatient clinics or emergency departments.

- **Associate.** New applicants are generally appointed as associate staff members for a period of two to four years, after which they become members of the attending staff.

- **Courtesy**. Certain doctors are designated as courtesy members when they have retired. They have privileges consistent with their abilities and qualifications.

- **Consulting**. Physicians of recognized professional ability in their specialty but who are not members of the attending staff.

- **House Staff**. Licensed physicians who are employed by the hospital to provide service to all patients, according to need, and are subject to the approval of the patients' own physicians.

Medicare. Federal program paying for health care for the elderly.

Medicare Part A. The portion of the Medicare program applicable to the reimbursement of hospitals for hospital costs.

Medicare Part B. The portion of the Medicare program which is payable to physicians (or to hospitals for services of hospital-based physicians) for the professional component of services the physicians render to Medicare patients.

Medicaid. Program involving federal and state partnership that pays for health care for the poor.

Member Month. One member enrolled in an HMO for one month.

Merger. The joining of two or more businesses into a single economic entity. See pooling of interest method and purchase method.

Minority Interest. A balance sheet account on consolidated statements showing the equity in a subsidiary company allocable to those who are not part of the controlling (majority) interest.

Minutes Book. A record of all actions authorized at corporate board of directors' or stockholders' meeting.

Mixed Cost. A semi-fixed or a semi-variable cost.

Modified Cash Basis. The cash basis of accounting with long-term assets accounted for using the accrual basis of accounting.

Monetary Assets, Liabilities. See monetary items.

Monetary Gain or Loss. The gain or loss in general purchasing power as a result of holding monetary assets or liabilities during a period when the general purchasing power of the dollar changes.

Monetary Items. Amounts fixed in terms of dollars by statute or contract. Cash, accounts receivable, accounts payable, and debt.

Money Market. Financial market in which funds are borrowed or loaned for short periods. (The money market is different from the capital market, which is the market for long-term funds).

Mortality Table. Data on life expectancies or probabilities of death for persons of specified ages and sex.

Mortgage. A claim given by the borrower to the lender against the borrower's property in return for a loan.

Moving Average. An average computed on observations over time. As a new observation becomes available, the oldest one is dropped so that the average is always computed for the same number of observations using only the most recent ones.

Municipal Bond. A bond issued by a village, town, city, country, state, or other public body.

Mutual Fund. An investment company that issues its own stock to the public and uses the proceeds to invest in securities of other companies.

Natural Business Year. A twelve month period chosen as the reporting period so that the end of the period coincides with a low point in activity or inventories.

Natural Classification. Income statement reporting form in which expense are classified by nature of items, that is materials, wages, salaries, insurance, and taxes, as well as depreciation.

Negotiation. Any behavioral exchange designed to induce the other party to change their minds, or prior decisions.

Negotiable. Checks, notes, stocks, and bearer bonds that are legally capable of being transferred by endorsement.

Net. Reduced by all relevant deductions.

Net Accounts Receivable. Gross accounts receivable minus allowances for uncol-lectible accounts.

Net Assets. Owners' equity = total assets minus total liabilities.

Net Current Assets. Net working capital = current assets – current liabilities.

Net Income. The excess of all revenues for the reporting period over all expenses of the period.

Net Income Ratio. Profitability ratio used to evaluate the relationship between net income and patient revenue. Calculated by dividing net income by patient revenue. Also related to **operating margin ratio.**

Net Loss. Negative net income. The excess of all expenses for the reporting period over all revenues of the period.

Net Present Value. Discounted or present value of all cash inflows and outflows of a project at a given discount rate.

Net Realizable Value. Selling price of an item less reasonable out-of-pocket costs to make the item ready for sale.

Net Sales. Sales less returns, allowances, and discounts taken.

Net Variance. Refers to the sum of several variances. For example, may refer to the sum of two labor variances, as in the net labor variance is the sum of the labor rate variance and the labor efficiency variance.

Net Working Capital. Current assets-current liabilities.

Net Worth. Owners' equity.

Nominal Accounts. Temporary accounts such as income statement accounts as opposed to balance sheet accounts. Nominal accounts are normally closed at the end of each accounting period.

Nominal (stated) Interest Rate. The rate of interest charged by the lender of funds and paid by the borrower.

Noncash Charges. Accounting expenses deducted on the income statement that do not involve an actual outlay of cash during the period.

Noncontributory. A pension plan where only the employer makes payments to a pension fund.

Noncontrollable Cost. A cost whose amount can not be easily influenced by the way in which operations are carried out or by particular managerial decisions. Contrast with **controllable costs.**

Non-covered Charges. Charges which are not covered under contractual agreements with third-party payers. For example television and telephone charges.

Noncurrent. Liability accounts that are not due within one year.

Nonexpendable Fund. A governmental fund whose principal may not be spent.

Noninterest-Bearing Note. A note which bears no explicit interest note. The present value of such a note at any time before maturity is less than the face value so long as interest rates are positive.

Nonoperating. Revenues and expenses arising from transactions incidental to the company main line(s) of business.

Nonprofit Corporation. An incorporated entity, where the profits do not accrue to the owners or managers of the company.

Nonrecurring. A revenue expense that is not expected to occur on a continuing basis.

No Par. Capital stock without a par value.

Normal Volume. The volume planned to be produced for the year.

Not-For-Profit Firm. Firms organized to serve purposes other than wealth maximization.

Note. An unconditional written promise by the maker to pay a certain amount on demand or at a specified time.

Note Receivable Discounted. A note assigned by the holder to another. For value received, usually less than the full amount plus interest. If the note is assigned with recourse, it is the contingent liability of the assignor until the debt is paid.

Notes. More detailed information than that provided in the income statement, balance sheet, statement of retained earnings, and cash flow statement. These are considered an integral part of the statements and are covered by the auditor's report. Also known as **footnotes**.

OAS(H)I. Old Age, Survivors, Disability, and (Hospital) Insurance.

OB-GYN. Denotes the **obstetric and gynecology** departments of the hospital.

Objectivity. An accounting principle stressing that recognition not be given to an event in financial statements until the magnitude of the events can be measured with reasonable accuracy and is subject to independent verification.

Obsolescence. A decline in market value of an asset caused by technological changes or improved versions becoming available that are more cost-effective.

Occupancy Percentage. The ratio of actual patient days to the total patient days available, as determined by bed capacity, during a given period of time.

OCHAMPUS. An insurance program sponsored by the Department of Defense to cover military dependents and retirees at nonmilitary or VA hospitals. agencies. Was known as **CHAMPUS**; most operations have been transferred to the private sector.

Off-Balance Sheet Financing. A description used for financing sources that are not shown on the balance sheet. Many operating leases fell into this category in the past.

Official Statement (Prospectus). Formal offering document for securities containing information potential investors need for decision making.

Old Age, Survivors, Disability and (Hospital) Insurance. The technical name for Social Security under the Federal Insurance Contribution Act (FICA).

Open Account. Any account with a non-zero debit or credit balance.

Operating. An adjective used to refer to revenue and expense items relating to the company's main line(s) of business.

Operating Accounts. Revenue and expense accounts.

Operating Budget. Consists of revenue and expense budgets. Is equivalent to a projected income statement.

Operating Cycle. The earnings cycle, usually one year or less, which represents that amount of time for the cash-out flows for resources to the cash inflow for services provided.

Operating Expenses. Expenses incurred in accomplishing the ordinary activities of the organization.

Operating Lease. A lease accounted for by the lessee without showing an asset for the lease rights (leasehold) or a liability for the lease payment obligations. Payments of the lessee are shown as expenses of the period.

Operating Margin Ratio. Profitability ratio used to evaluate the relationship between operating income and operating revenue. Calculated by dividing operating income by operating revenue. Also related to **net income ratio**.

Operating System. Instructions used by the control unit of the central processing unit in directing the operations of the computer system. Its functions are: job control, job scheduling, library management, memory management, and peripheral management.

Operations Research. Application of scientific principles to business management. This may involve setting up mathematical equations to simulate management problems.

Opinion. The auditor's report containing an attestation.

Opportunity Cost. The value foregone by selecting one alternative over another.

Opportunity Cost of Funds. Rate of return that could be earned from alternative investments.

Optimal Capital Structure. Mix of long-term debt and equity that minimizes the firm's overall cost of capital.

Option. The legal right to buy stock during a specified period at a specified price.

Ordinary Annuity. An annuity in arrears. The payment arrives at the end of each time period.

Ordinary Income. Reportable income not qualifying as capital gains for tax purposes.

Organization Costs. The costs incurred in planning and establishing an organization. These intangible assets should be capitalized and put on the balance sheet if material.

Original Cost. Acquisition cost or historical cost of the asset.

Original Entry. Formal entry in a journal or book of record.

Outlay. The amount of an expenditure.

Out-of-Pocket. An expenditure made by a patient rather than a third party payer.

Outpatient. An ambulatory patient who visits the hospital for services; but who is not admitted to a hospital bed.

Outpatient Services. Outpatient services are those service offered by a hospital to ambulatory patients on a scheduled or referral basis.

Output. Physical quantity or monetary measurements of goods and services produced or relating to devices or programs which record processed information on some type of media such as a business form or magnetic tape.

Outside Director. A member of a corporate board of directors who is not a company officer and does not participate in the corporation's day-to-day management.

Outstanding. Unpaid or uncollected obligations of the organization.

Over-and-Short. Title for an expense account used to account for small differences between book balances of cash and actual cash and vouchers or receipts in petty cash or change funds.

Overapplied (Overabsorbed) Overhead. The costs applied, or charged, to the product for a period of time over actual overhead costs during the period. This would create a credit balance in an overhead control.

Overdraft. A check written on a checking account containing less funds than the amount of the check.

Overdraft Account. Bank accounts that automatically issue loans to cover the amount of overdrafts.

Overhead Costs. Any cost not specifically or directly associated with the providing of products of services. Typically, indirect costs fall into this category.

Overhead Rate. Standard or other predetermined rate at which overhead costs are applied to services.

Owner's Equity. Assets minus internal liabilities.

Paid-In Capital. Sum of balances in capital stock and capital contributed in excess of par (or stated) value accounts.

Paper Profit. A gain not yet realized through a transaction.

Par. Said of a bond or preferred stock issued or selling at its face amount.

Part A. The portion of the Medicare program applicable to the reimbursement of hospitals for hospital care.

Part B. The portion of the Medicare program which is payable to physicians (or to hospitals for services of hospital based physicians) for the professional component of services the physicians render to Medicare patients.

Partially Funded. Pension plan where not all earned benefits have been funded.

Partially Vested. A pension plan where not all employee benefits are vested.

Participating Dividend. Dividend paid to preferred stockholders in addition to the minimum preferred dividends.

Participating Preferred Stock. Preferred stock with rights to participating dividends.

Partner's Drawing. A payment to a partner to be charged against his or her share of income or capital.

Partnership. Contractual arrangement between individuals to share resources and operations in a jointly run business.

Par Value. Face amount of a security.

Par Value Method. The method of accounting for treasury stock that debits a common stock account with the par value of the shares reacquired and allocates the remaining debits between the additional paid-in capital and retained earnings accounts.

Past Service Cost. Present value at a given time of a pension plans' unfunded benefits owed employees for service rendered before the inception of the plan.

Patent. Exclusive right granted by the government to an inventor for seventeen years to enjoy the fruits of an invention.

Patient Day. A common statistical measurement of hospital activity. It represents one patient in the hospital overnight when the official patient census is taken.

Patients. A hospital patient is a person receiving services in a hospital.

Payable. Unpaid but not necessarily due or past due.

Payback Period. Amount of time that must elapse before the cash inflows from a project equal the cash outflows.

Payback Reciprocal. One divided by the payback period. This number approximates the internal rate of return on a project when the project life is more than twice the payback period and the cash inflows are identical in every period after the initial investment.

Payee. The entity to whom a cash payment is made or who will receive the stated amount of money on a check.

Payers. Third party payers such as insurance companies, health maintenance organizations, and governmental programs.

Payout Ratio. Common stock dividends declared for a year divided by net income to common stock for the year.

Payroll Taxes. Taxes levied because salaries or wages are paid, (e.g., FICA and unemployment compensation insurance taxes).

Pediatric Day. The day that each patient 13 years of age and younger is in the hospital, excluding newborn days.

Pension Fund. A fund, the assets of which are to be paid to retired ex-employees, usually as a life annuity. It should be held by an independent trustee and would not be an asset of the firm.

Pension Plan. The provisions of employer's contract with employees for paying retirement annuities or other benefits.

Per Books. An expression used to refer to the book value of an item.

Per-Unit-of-Time Approach. See **Time-Based Techniques.**

Percentage of Completion Method. The practice of recognizing revenues and expenses on a job, order, or contract in proportion to the costs incurred for the period, divided by total costs expected to be incurred for the job or order.

Percentage Statement. A statement containing, in addition to dollar amounts, ratios of dollar amounts to some base, usually total assets for balance sheets and the total revenues for the income statement.

Performance Ratios. Performance ratios are used to evaluate a firm's profitability. May be called **profitability ratios**. They indicate how effectively assets are used. They indicate how much better off the organization is, as a result of profits or changes in net assets. Two ratios that are closely related are the **operating margin** and the **return on assets**.

Period Cost. Period expense. Contrast with **product costs**.

Period Expense (Charge). An expenditure usually based upon the passage of time and charged to operations of the accounting period rather than capitalized as an asset.

Periodic Interim Payment (PIP). A plan under which the hospital receives advance cash payments from third-party payers for services estimated to be provided to subscribers covered by the plan. The PIP payments are compared to the actual costs after the close of the year and adjustments made if necessary.

Periodic Inventory. A method of recording inventory that uses data on beginning inventory, additions to inventories, and ending inventory in order to find the cost of withdrawals from inventory.

Permanent Account. An account which appears on the balance sheet.

Permanent Current Assets. Current assets whose level does not fluctuate with seasonal or other demand factors.

Perpetual Annuity. See perpetuity.

Perpetual Inventory. Entries are made on the quantity and amounts of inventory with each physical addition to or withdrawal from the stock of goods. The records will show the physical quantities and the dollar valuations that should be on hand at any time.

Perpetuity. An annuity whose payments continue forever. The present value of a perpetuity in arrears is p/r where p is the periodic payment and r is the interest rate per period.

Personal Account. Drawing account, used by sole proprietors or partners.

Personal Health Services. Health care services consumed by individuals.

Petty Cash Fund. Currency maintained for expenditures that are conveniently made with cash on hand.

Philanthropic Financing. Contributions.

Physical Verification. Verification by an auditor, performed by actually inspecting items in inventory, plan assets, and the like.

Plant Assets. Physical properties used for hospital purposes, (i.e., land, buildings, improvements, equipment), etc. The term does not include real estate or properties of restricted or unrestricted funds not used for hospital operations.

Pledging. The borrower assigns assets as security or collateral for repayment of a loan.

Pledging of Receivables. The process of using expected collections on amounts receivable as collateral for a loan.

Plow Back. To retain earnings for continued investment in the business.

Point of Equality (dollars). The point of intersection of the Total Revenue line with the Total Cost line on cost-volume-profit chart. May be called the breakeven point. Where total revenues exactly equal total costs, that point of equality can be defined as breakeven. This point is not necessarily a goal, but it is a point of reference that managers might use as a way to evaluate various alternative plans. When a desired profit goal is specified, then the point of intersection is not breakeven, it is merely a point where revenues equal costs.

Points. The same as percentage or tenths of percents. In the case of a bond, a point means $10 since a bond is quoted as a percentage of $1,000. A bond or bond issue that is discounted two points is quoted at 98% of its par value.

Pooled Investments. Assets of two or more funds combined for investment purposes.

Pooling of Interests Method. Accounting for a business combination by merely adding together the book value of the assets and equities of the combined firms.

Post. To record entries in an account in a ledger.

Post-Closing Trial Balance. Trial balance taken after all temporary accounts have been closed.

Post-Statements Events. Events with material impact that occur between the end of the accounting period and the formal publication of the financial statements. Such events must be disclosed in notes for the auditor to give a clean opinion, even though the events are subsequent to the period being reported on.

Pre-Closing Trial Balance. A trial balance taken at the end of the period before closing entries.

Pre-emptive Right. The privilege of a stockholder to maintain a proportionate share of ownership by purchasing a proportionate share of any new stock issues.

Preference as to Assets. The rights of preferred stockholders to receive certain payments in case of dissolution before common stockholders receive payments.

Preferred Provider Organization (PPO). Firm that contracts with participating providers to provide services for covered beneficiaries.

Preferred Stock. Capital stock with a claim to income or assets after bondholders but before common stock. Dividends on preferred stock are income distributions, not expenses, such as interest on debt.

Prefinancing Return on Net Assets and Long-term Debt. A performance or profitability ratio used to evaluate a firm's income before deducting interest expense. Calculated by dividing income before interest expense by long-term debt plus owners' equity.

Preliminary Official Statement. Preliminary version of official offering statement for securities. Contains information investors need for decision making. Also called a **red herring** because of red lettering of a cautionary phrase indicating the information contained in the statement is preliminary.

Premium. The excess of issue (or market) price over par value.

Premium on Capital Stock. An alternative title for capital
contributed in excess of par (or stated) value.

Prepaid Expense. An expenditure that leads to a deferred charge or prepayment and entry on the balance sheet.

Prepayment. Method of payment whereby estimated or budgeted costs are determined before the start of the year and these costs are the basis for (1) payment to the provider for services provided. Also related to **Periodic Interim Payment.**

Prepayments. Deferred charges and prepaid expenses such as insurance premiums or advance payments of rent.

Present Value. Value today of an amount or amounts to be paid or received later, discounted at an appropriate rate.

Price Adjustments. The heavy fixed costs of most health care providers make individual prices extremely sensitive to changes in mix and volume of services offered. Many health care providers now only adjust their prices on an annual basis. Annual adjustments are usually insufficient for proper management of the financial resources of the organization. For example, more frequent price adjustments would mean a smaller percentage increase each time rather than a single adjustment each year. The advantages of frequent price increases, especially from a political perspective, but also from a fairness and financial perspective, should be seriously considered.

Price-Earnings Ratio. At a given time, the market value of a company's common stock, per share, divided by the earnings per common share for the past year.

Price Index. A series of numbers relative to a base period.

Price Level Adjusted Statements. Financial statements expressed in terms of dollars of uniform purchasing power.

Price Risk. The risk that the price of a debt security will change because of a change in interest rates.

Price Setter. Firm that has the ability to set its prices rather than take market or regulated prices.

Price Taker. Firm that must accept market or regulated prices. It does not control the price it receives.

Price Variance. In accounting for standard costs, actual cost per unit or standard cost per unit times quantity purchased.

Pricing Strategies. Both for-profit and not-for-profit providers should develop pricing strategies, since both provide services that recognize the quasi-regulatory nature of the health care sector as well as recognizing the market forces that result from competition with each other. Such strategies (e.g., always meeting the competition's price, being the low-cost provider in the community, or, conversely, being the price leader) can provide the resources necessary to meet the firm's financial goals. There are three major pricing strategies: cost-based, negotiated, and market-driven.

Primary Earnings per Share. Net income to common stockholders plus interest (net of tax effects) or dividends paid on common stock equivalents. Weighted-average of common shares outstanding plus the net increase in the number of common shares that would become outstanding if all common stock equivalents were exchanged for common shares with cash proceeds, if any, used to retire common shares. A required earnings per share number for companies with a more complex capital structure, having not only stocks but also convertible securities. It shows the effect the conversions of current viable convertible securities would have on the earnings per share number.

Primary Market. Term that describes the market when securities are first issued.

Prime Cost. Sum of direct materials plus direct labor costs assigned to product.

Prime Rate. The rate for loans charged by commercial banks to their most preferred risks.

Principal. Amount invested in a financial security.

Principle. See generally accepted accounting principles.

Prior-Period Adjustment. A debit or credit made directly to retained earnings (which does not affect income for the period) to adjust retained earnings for such things as lawsuit settlements and changes in income tax expense of prior periods.

Prior Service Cost. Present value at a given time of a pension plan's unrecognized benefits owed to employees for their service before that given time.

Private Placement. The direct sale of a new security issue to a selected investor or group of investors.

Procedure. A unit of activity in an ancillary department.

Procedure-based Standard Costing. Standard costs associated with health or medical procedures. The unit of activity is medical treatment or procedure.

Proceeds. The funds received from disposition of assets or from the issue of securities.

Process Costing. A method of cost accounting based on average costs (total cost divided by the equivalent units of work done in a period).

Processing Float. The time it takes a payee to process a check and deposit it in the bank.

Product Cost. Costs that are associated with inventories; costs that are not charged as **period costs**.

Professional Component. The professional services provided to patients by hospital based physicians, as opposed to the administrative duties performed by the HBP.

Professional Standards Review Organizations. A professional peer review group, either staffed for the purposes of monitoring the quality of patient care and to encourage the most economic, medically appropriate models and sites of treatment.

Profit. Excess of revenues over expenses for a transaction. Sometimes used synonymously with net income for the period.

Profitability Accounting. Responsibility accounting.

Profitability Ratios. Profitability ratios are used to evaluate a firm's performance. May be called **performance ratios.** They indicate how effectively assets are used. They indicate how much better off the organization is, as a result of profits or changes in net assets. Two ratios that are closely related are the **operating margin** and the **return on assets.**

Profit and Loss Sharing Ratio. The fraction of net income or loss allocable to a partner in a partnership.

Profit and Loss Statement. Income statement.

Profit Center. A segment of a business responsible for its own revenues and expenses.

Profit Margin. Sales minus all expenses. As a ratio, it is computed as sales minus all operating expenses divided by sales.

Profit-Volume Ratio. Net income divided by net sales in dollars.

Pro Forma Statements. Projected financial statement as they would appear if the budget of the organization was accomplished as planned. It can also be used to illustrate the financial statements as they would appear after the planned event takes force.

Progressive Tax. Tax for which the rate increases as the tax base, such as income, increases.

Promissory Note. An unconditional written promise to pay a specified sum of money on demand or at a specified date.

Proof of Journal. The process of checking arithmetic accuracy of journal entries by testing for the equality of all debits with all credits since the last previous proof.

Property Dividend. A dividend in kind.

Prorate. To allocate in proportion to some base. For example, to allocate service department costs in proportion to hours of service used by the benefited departments.

Prospective Payment. Medicare switched to a prospective payment system (PPS) using diagnosis-related groups (DRGs) in 1985 as a payment mechanism for services furnished to government-sponsored patients. Under PPS, the rate per unit of service is set in advance, as compared to retrospective payment systems.

Prospectus. Formal written document describing securities to be issued.

Protest Fee. Fee charged by banks or other financial agencies when items such as checks presented for collection cannot be collected.

Provider. Any health care organization that has been licensed to provide services to patients.

Provider Reimbursement Review Board. Five member board established by Public Law 92-603 for the purpose of reviewing Medicare cases appealed to it involving cost reporting periods ending on or after June 30, 1973.

Provision for Bad Debt. See allowance for bad debt.

Proxy. Written authorization given by one person to another so that the second person can act for the first, such as to vote shares of stock.

Public Accountant. Generally, this term is synonymous with certified public accountant. In some jurisdictions individuals have been licensed as public accountants without being CPA's, however these public accountants may not perform the attest function.

Public Accounting. That portion of accounting primarily involving the attest function and culminating in the auditor's report.

Public Law 92-603. Officially titled the "Social Security Amendments of 1972" approved and signed by the President on October 30, 1972. Significant provisions of this amendment are: providers to be reimbursed at the lower of cost or charges; established a provider reimbursement review board; established cost limitations on inpatient general routine service cost.

Public Law 93-641. Officially titled the "National Health Planning and Resources Development Act of 1974." This act calls for the establishment of State Health Planning and Development Agencies and local Health Systems Agencies.

This program replaces the Comprehensive Health Planning, Regional Medical Programs, and the Hill-Burton Facilities Construction Authorities. The Act requires each state to have certificate of need laws and requires each Health System Agency to be responsible for area-wide health planning and development in health services areas (HSA's) designated by each state governor.

Purchase Method. Accounting for a business combination by adding the acquired company's assets at the price paid for them to the acquiring company's assets.

Qualified Report (Opinion). Auditor's report containing a statement that the auditor was unable to complete a satisfactory examination of all things considered relevant or that the auditor has doubts about the financial impact of some item reported in the financial statements.

Qualified (Stock) Option (Plan). A compensation scheme in which options to purchase stock are granted to employees and in which the implicit compensation is neither tax deductible as an expense by the employer nor taxable income to the employee.

Quantity Discount. A reduction in purchase price. As quantity purchased increases the amount of the discount is constrained by law (Robinson-Patman Act).

Quantity Variance. The standard price per unit times actual quantity, used minus standard quantity that should be used.

Quasi-Reorganization. A reorganization where no new company is formed or no court has intervened, as would happen in bankruptcy. The primary purpose is to absorb a deficit and get a "fresh start."

Quick Assets. Assets readily convertible into cash, such as marketable securities and receivables in addition to cash.

Quick Ratio. Acid test ratio.

Rate of Return (On Total Capital). Net Income divided by total assets.

Rate Variance. Price variance.

Ratio. The number resulting when one number is divided by another.

Ratio Analysis. Also called financial analysis. Includes all of the techniques used to calculate ratios from the firm's financial statements and evaluate its liquidity, profitability, capitalization, etc.

RCC. (Ratio of charges to charges) the ratio of expenses to revenues in an organizational unit such as a revenue center or department.

RCCAC. The **ratio of charges to charges applied to costs,** i.e., the ratio of program charges (Medicare, Blue Cross, etc.) to total patient charges, multiplied by allowable costs to determine reimbursement in a cost-based system where actual costs by patient programs are not debt.

Real Accounts. Balance sheet account, as opposed to nominal or income accounts.

Real Estate. Land and its improvements, such as landscaping and roads but not buildings.

Realizable Value. Market value.

Realization Convention. The accounting practice of delaying the recognition of gains and losses from changes in the market price of assets until the assets are sold. As a general rule, unrealized losses on inventory and marketable securities are recognized prior to sale when the lower of cost, or market valuation basis is used.

Recapitalization. Reorganization.

Receivable. Any collectible whether or not it is currently due.

Reciprocal Method. Uses the simultaneous solution of a series of equations representing the patterns of services between cost centers. Called the reciprocal method because it recognizes all services that cost centers provide to, and receive from, other cost centers. Conversely, other methods, such as the direct or step-down method, do not recognize patterns of reciprocal services. The reciprocal method is considered to be more accurate and objective than the other methods because it recognizes service interdependencies. It does not rely on an arbitrary starting point. No order of allocation is necessary because this method is a simultaneous solution, using matrix algebra, of **all** the cost flows between cost centers. Since it captures all of the service relationships, no information is ignored and no bias is introduced by the choice of a cost allocation method.

Record. To record a transaction in appropriate journals and ledgers.

Record Date. Dividends are paid on payment date to those who own the stock on the record date.

Recourse. The firm selling accounts receivable remains liable for paying receivables to the buying firm if the receivable turns out to be a bad debt. The amount of accounts receivable remains on the selling firm's balance sheet.

Red Herring. Preliminary version of official offering statement for securities. Contains information investors need for decision making. Called a **red herring** because of red lettering of a cautionary phrase indicating the information contained in the statement is preliminary.

Redemption. Retirement by the issuer of stocks or bonds.

Redemption Value. The price paid to retire bonds if called before maturity.

Refinancing. Extending the maturity date or retiring existing debt and issuing new debt.

Refunding Bond Issue. A bond issue whose proceeds are used to retire bonds outstanding from another issue.

Registered Bond. The principal and interest is paid to the owner listed on the books of the issuer.

Registrar. An agent appointed by a corporation to keep track of the names of stockholders and distributions of earnings.

Registration Statement. Statement required by the Securities Act of 1933 and 1934 of companies wishing to issue securities to the public or companies wishing to have its securities traded in public markets. Statement primarily discloses financial data and related activities.

Regressive Tax. Tax for which the rate decreases as the tax base increases.

Regulation S-X. The SEC's regulation specifying the form and content of financial reports to the SEC.

Relative Value Units. Units of service intensity based on average resources necessary to complete particular tests or procedures. Used primarily in ancillary services. Called **Resource-based Relative Value Units(RBRVS)** when referring to physician services. Relative value units (RVUs) have also been developed for laboratory procedures by the American College of Pathology and for radiology procedures by the American College of Radiology. The relative value approach depends upon developing some common element of resources required. Each procedure or test is then expressed in terms of this common factor. The total quantity of each procedure is multiplied by the weighted value to obtain the total weighted units to be performed. Dividing the financial goals for the department by the total weighted unit gives an average cost for each common factor. Multiplying the average common factor cost by the number of factors in each procedure yields the price to be charged for specific examinations.

Relevant Cost. Incremental or differential cost.

Relevant Range. Activity levels over which variable costs are linear or certain costs remain fixed.

Remittance Advice. Information on a check stub or on a document attached to a check by the drawer which tells the payee why a payment is being made. Also, the documentation that accompanies each payment from the fiscal intermediary for the Medicare or Medicaid programs and indicates what amounts were paid for each patient and for what purposes.

Rent. A charge for the use of land, buildings, or other assets.

Re-order Point. The inventory level at which the supplies must be ordered to avoid stockouts.

Reorganization. A major change in the capital structure of a corporation that leads to changes in the rights, interests, and implied ownership of the various security owners.

Replacement Cost. The current market price to purchase a similar asset (with the same service potential). Current cost.

Replacement Method of Depreciation. The original-cost depreciation charge is augmented by an amount based upon a portion of the difference between the current replacement cost of the asset and its original cost.

Reproduction Cost. The cost necessary to construct an asset similar in all important respects to another asset for which a current value is wanted but not readily available from market prices.

Repurchase Agreement. An agreement whereby a bank or security dealer sells specific securities and agrees to repurchase them at a specific price and time.

Required Rate of Return. The minimum rate of return required before making an investment. A normative target.

Required Return on Assets. The minimum rate of return required before making an investment. A normative target.

Requisition. A formal written order or request, such as for withdrawal of supplies from the storeroom.

Resale Value. Exit value expected to be received upon sale.

Research and Development. An expense aimed at creating or improving new products, processes, or service. The FASB requires that costs of such activities be expensed as incurred on the grounds that the future benefits are too uncertain to warrant capitalization as an asset.

Reserve. Refers to an account that appropriates retained earnings and restricts dividend declarations. In addition, used in the past to indicate an asset contra (for example, "reserve for depreciation") or an estimated liability (for example, "reserve for warranty costs"). Reserve accounts have credit balances and are not pools of funds as the term implies. Cash has been set aside, the cash itself should be called a fund.

Residual Value. The estimated, or actual, net realizable value of an asset. Also known as **salvage value.**

Resource Costing. See standard cost and standard cost system.

Resource Requirements. As a first step in developing standard costs, knowledgeable individuals must estimate the resources required to provide a quality outcome. In a health care organization, health professionals or care-givers are usually the most appropriate individuals to determine the required resources.

Responsibility Accounting. Accounting information that focuses on the management control uses of accounting information.

Responsibility Management. Management that includes staff at numerous points it the budgeting process. Authority and responsibility are delegated to the lowest level of management in the organization.

Restricted Assets. Resources restricted by legal or contractual requirements for specific purposes. Some Board restricted funds are erroneously listed in this category.

Restricted Funds. Funds which have been contributed by external parties with a specific restriction as to their use. Either principal or interest or both may be restricted.

Restricted Retained Earnings. Retained earnings not legally available for dividends.

Restrictive Covenants. Promises that are part of a bond indenture to perform certain acts and avoid others.

Retained Earnings. The amount of earnings retained in the organization. It is computed by subtracting all liabilities plus contributed capital from total assets.

Retained Earnings, Appropriated. Similar to restricted retained earnings. It is used to indicate that a portion of retained earnings is not available for dividends.

Retained Earnings Statement. Generally accepted accounting principles require that whenever comparative balance sheets and an income statement are prepared, a reconciliation must also be shown of the beginning and ending balances in the retained earnings account.

Retrospective Payment (or Reimbursement). Method of paying providers for actual costs incurred during the year after the end of the year.

Return on Assets Ratio. Expresses the net income (increase in unrestricted net assets) as a percentage of the assets employed to provide services. This is an overall profitability ratio because it uses the "bottom line" on the income statement. Provides managers with an indication on how revenues, expenses, and assets were used to provide health care services. If the result is too low, management has the option of raising rates or reducing expenses. If the return on assets is low, management can either increase the operating margin or reduce the amount of assets utilized.

Return of Capital Investment. A payment to owners from an owners' equity account other than retained earnings.

Return on Equity. A profitability ratio used to evaluate the returns to owners. Calculated by dividing net income by owners' equity. In a non-profit setting, used to evaluate returns on net assets, regardless of their source.

Return on Investment. Income for a period of time divided by total assets.

Revenue. The dollar amount of a service or procedure rendered.

Revenue Budget. Planned revenues.

Revenue Center. An organizational unit that provides services or products to patients or clients. Revenues are earned when such services are provided.

Revenue Maximization. Management policies designed to maximize revenues from government patients. Such policies ensure that the full costs were recovered from government payers. These policies led to many unintended consequences and illustrated the **perverse incentives** often associated with cost-based reimbursement systems. To alleviate these perverse incentives, many payers designed payment systems that were not based on CBR.

Revenue Received in Advance. Advances from customers.

Reversing Entry. An entry used to reverse a previous adjusting entry, usually an accrual.

Reverse Stock Split. A stock split in which the number of shares outstanding is decreased.

Revolving Fund. A fund whose amounts are continually expended and then replenished; for example, a petty cash fund.

Revolving Loan. A loan which is expected to be renewed at maturity up to a prearranged amount.

Right. The privilege to subscribe to new stock issues or to purchase stock.

Risk. A measure of the variability of the return on investment not to be confused with uncertainty. Therefore, in rational markets, investments with more risk usually promise or are expected to yield, a higher rate of return than investments with lower risk. "Risk" is used when the probabilities attached to the various outcomes are known. "Uncertainty" refers to an event where the probabilities of the outcomes, can only be estimated.

Risk-Adjusted Discount Rate. A discount rate usually the cost of capital which is adjusted for the perceived amount of risk in the investment.

Risk-Averse. The attitude toward risk in which an increase in risk requires an increased return.

Risk-Free Rate of Interest. The rate of return earned on a virtually riskless investment such as a U.S. Treasury Bill.

Risk Premium. The amount by which the required discount rate for a project exceeds the risk-free rate.

Risk-Return Trade-Off. The expectation that investors must be compensated with greater returns for accepting greater risk.

Rolling Budget. Budget that is continually updated.

Routine Services. Daily nursing care and room and board provided for inpatients.

Royalty. Compensation for the use of property, a property right or natural resources.

Rule of 69. An amount of money invested at r percent per period will double in 69/r plus .35 periods. At 10 percent per period, a given sum doubles in 7.27 plus periods.

Rule of 72. An amount of money invested at r percent per period will double in 72/r periods. For example, at 10 percent per period, the rule says a given sum will double in 72/10 = 7.2 periods.

Rule of 78. The rule followed by lenders for determining interest on loans among the month of a year on the sum-of-the-months-digits basis. The sum of the digits from 1 through 12 is 78, so 12/78 of the year's earnings are allocated to the first month, 11/78 to the second month, and so on.

Ruling an Account. The process of summarizing a series of entries in an account by computing a new balance and drawing double lines to indicate the information above the double lines has been summarized in the new balance.

Salary. Compensation earned by managers, administrators, professionals that is not based on an hourly rate.

Sale. A revenue transaction where goods or services are delivered to a customer in return for cash or a contractual obligation to pay.

Sale and Leaseback. A financing transaction where improved property is sold with the understanding the seller can use it as a long-term lease.

Sales Basis of Revenue Recognition. Revenue is recognized only when the sale has been consummated and cash or a legal receivable obtained.

Salvage Value. The estimated value of a physical asset of the time of disposal.

Schedule. Supporting set of calculations which show how figures in a statement or tax return are derived.

Scrap Value. Salvage value of a physical asset that is being sold for scrap or otherwise disposed of.

SEC. Securities and Exchange Commission, an agency authorized by the U.S. Congress to regulate the financial reporting practices of most public corporations. The requirements are stated in its Accounting Series Releases (ASR) and Regulation S-X.

Secondary Market. Market in which outstanding securities are resold.

Secured Debt. Debt that is guaranteed by the pledge of assets of collateral.

Securitization. Process of converting or repackaging assets into securities for investors.

Segment (of a business). A component of an entity whose activities represent a separate major line of business or class of customer.

Self-Balancing. A set of records with equal debits and credits such as the balance sheet, and a fund in nonprofit accounting.

Semi-fixed Costs. Costs that increase with volume of activity as a step function.

Semi-variable Costs. Costs that increase linearly with volume of activity but that are greater than zero at zero activity level. For example, commission of four percent of sales is variable; Commission of $5000 per year plus four percent of sales is semi-variable.

Serial Bonds (Debt). An issue of bonds that have definite amounts maturing at different times over the life of the debit.

Service Department. A department, such as personnel, that does not directly provide patient services but services to other departments that do.

Service Life. Period of expected usefulness of an asset. Sometimes considered to be economic life.

Setup. The time or costs required to prepare equipment to provide a service.

Share. A unit of stock representing ownership in a corporation.

Short-Term. Current assets or liabilities.

Should Cost Approach. Refers to standard costing where standards are set according to normative goals.

Shrinkage. The amount of inventory shown on the books does not agree with the actual physical quantities on hand.

Simple Interest. Interest = (principal) times (interest rate) times (time).

Single-Entry Accounting. Accounting that is not self-balancing.

Sinking Fund. Assets and their earnings earmarked for the retirement of bonds or other long-term obligations.

Sinking Fund Method of Depreciation. The depreciation expense is calculated similar to an annuity so that the value at the end of depreciable life is equal to the acquisition cost of the asset.

Skeleton Account. T-account.

Social Security Taxes. Taxes levied by the federal government on both employers and employees to provide funds to pay persons who are entitled to receive such payments.

Software. A set of computer programs and routines concerned with the operation of the entire system.

Sole Proprietorship. A single owner type of enterprise.

Solvent. Able to meet debts when due.

Source of Funds. Any transaction that increases working capital.

Sources and Uses Statement. Statement of changes in financial position, generally obsolete and not used.

Special Assessment. A mandatory levy made by a governmental unit or taxing district on property to pay the costs of a specific improvement, or service, presumed to benefit primarily the owners of the property so assessed.

Special Journal. A journal, such as sales journal or cash disbursements journal for frequent similar transactions.

Specific Purpose Funds. Funds restricted by the donor for a specific purpose or project. Board-Designated funds do not constitute specific purpose funds.

Speculative Motive. Holding cash for potential investment in physical or financial assets.

Spending Variance. In standard cost systems, the price variance for overhead costs.

Split Billing. A bill submitted to the intermediary for all patients still in the hospital at the end of the hospital's accounting year which contains the charges for all un-billed services furnished to the patient through the end of the year.

Split-off Point. The point where all costs are no longer joint costs but can be identified with individual products.

Spread Sheet. A work sheet organized like a matrix that provides a two-way classification of accounting data. The rows and columns are both labeled with account titles.

Stabilized Accounting. General price-level adjusted accounting.

Standard Cost. Estimate of producing a unit of output.

Standard Cost System. A costing system using standard costs rather than actual costs.

Standard Price (Rate). Unit price established for materials or labor used in standard cost systems.

STAT. A term used when requesting services, meaning "immediately."

Stated Capital. Amount of capital contributed by stockholders.

Stated Value. A term used for capital stock only if no par value is indicated.

Statement. A programming term, referring to an expression or instruction written in a source language.

Statement of Changes in Financial Position. A statement which explains the changes in working capital balances during a period and may show the changes in the working capital accounts themselves, generally obsolete and not used frequently.

Statement of Operations. Also called in income statement or operating report.

Statement of Retained Earnings. A statement that reconciles the beginning-of-period and end-of-period balances in the retained earnings account.

Static Budget. A budget unadjusted for volume or activity changes.

Step Cost. Semi-fixed cost.

Step Down. A cost finding technique involving a series of distributions of the costs of nonrevenue producing departments to each other and to the revenue producing departments.

Step-Down Method. The method for allocating service department costs that starts by allocating one service department's cost to revenue departments and to all other service departments. Then a second service department's costs, including costs allocated from the first, are allocated to revenue departments and to all other service departments except the first one. This is continued until all the service department costs have been allocated to the revenue department.

Stock Dividend. A dividend where additional shares of capital stock are distributed to existing shareholders.

Stockholder's Equity. Owners' equity of a corporation.

Stock Option. The right to purchase a specified number of shares of stock for a specified price at specified times.

Stock Split. An increase in the number of common shares outstanding resulting from the issuance of additional shares to existing stockholders without additional capital contributions by them. Stock splits are usually limited to distributions that increase the number of shares outstanding by 20 percent or more. Distributors of less than 20% are called stock dividends.

Straight Debt Value. An estimate of what the market value of a convertible bond would be if the bond did not contain a conversion privilege.

Straight-Line Depreciation. If the depreciable life is n periods, then the periodic depreciation charge is $1/n$ of the depreciable cost. Results in equal periodic charges for depreciation expense.

Subject To. Qualifications in an auditor's report usually caused by a material uncertainty in the valuation of an item or an amount shown on the financial statements.

Subscribed Stock. A stockholder's equity account showing the capital that will be contributed as soon as the subscription price is collected. A subscription is a legal contract.

Subscription. Agreement to buy a security.

Subsidiary. A company where 50 percent of the voting stock is owned by another organization.

Subsidiary (Ledger) Accounts. The accounts in a subsidiary ledger.

Subsidiary Ledger. The ledger that contains the detailed accounts whose total is shown in a controlling account of the general ledger.

Summary of Significant Accounting Principles. APB Opinion No. 22 requires that every annual report summarize the significant accounting principles used in compiling the annual report.

Sum-of-the-Year's-Digits Depreciation. An accelerated depreciation method for an asset with depreciable life of n years where the charge in period i (i = 1, . . . , n) is the fraction (n = 1 i)/[n(n = 1)/2] of the depreciable cost. If an asset has a depreciable cost of $10,000 and a five-year depreciable life, for example, the depreciation charges would be $6,000 (= 5/15 x $18,000) in the first year, 4/15 in the second, 3/15 in the third, 2/15 in the fourth, and 1/15 in the fifth.

Sunk Cost. Costs incurred in the past that are not affected by, and not relevant in current decisions.

Surcharge Techniques. Pricing technique based on surcharges, which is similar to mark-ups in a retail store. For example, in a pharmacy or central supply setting where many low-cost individual units are issued or dispensed, the development of individual prices would be very time-consuming. In this type of setting, the surcharge or average mark-up on costs is used to accomplish the goals of recovering costs, while minimizing the impact of record keeping.

Supplementary Statements (Schedules). Statements in addition to the four basic financial statements.

Syndicate. A group of investment bankers jointly underwriting debt.

T-account. Basic accounting tool shaped like the letter T with the title above the horizontal line. Debits are shown to the left of the vertical line; credits, to the right.

Table Showing Procedures and Standard Costs per-Unit. Used to show how procedure-based standard costs comprise fixed and variable per-unit costs in a table, where costs are viewed as rows in a table and procedures can be viewed as the columns.

Tangible. Physical assets.

Target Cost. Standard cost.

Taxable Bonds. Bonds whose interest income is taxable for investors.

Tax Credit. A subtraction from taxes payable.

Tax Deduction. A subtraction from revenues to arrive at taxable income.

Tax Evasion. A fraudulent activity designed to avoid the payment of taxes.

Tax-Exempt Bond. A bond on which the interest is exempt from federal and sometimes state and local income taxes for investors.

Tax Shield. The amount of an expense that reduces taxable income but does not require working capital, such as depreciation.

Temporary Account. Nominal accounts, that do not appear on the balance sheet such as revenue, expense accounts, and cost accounts.

Temporary Current Assets. Current assets that are needed to cover seasonal and other demand fluctuations.

Temporary Investments. Investments in marketable securities that the owner intends to sell within a short time, usually one-year, and are classified as current assets.

10-K. The name of the annual report required by the SEC of nearly all publicly-held corporations. It is usually more detailed than the annual report given to stockholders. Corporations must send a copy of the 10-K to any stockholders requesting it.

Term Bonds. A bond issue whose component bonds all mature at the same time.

Term Loan. A loan with a maturity date, as opposed to a demand loan which is due when the lender requests payment.

Terms of Sale. The conditions governing payment for a sale. For example, the terms /10, net /30 mean that if payment is made within ten days of the invoice date, a discount of one percent from invoice price can be taken. The full invoice amount is due within thirty days.

Third Party Payer. An agency which contracts with hospitals and patients to pay for the care of insured patients.

Time-Adjusted Rate of Return. Internal rate of return.

Time-Based Techniques. When the major determinant of cost is the time involved, an hourly or per-minute rate pricing model can be developed. For example, in an operating room, most of the costs are relatively fixed for most surgical procedures. Dividing the financial goal of the operating room by the number of hours or minutes available gives the average charge per unit of time. Multiplying this average charge by the units of time for specific procedures gives the operating room charge to be established for individual procedures.

Times-Interest Earned. Ratio of pre-tax income plus interest charges to interest charges. This ratio is of particular interest to bondholders of bonds in corporations with a high ratio of debt to stockholders' equity as an indicating of financial strength.

Timing Difference. A difference between taxable income and pre-tax income reported to stockholders that will be reversed in a subsequent period and requires an entry in the deferred income tax account.

Title XVIII. Health insurance for the aged and disabled (Medicare) as established by the Social Security Amendments of 1965 (Public Law 89-97).

Title XIX. Officially titled "Grants to States for Medical Assistance Programs" (Medicaid) as established by the Social Securities Amendments of 1965 (Public Law 89-97) as amended by Public Law 93-233. This Act provides for Federal grants to states for assistance in providing medical care for the needy. Medicaid is a state administered program as constructed to Medicare which is a federally administrative program.

Total Asset Turnover Ratio. See asset turnover.

Total Cost Approach. Decision making approach that compares the total costs of each alternative or program. Contrast with the **incremental cost approach's** perspective that, "Given that we are committed to

spending about x dollars over the long run, how much *more* are we going to spend with one alternative than with the others?"

Trade Acceptance. A draft drawn by a seller which is presented for signature to the buyer at the time goods are purchased.

Trade Credit. Credit with no explicit interest rate provided by suppliers.

Trade Discount. A discount from list price offered to all customers of a given type.

Trademark. A distinctive name, sign, or a symbol. Exclusive rights to use a trademark are granted by the federal government for twenty-eight years and can be renewed for another twenty-eight years.

Trade Payables (Receivables). Payable (receivables) arising in the ordinary course of business transactions.

Trading on the Equity. The use of debt financing.

Transaction. Any event that requires a journal entry.

Transfer Agent. A bank of trust company designated by a corporation to make legal transfers of stock or (bonds) and to pay dividends.

Transfer Price. The price used in profit center or responsibility accounting when one segment of the business "sells" to another segment.

Treasury Bill. Debt security issued by the U.S. government with a maturity of a year or less.

Treasury Stock. Capital stock issued and then reacquired by the corporation. Such reacquisitions result in a reduction of stockholders' equity, and are usually shown on the balance sheet as contra to stockholders' equity unless retired.

Triage. The process of screening emergency patients to determine the severity of the medical emergency and type of care necessary.

Trial Balance. A listing of account balances. All accounts with debit balances are totaled separately from accounts with credit balances. The two totals should be equal.

Trustee. Usually a bank that administers the bond indenture agreement and enforces its various provisions.

Turnover. The number of times that assets, such as inventory or accounts receivable, are replaced on average during the period. Accounts receivable turnover, for example, is total revenues on account for a period divided by average accounts receivable balance for the period. Turnover ratios, in general, are used to link the income statement to the balance sheet.

Unadjusted Trial Balance. Trial balance before adjusting and closing entries are made at the end of an accounting period.

Unappropriated Retained Earnings. Retained earnings not appropriated and against which dividends can be charged.

Uncertainty. Refers to an event where the probability of the outcome can only be estimated.

Uncollectible Account. An account receivable that will not be paid by the debtor.

Uncontrollable Cost. A cost which is not under the control of the responsibility center.

Underapplied (Underabsorbed) Overhead. An excess of actual overhead costs for a period over costs applied, or charged to products produced, or services provided during the period.

Underlying Document. The record, memorandum, voucher, or other signal or source document that is the authority for making an entry into a journal.

Underwriter. One who agrees to purchase an entire security issue for a specified price, usually for resale to others.

Unearned Income (Revenue). Advances from customers.

Unemployment Tax. See FUTA.

Unencumbered Appropriation. In governmental accounting, portion of an appropriation not yet spent or encumbered.

Unexpired Cost. An asset.

Unfavorable Variance. In standard cost accounting, an excess of actual cost over standard cost assigned to product.

Unfunded. An obligation or liability, usually for pension costs, that exists due to company policy but for which no funds have been set.

Uniform Partnership Act. A model law, enacted by many states, to govern the relations between partners where the partnership agreement fails to specify the agreed-upon treatments.

Unissued Capital Stock. Stock authorized but not yet issued.

Unlimited Liability. The liability of general partners or a sole proprietorship for all debts of the partnership or sole proprietorship.

Unrecovered Cost. Book value of an asset.

Unrestricted Funds. Funds which have no external restrictions as to use or purpose by donors or grants, i.e., funds which can be used for any legitimate purpose designated by the Governing Board.

Unsecured Debt. Debt not secured by collateral.

Usage Variance. Quantity variance.

Useful Life. Service life.

Use of Funds. Any transaction that reduces working capital.

Utilization (Third-Party). The ratio of hospital services provided to third-party beneficiaries in relation to services provided to all patients of the hospital.

Utilization Review (UR). A hospital procedure in which after a certain length of stay, depending upon the patient's age, primary diagnosis and other factors, the attending physician must complete a short note specifying the length of time he plans to keep the patient hospitalized and the reasons for his returns. The hospital's utilization review committee will review the appropriateness of the request. If determined not medically necessary, certain insurance benefits may be denied.

Value. A monetary worth, however, it is a subjective term with many meanings.

Value Added. Cost of a product or work in process, minus the cost of the materials purchased for the product or work in process.

Variable Annuity. An annuity whose periodic payments depend upon some uncertain outcome, such as stock market prices.

Variable Budget. Flexible budget.

Variable Costing. Direct costing.

Variable Costs. Costs that change at a linear rate as activity levels change.

Variable Cost Ratio (VCR). The ratio of variable costs to revenues. Calculated as:

$$\text{Variable Cost Ratio} = \frac{\text{Variable Costs}}{\text{Total Revenues}} = \frac{VC}{TR} = VCR$$

Alternatively, using per unit data:

$$\text{Variable Cost Ratio} = \frac{\text{Variable Cost per Unit}}{\text{Revenue per Unit}} = \frac{VCU}{RU} = VCR$$

Variable Interest Rate. Interest rate on debt that changes with market interest rates.

Variance. Difference between actual and standard costs or between budgeted and actual expenditures or expenses.

Variance Analysis. Analysis of the causes of changes between planned and actual amounts.

Verifiable. A qualitative objective of financial reporting specifying that items in financial statements can be checked by referring to original source document.

Verification. The auditor's act of reviewing or checking items in financial statements by referring to original source documents or other physical measures.

Vertical Analysis. Analysis of percentage composition of a firm's financial statements, as opposed to horizontal or time series analysis where items are compared over time (or across firms).

Vertical Integration. With respect to health care, a firm that provides a continuum of health care services.

Vested. Said of pension plan benefits that are not contingent on the employee continuing to work for the employer.

Volume. Quantity of output or services.

Volume Variance. Capacity variance or the difference between planned and actual volume.

Voucher. A document that recognizes a liability and authorize the disbursement of cash.

Voucher System. A method for controlling cash that requires each check to be authorized with an approved voucher and specified signatures.

Wage. Compensation of employees based on time worked or output of product for manual labor.

Warrant. A certificate entitling the owner to buy a specified amount of stock at a specified time for a specified price.

Warranty. A promise by a seller to correct deficiencies in items sold.

Wash Sale. The sale and purchase of the same or similar asset within a short time period.

Watered Stock. Stock issued for assets with fair market values less than par value.

Window Dressing. The attempt to make financial statements show operating results, or financial position, as favorable as possible by using favorable accounting practices.

With Recourse. See recourse.

Without Recourse. Firm that sells accounts receivable has no further responsibility for collecting or paying funds to the buyer. The accounts receivable are no longer shown on the seller's balance sheet.

Working Capital. Current assets.

Working Capital per Bed Ratio. Liquidity ratio from the balance sheet used to identify the amount of working capital associated with each bed. Calculated by dividing working capital by the number of licensed, or available, beds.

Working Capital Provided by Operations. Funds provided from the primary business of the company.

Working Papers. The schedules and analyses prepared by the auditor in carrying out investigations prior to issuing an opinion on financial statements.

Work Sheet. A tabular schedule for convenient summary of adjusting and closing entries.

Write-Up. To increase the recorded cost of an asset without a corresponding disbursement of funds.

Yield. Internal rate of return on a stream of cash flows.

Yield to Maturity. The rate of return an investor receives if a debt security is held to maturity.

Zero-Balance Account. Account in which a zero balance is maintained until the bank notifies the firm of the amount of checks outstanding. Then the amount is transferred into the account.

Index